DEDICATION

To our mentors, past and present

Dorothy Rice, Katherine Wiley, Carol Andrews, Janet Rueff, Barbara Heater,
Bonnie Flood Chez, Margaret Comerford Freda, and Louis Flick
KRS

Ruth Creehan, Jacqueline Creehan, Jean Kline, Patricia Murray,
Edna Lalli, Vanessa Butcher, and Diane Palaces
PAC

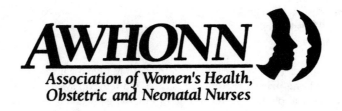

Competence Validation for Perinatal Care Providers: Orientation, Continuing Education, and Evaluation

Kathleen Rice Simpson, PhD, RNC
Perinatal Clinical Nurse Specialist
Women and Children's Care Center
St. John's Mercy Medical Center
St. Louis, Missouri

Patricia A. Creehan, MS, MA, RNC, ACCE
Perinatal Clinical Nurse Specialist
Palos Community Hospital
Palos Heights, Illinois

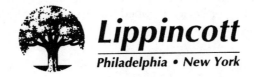

Acquisitions Editor: Jennifer Brogan
Coordinating Editorial Assistant: Susan V. Barta
Production Manager: Helen Ewan
Production Service: Michael Bass & Associates
Compositor: JR Bidwell/Tactical Graphics
Printer/Binder: Victor Graphics, Inc.

Copyright © 1998 by Association of Women's Health, Obstetric, and Neonatal Nurses. All rights reserved. This book is protected by copyright. No part of it may be reproduced, stored in a retrieval system, or transmitted, in any form or by any means—electronic, mechanical, photocopy, recording, or otherwise—without the prior written permission of the publisher, except for brief quotations embodied in critical articles and reviews and testing and evaluation materials provided by the publisher to instructors whose schools have adopted its accompanying textbook. Printed in the United States of America. For information write Lippincott–Raven Publishers, 227 East Washington Square, Philadelphia, PA 19106.

9 8 7 6

Library of Congress Cataloging-in-Publication Data

AWHONN's competence validation for perinatal care providers : orientation, continuing education, and
    evaluation / [edited by] Kathleen Rice Simpson, Patricia A. Creehan
        p. cm.
    Includes bibliographical references and index.
    ISBN 0-397-55462-1
    1. Maternity nursing—Study and teaching (Continuing education)   2. Maternity nursing—Ability testing.
 3. Clinical competence.   I. Simpson, Kathleen Rice.   II. Creehan, Patricia A.   III. Title: Competence
validation for perinatal care providers.
        [DNLM: 1. Maternal-Child Nursing—standards.   2. Maternal-Child Nursing—education.   3. Education,
Nursing, Continuing.   4. Staff Development.   5. Clinical Competence.   WY 157.3   A959 1998]
RG971.A95   1998
362.1'9832—DC21
DNLM/DLC
for Library of Congress   98–12234
                                                                                                                             CIP

Care has been taken to confirm the accuracy of the information presented and to describe generally accepted practices. However, the authors, editors, and publisher are not responsible for errors or omissions or for any consequences from application of the information in this book and make no warranty, express or implied, with respect to the contents of the publication.

The authors, editors, and publisher have exerted every effort to ensure that drug selection and dosage set forth in this text are in accordance with current recommendations and practice at the time of publication. However, in view of ongoing research, changes in government regulations, and the constant flow of information relating to drug therapy and drug reactions, the reader is urged to check the package insert for each drug for any change in indications and dosage and for added warnings and precautions. This is particularly important when the recommended agent is a new or infrequently employed drug.

Some drugs and medical devices presented in this publication have Food and Drug Administration (FDA) clearance for limited use in restricted research settings. It is the responsibility of the health care provider to ascertain the FDA status of each drug or device planned for use in their clinical practice.

CONTRIBUTORS

Debra D. Biggs, RN, MA
Human Resources Specialist
St. John's Mercy Medical Center
St. Louis, Missouri

Barbara Buchko, RN, MS
Maternal-Newborn Clinical Nurse Specialist
York Hospital
York, Pennsylvania

Theresa Peters Buell, RN
Sioux Valley Hospital
Sioux Falls, South Dakota

Mary Burroughs, MSN, RNC
Perinatal Clinical Nurse Specialist
Northwest Hospital
Seattle, Washington

Vicki Calvin, RNC, MSN
Nurse Educator
St. Elizabeth's Health Center
Youngstown, Ohio

Gwen Chute, MS, RN, IBCLC
Educator, Education Department
Westmoreland Regional Hospital
Greensburg, Pennsylvania

Patricia A. Creehan, MS, MA, RNC, ACCE
Perinatal Clinical Nurse Specialist
Palos Community Hospital
Palos Heights, Illinois

Beverly J. Deaton, MSN, FACCE, RNC
Director of Maternity and Emergency Services
St. Francis Hospital
Litchfield, Illinois

Helen Essenpreis, RNC, MSN
Director, Women and Infants
St. Joseph's Hospital
Breese, Illinois

Mary Kay Fallon, RNC, MS, MAEd
Perinatal Nurse Coordinator
Department of Obstetrics and Gynecology
St. John's Mercy Medical Center
St. Louis, Missouri

Barbara Fontanazza, RN, MS
Assistant Professor
York College of Pennsylvania
York, Pennsylvania

Joy Grohar, RNC, MS, CNM
University of Illinois
Midwifery Program
Chicago, Illinois
President, Comprehensive Perinatal
  Consultants
Lockport, Illinois

Susan D. Guild, RNC, MS, NNP, PNP
Neonatal Nurse Practitioner, NICU
Perinatal Clinical Nurse Specialist, Birth Center
  Newborn Nursery
University of Rochester Medical Center
Strong Memorial Hospital
Rochester, New York

Joan Harper, RNC, BS, FACCE
Manager of Maternal-Child Education and
  Perinatal Center
St. John's Mercy Medical Center
St. Louis, Missouri

Mildred G. Harvey, RNC, BSN, MSN
Obstetrical Clinical Nurse Specialist
Perinatal Nursing Consultant
Senior Consultant, Harvey, Troiano, and
  Associates, Inc.
Dallas, Texas

Beth Hindbjorgen, RN, MS
Education Specialist
Education and Development Center
Sioux Valley Hospital
Sioux Falls, South Dakota

Karen Huskey, RNC, IBCLC
Nurse Clinician/Lactation Consultant
Maternity Services
Lake Forest Hospital
Lake Forest, Illinois

Dotti C. James, PhD, RN
Assistant Professor
Maternal-Child Nursing Department
Saint Louis University School of Nursing
St. Louis, Missouri

Mary Beth Johnson, RNC, MS
Clinical Nurse Specialist
Sioux Valley Hospital
Sioux Falls, South Dakota

Susan Kendig, RNC, MSN, WHCNP
Vice-President, Women's Healthcare
  Partnership
St. Louis, Missouri
Coordinator, Women's Health Nurse
  Practitioner Program
Barnes College of Nursing
University of Missouri, St. Louis
St. Louis, Missouri

Jo M. Kendrick, RNC, MSN
Manager, Nurse Practitioner Services
Department of Obstetrics and Gynecology
University of Tennessee Medical Center
Knoxville, Tennessee

Ermalynn Kiehl, PhD, ARNP
Assistant Professor
University of Central Florida
Orlando, Florida

Linda Closs Leoni, MS, RN
Perinatal Loss Coordinator
Pregnancy Loss Support Service
Coordinator, Obstetrics and Gynecology
  Department Quality Assurance Program
University of Rochester Medical Center
Strong Memorial Hospital
Department of Obstetrics and Gynecology
Rochester, New York

Carol J. Luppi, RNC, BSN
Co-Chair, Critical Care Obstetric Nursing Team
Brigham and Women's Hospital
Harvard University
Boston, Massachusetts

Cydney Afriat Menihan, CNM, MSN, RDMS
Nurse-Midwife
Women and Infants Hospital
Clinical Teaching Associate
Brown University School of Medicine
Providence, Rhode Island
Adjunct Assistant Professor
University of Rhode Island
College of Nursing
Kingston, Rhode Island

Alison Benzies Miklos, RNC, MSN
Neonatal Clinical Nurse Specialist
Christ Hospital and Medical Center
Oak Lawn, Illinois

Bette-Jo Moore, BSN, RNC
HealthEast Competency Project Manager
St. Paul, Minnesota

Karen Sanders Moore, RNC, MSN, IBCLC
Perinatal Clinical Nurse Specialist
St. John's Mercy Medical Center
St. Louis, Missouri

Mary Lou Moore, PhD, RNC, FACCE, FAAN
Research Assistant Professor
Wake Forest University
Bowman Gray Medical Center
Winston-Salem, North Carolina

Patricia L. Nash, RNC, MSN, NNP
NNP-Manager, Neonatal Services
Cardinal Glennon Children's Hospital and St.
  Mary's Health Center
St. Louis, Missouri

Mary Neuman, RNC, MS
Perinatal Outreach Coordinator
Methodist Hospital
Omaha, Nebraska

Mary Nordquist, RN
Sioux Valley Hospital
Sioux Falls, South Dakota

Nancy O'Brien-Abel, MN, RNC
Perinatal Clinical Nurse Specialist
Northwest Regional Perinatal Program
Department of Obstetrics and Gynecology
University of Washington School of Medicine
Seattle, Washington

Sister Jean Orsuto, HM, RNC, MSN
Director of Women and Children's Services
St. Elizabeth's Health Center
Youngstown, Ohio

Nancy E. Pea, RN, BSN
Instructor
Department of Organizational Development
St. John's Mercy Medical Center
St. Louis, Missouri

Patricia Petry, RNC, MS, FNP
Director of Maternity Services
Lake Forest Hospital
Lake Forest, Illinois

Celeste R. Phillips, RN, EdD
President
Phillips and Fenwick
Scotts Valley, California

Judith Poole, RNC, MN, FACCE
Coordinator of Perinatal Outreach Education
Carolinas Medical Center
Department of Obstetrics and Gynecology
Charlotte, North Carolina

Dawn E. Reimann, RNC, MS
Education Coordinator
Perinatal Center
Chicago, Illinois

Judy Schroeder, MN, RNC
Perinatal Educator
Valley Medical Center
Renton, Washington

Linda J. Seibold, RN
Executive Vice President and Co-Founder
Healthy Homecomings, Inc.
St. Louis, Missouri

Kathleen Rice Simpson, PhD, RNC
Perinatal Clinical Nurse Specialist
Women and Children's Care Center
St. John's Mercy Medical Center
St. Louis, Missouri

Mary Ellen Burke Sosa, RNC, MS
Clinical Teaching Associate
Brown University School of Medicine
Staff Nurse, Labor/Delivery/Recovery
Women and Infants' Hospital
Providence, Rhode Island

Lyn Vargo, RNC, MSN, NNP
Neonatal Nurse Practitioner
St. John's Mercy Medical Center
St. Louis, Missouri

Susan Weekly, MS, RNC
Perinatal Outreach Educator
Methodist Hospital
Omaha, Nebraska

Julie Wehmeyer, MN, RNC
Director, Women and Infant Services
Overlake Hospital Medical Center
Bellevue, Washington

Sara Wheeler, RN, MSN
Certified Grief Counselor
Clinical Faculty
University of Illinois at Chicago-Urbana
    Regional Campus
Urbana, Illinois

Lynn G. Wellman, MS, RNC
Educator
March of Dimes
White Plains, New York

Lenore R. Williams, MSN, RN
President/Director
Professional Nurse Associates, Inc.
Cleveland, Ohio

Yvonne Zastrow, RNC
Nurse Clinician
Maternity Services
Lake Forest Hospital
Lake Forest, Illinois

Marge Zerbe, RNC, BS
National Lecturer
Obstetrical Seminars and Consulting
Staff Nurse, High Risk Perinatal Unit
Florida Hospital
Orlando, Florida

REVIEWERS

Linda Bertucci, CNM, MS
Associate Clinical Professor
University of California—Irvine School of Medicine
Irvine, California
Orange Coast Women's Medical Group
Laguna Hills, California

Paul Craig, RN, JD
Risk Consultant
MMI Risk Management Resources
MMI Companies, Inc.
San Francisco, California

Ann Flores, RNC, MN
Special Projects Manager
Women's and Children's Services
Via Christi Medical Center
St. Francis Campus
Wichita, Kansas

Margaret Comerford Freda, EdD, RN, CHES, FAAN
Associate Professor
Director of Patient Education Programs
Department of Obstetrics, Gynecology, and Women's Health
Albert Einstein College of Medicine
Montefiore Medical Center
Bronx, New York

Linda Grossglauser, MSN, RNC, NNP
Neonatal Nurse Practitioner
St. John's Mercy Medical Center
St. Louis, Missouri

G. Eric Knox, MD
Medical Director
MMI Companies, Inc.
Deerfield, Illinois
Director, Perinatal Center
Abbott Northwestern Hospital
Professor, Department of Obstetrics and Gynecology
University of Minnesota
Minneapolis, Minnesota

Nancy O'Brien-Abel, MN, RNC
Perinatal Clinical Nurse Specialist
Clinical Faculty
University of Washington School of Medicine
Northwest Regional Perinatal Program
Seattle, Washington

Liz Phillips, RN, BSN
Nurse Manager
Women and Newborns Services
Women and Children's Care Center
St. John's Mercy Medical Center
St. Louis, Missouri

Mary Ellen Burke Sosa, RNC, MS
President, Perinatal Resources
Rumford, Rhode Island

Michelle Teschendorf, RNC, BSN
Labor, Delivery, Recovery Staff Nurse
Women's and Children's Care Center
St. John's Mercy Medical Center
St. Louis, Missouri

Kathleen Thorman, BSN, MA, PhD
Administrator, Women's and Children's Care Center
St. John's Mercy Medical Center
St. Louis, Missouri

FOREWORD

Perhaps the most characteristic feature of nurses' lives during the past decade has been the rapid increase in the rate of change in the healthcare system. Challenged to do more with less, nurses today need to manage the cost of care while improving its quality.

In the provision of perinatal care there are many unique challenges. These include the unpredictability of the birthing process, wide swings in census from day to day and sometimes hour to hour, and the legal climate surrounding contemporary perinatal practice.

Cross-training of perinatal staff facilitates staffing as census fluctuates and thus increases productivity. Utilizing unlicensed assistive personnel (UAPs) to perform noncaregiver tasks can free the professional nurse to spend more time providing nursing care. The resultant nursing model requires a decreased emphasis on tasks and an advanced level of clinical management and supervision skills. There is an increase in intellectual activities and professional accountability.

Perinatal nurses have a unique opportunity to make a positive difference in a woman's life. This caring and supportive relationship must not be compromised. Continuity of care across the childbearing experience can be enhanced by flexible utilization of multiskilled perinatal nurses and appropriate delegating of activities to unlicensed care providers. The result is an increase in nursing's accountability, its professionalism, and control over day to day practice.

Ironically, when the pressure to reduce costs increases, nursing education within the hospital is often the first service to be jettisoned. What a mistake! In these difficult times, investment in human capital has the potential to pay dividends for healthcare organizations.

This text provides the tools needed to develop an individualized approach to staff development that is evidence-based and cost-effective. There are creative strategies for use across the spectrum of perinatal care for acute care to homecare settings. Both professional staff education and skills and practices for unlicensed care providers are included. The timing for this text couldn't be better. Use it well.

Celeste Phillips, EdD, RN

INTRODUCTION TO COMPETENCE VALIDATION FOR PROVIDERS OF PERINATAL CARE

We began this process intending to develop a small manual to accompany our previous text, *AWHONN's Perinatal Nursing*, that could be used as part of a comprehensive orientation and competence validation program. As the project progressed and we heard from many educators, managers, and clinical nurse specialists who were involved in staff development, it was evident that there was a need for a more complete resource for competence validation for perinatal care providers. Standards from regulatory agencies and professional organizations, decreasing financial and human resources, and limited time to accomplish the educational goals and objectives that are critical to quality staff development programs are factors that contribute to this need.

The purpose of this text is to provide examples of excellence in orientation, competence validation, and continuing education and stimulate ideas for new programs that are meaningful and meet the requirements of individual nurses and their employers. Multiple individuals and institutions contributed to this effort. As with *AWHONN's Perinatal Nursing*, we solicited examples from around the country. A call for contributions on the Internet and from professional contacts provided the many excellent ideas and resources that are included in the appendices.

There are two essential components of competence validation: clinical skills verification and knowledge base evaluation. Multiple approaches can be used to meet these criteria. Traditional skills checklists and paper and pencil tests are not the only answer. Innovative strategies can be developed and implemented to achieve education and competence validation goals. Ideally, competence validation is an ongoing process that begins with a thoughtful self-assessment before initial orientation to the unit and includes intermediate evaluations at the completion of orientation and periodically thereafter as needed or at least on an annual basis. Continuing education should be developed based on data gathered through the competence validation process. Specific needs assessment and identified areas of additional required knowledge and skills should be the focus of continuing education programs. Competence validation is a learning process both for the nurse who is being evaluated and for the employing institution.

An integrated approach to competence validation following the AWHONN framework, which combines knowledge evaluation and clinical skills verification rather than isolating the two components, seems to work best. For example, the ability to correctly interpret fetal heart rate monitoring tracings is of little value if the nurse does not know the physiologic principles underlying FHR monitoring and appropriate nursing interventions for the FHR pattern displayed. The ability to monitor maternal vital signs during epidural administration is meaningless without the additional knowledge related to maternal-fetal responses to analgesia/anesthesia and appropriate nursing interventions. Newborn physical assessment skills must be combined with a thorough knowledge of physiology and the subtle signs of evolving newborn sepsis or respiratory distress. Nursing care of the woman during the postpartum period is guided by the knowledge of nursing theory about the timing of appropriate maternal self-care teaching and the ability of the new mother to learn how to care for her newborn.

Technical expertise and adequate knowledge cannot exist in isolation. Competent perinatal nurses have both clinical skills and a thorough understanding of the basis of nursing practice. Possession of a thorough knowledge base does not necessarily translate into the ability to apply that knowledge to clinical practice. Proficiency in clinical tasks does not ensure an understanding of the rationale for essential nursing interventions. Although labor and birth are natural physiologic processes and most women do well with minimal interventions, emergent situations can and do occur in any type of clinical practice setting. The type and amount of nursing orientation and continuing education combined with the depth of acquired knowledge provide the foundation for clinical judgment and critical thinking when patient care decisions need to be made in the practice setting in a timely manner. There is a fundamental interrelationship between the requisite clinical skills for perinatal nurses and the knowledge of nursing theories, and the physiologic, pathophysiologic, and psychosocial foundations of what we do everyday for the women and newborns who are the recipients of perinatal nursing care. Quality perinatal nursing care is provided by nurses who are highly knowledgeable and technically skilled. The challenge is to develop a systematic approach to competence validation that truly evaluates both essential components.

Methods to verify clinical skills include

- preceptor and/or peer evaluation via skills checklists,
- manager evaluation,
- patient and family feedback,
- multidisciplinary team member feedback,
- clinical skills simulation, and
- medical record audits.

Methods to evaluate the requisite knowledge base can be written or verbal and include

- computer-assisted instructional (CAI) programs and videotape viewing followed by self-assessment,
- learning modules with self-assessment,
- paper and pencil tests,
- medical record audits,
- case presentations,
- case study evaluations, and
- electronic fetal heart rate monitoring strip reviews.

Knowledge acquisition and evaluation do not have to occur in the institution setting. Many activities can be done at home at the convenience of the learner, such as videotape viewing, module completion, and computer-assisted instructional programs.

Current Issues Related to Competence Validation

No one way is superior. Each institution must design a program to meet individual needs. Current issues related to this process are

- how to develop meaningful programs that are appropriate in depth and scope both for nurses new to the specialty and for those with years of experience,
- how often it should occur,
- how it should be documented,
- how the needs of hospitals that care for a small number of childbearing women and the needs of large volume perinatal centers differ,
- how to meet the unique challenges of competence validation for perinatal nurses in the homecare setting and those who are triaging women via telephone, and
- determining what types of skills and practices are appropriate for unlicensed care providers.

At some institutions the person responsible for competence validation must "reinvent the wheel" every year. Many times what results is a program that has little real value in assessing the requisite knowledge base and verifying essential clinical skills. One limitation of using traditional skills checklists year after year is that little data are generated that can be used to promote meaningful changes in practice. Research about use of skills checklists for experienced nurses suggest no benefits for the individual nurse or employer.

Considerable time and energy is spent on annual competence validation, so the process and the data collected should serve more than one purpose. Medical record audits are useful because they provide verification of clinical skills and evaluation of knowledge. They can also motivate nurses to be accurate in assessments and documentation and provide important information for risk management programs. Soliciting patient feedback provides valuable information about ways to enhance patient satisfaction and can be used to share positive comments with nurses about their ability to make a difference in the childbirth experience for their patients. Use of learning modules is effective because nurses have the opportunity to learn new practice concepts before completing the self-assessment sections that provide evidence of knowledge base evaluation. Learning modules, videotape series, and computer-assisted instructional programs have the added benefit of being able to be used at home at the convenience of the learner. EFM strip reviews with nurses and physicians participating foster communication and promote collaboration in practice.

Staff education programs can be fun and provide worthwhile information. The competence validation process should allow opportunity for enhanced learning and professional growth. Nontraditional methods can be used to develop meaningful programs that are consistent with published standards. Any program today must be evidence-based, cost-effective, and contribute to quality clinical, financial, and patient satisfaction outcomes. We hope that this text will be helpful in meeting these goals.

Kathleen Rice Simpson, PhD, RNC
Patricia A. Creehan, MS, MA, RNC, ACCE

CONTENTS

PART I ORIENTATION, COMPETENCE VALIDATION, AND CONTINUING EDUCATION FOR REGISTERED NURSES ... 1

1. Using Guidelines and Standards of Care from Professional Organizations as a Framework for Competence Validation ... 2
   Kathleen Rice Simpson, PhD, RNC

2. Developing a Competence-Based Orientation and Cross-Training Program for Nurses in the Inpatient Setting ... 12
   Susan D. Guild, MS, RNC and Linda Closs Leoni, MS, RN

3. Meeting the Unique Needs of Nurses in Small Rural Hospitals ... 33
   Bev Deaton, MSN, RNC, Helen Essenpreis, MSN, RNC, and Kathleen Rice Simpson, PhD, RNC

4. Challenges of Perinatal Outreach: Identifying and Meeting Educational Needs of Nurses in Network Hospitals ... 43
   Mary Neuman, MS, RNC and Susan Weekly, MS, RNC

5. The Perinatal Education Consortium: A Regional Approach to Nursing Education and Collaboration ... 62
   Nancy O'Brien-Abel, MN, RNC, Judy Schroeder, MN, RNC, Mary Burroughs, MSN, RNC, and Julie Wehmeyer, MN, RNC

6. Competence Assessment for Nurses Providing Mother-Baby Home Care ... 83
   Lenore Williams, MSN, RN

7. Competence-Based Orientation and Education: A Working Perinatal Model ... 96
   Bette-Jo Moore, CNS, BSN, RNC

PART II PROFESSIONAL ROLES AND RESPONSIBILITIES AND COMPETENCE VALIDATION FOR UNLICENSED ASSISTIVE PERSONNEL — 105

8. Registered Professional Nurses and Unlicensed Assistive Personnel: Delegation, Supervision, and Staffing Resources — 106
   Kathleen Rice Simpson, PhD, RNC

9. Unlicensed Assistive Personnel: Orientation and Competence Validation in the Perinatal Clinical Setting — 116
   Kathleen Rice Simpson, PhD, RNC

PART III APPENDICES — 135

A. Item Bank with Answer Key — 136
B. Core Competence Checklist for Perinatal Units — 177
C. Suggested Perinatal Nursing Resources for Orientation and Continuing Education: Computer-Assisted Instructional Programs, Videotape Series, Self-Assessment Learning Modules, and Current Perinatal Textbooks — 181
D. Culturally Competent Caregiving Tools — 184
E. Age-Specific Care-Competence Assessment Tools — 198
F. Interpersonal Skills-Assessment Tools — 223
G. Critical Thinking Skills-Assessment Tools — 225
H. Antepartum/Intrapartum Competence Assessment Tools and Skills Checklists — 228
I. Competence Assessment Tool for Nurses Providing Care to Critically Ill Pregnant Women — 238
J. Fetal Monitoring Resources — 247
K. Perioperative Educational Programs and Competence Assessment Tools — 271
L. Mother-Baby Nursing: Competence Validation Tools and Skills Checklists — 290
M. Promoting and Assisting with Breastfeeding Competence Assessment Tools — 312
N. The Newborn: Healthy Full-Term Nursery, Special Care Nursery, and Neonatal Intensive Care Unit Competence Validation Tools and Skills Checklists — 317

O	Mother-Baby Homecare Competence Assessment Tools	341
P	Tool for Evaluation of Orientee by Preceptor	356
Q	The March of Dimes Nursing Modules Program: Continuing Education for Perinatal Nurses	358
R	Unlicensed Assistive Personnel: Position Descriptions, Competence Validation Tools, and Skills Checklists	363
S	Intrapartum Care	398
T	Newborn Care	431
U	Postpartum Care	469

INDEX 503

PART I

Orientation, Competence Validation, and Continuing Education for Registered Nurses

CHAPTER 1

Using Guidelines and Standards of Care from Professional Organizations as a Framework for Competence Validation

Kathleen Rice Simpson

Guidelines and standards of care from professional organizations such as the Association of Women's Health, Obstetric, and Neonatal Nurses (AWHONN), the American College of Obstetricians and Gynecologists (ACOG), the American Academy of Pediatrics, and the Joint Commission on Accreditation of Healthcare Organizations (JCAHO) provide a useful framework for evaluating perinatal nursing competence (see Display 1-1 for examples of professional organizations that publish guidelines and standards of care that have an impact on perinatal nursing practice). Institutional policy and procedures, protocols, care plans, and clinical pathways should reflect practice parameters outlined in publications by these professional organizations; therefore, it is reasonable to use this approach to develop a tool for competence validation.

REVIEW OF PUBLISHED GUIDELINES AND STANDARDS OF CARE

The first step in the process is a thorough review of published practice guidelines and standards of care. At a minimum, the guidelines and standards of care from the professional organizations listed in Display 1-1 should be reviewed, as well as applicable rules and regulations from the individual state's Department of Public Health. Most professional organizations provide copies of relevant publications for a nominal fee; however, in some cases these publications can be obtained at no cost. For example, AWHONN has a fax-on-demand service that can be used to order selected position statements, committee

DISPLAY 1-1

Professional Organizations with National Standards Related to Perinatal Nursing Practice

AWHONN	Association of Women's Health, Obstetric, and Neonatal Nurses
ANA	American Nurses' Association
AACN	American Association of Critical Care Nurses
ACOG	American College of Obstetricians and Gynecologists
AAP	American Academy of Pediatrics
ASPAN	American Society of Postanesthesia Nurses
ASA	American Society of Anesthesiologists
AORN	Association of Operating Room Nurses
NANN	National Association of Neonatal Nurses

Source: *AWHONN's Perinatal Nursing*, Simpson, 1996.

opinions, and clinical commentaries. The American Society of Anesthesiologists (ASA) will send copies of all current guidelines and standards of care at no cost following a phone or mail request. Many professional organizations have toll-free numbers that can be found by calling the 1-800 directory assistance operator. If the institution has a medical library, the librarian can act as a resource to help in locating telephone numbers and addresses.

An added benefit of assembling and reviewing all pertinent publications is the reassurance that institutional policies and procedures, protocols, care plans, and clinical pathways are consistent with current guidelines and standards of care. Through this process many institutions have discovered that revisions to their department manuals were needed. For example, many institutions have policies related to the care of women in labor who receive epidural analgesia/anesthesia that prescribe specific maternal blood pressure and fetal assessments prior to, immediately following, and for the duration of epidural analgesia/anesthesia administration that are not based on guidelines or standards of care from AWHONN, ASA, or ACOG. Some institutions require use of adjunct technologies such as automatic blood pressure devices, pulse oximetry, and cardiac monitoring for all women who receive regional analgesia/anesthesia. These professional organizations have not published specific frequencies or technologies for maternal-fetal assessments, but rather suggest assessments based on the individual clinical situation and risk status. Another example of policies and procedures that frequently could use an update are those for induction of labor. The ACOG (1995) Technical Bulletin, *Induction of Labor*, provides a detailed outline of clinical issues and oxytocin dosage rates that should be key components of any institutional policy about labor induction; however, many institutions have policies that are inconsistent with this ACOG publication. Fortunately, for most clinical issues there is no need to develop policies independently because professional organizations have publications that can serve as a useful framework for this process. Consistency with published guidelines and standards of care can decrease liability should the institution be involved in litigation related to care during childbirth.

Display 1-2 provides a summary of current guidelines and standards of care from professional organizations related to care during the labor, birth, and immediate postpartum period with references to specific publications. These summaries can be used as guidelines for developing a medical record audit tool; however, it is important to note that new editions of these documents are published frequently. For example, in 1997 the fourth edition of the *Guidelines for Perinatal Care* (AAP & ACOG) was published, and in 1998 the fifth edition of the *Standards and Guidelines for Professional Nursing Practice in the Care of Women and Newborns* (AWHONN) was published.

DEVELOPING A MEDICAL RECORD AUDIT TOOL

Medical record audits can be designed to cover both aspects of the competence validation process. Medical record audits provide substantial data about the requisite knowledge base and essential clinical skills during the intrapartum period. Comparison of fetal heart rate and uterine activity data documented in the medical record with the electronic monitor tracing provides valuable objective information about the nurse's ability to correctly interpret the patterns depicted. Medical record audits avoid observer bias inherent in the skills checklist approach.

Nursing interventions documented in the medical record related to the fetal heart rate and uterine activity displayed on the electronic monitoring tracing provide evidence of the nurse's knowledge of maternal-fetal physiology and can be used to verify clinical skills. For example, periods of uterine hyperstimulation with concurrent increases in oxytocin dosage administration may indicate that the nurse is unaware of the clinical signs of uterine hyperstimulation, the institutional policy on oxytocin administration, the pharmacokinetics of oxytocin, and/or the appropriate nursing interventions when there is excessive uterine activity during oxytocin administration. Prolonged periods on the electronic monitoring tracing where the fetal heart rate or

DISPLAY 1-2

Current Guidelines from Professional Organizations for Maternal-Fetal Assessments During Labor and Birth and Maternal-Newborn Assessments During the Immediate Postpartum Period

ASSESSMENTS FOR ANY HOSPITAL ADMISSION OF PREGNANT WOMEN

Pregnant women may come to the hospital's labor and delivery unit not only for obstetric care, but also for treatment of any sign or symptom of illness. Any pregnant woman presenting to a hospital for care should, at a minimum, be assessed for the following:

- fetal heart rate,
- maternal vital signs, and
- uterine contractions.

The responsible obstetric care provider should be informed promptly if any of the following findings are present: vaginal bleeding, acute abdominal pain, temperature of 100.4 F. or higher, preterm labor, preterm premature rupture of membranes, and hypertension (AAP & ACOG, 1997).

ASSESSMENTS DURING THE ADMISSION FOR LABOR PROCESS

When a pregnant woman is evaluated for labor the following factors should be assessed and recorded:

- blood pressure, pulse, temperature,
- frequency and duration of uterine contractions,
- fetal heart rate,
- clinical estimation of fetal weight,
- urinary protein and glucose,
- cervical dilatation and effacement, unless contraindicated (e.g., placenta previa),
- fetal presentation and station of the presenting part,
- status of the membranes, and
- date and time of the woman's arrival and notification of the provider (AAP & ACOG, 1997).

If the woman has had prenatal care and a recent examination has confirmed the normal progress of pregnancy, her admission evaluation may be limited to an interval history and physical examination directed at the presenting complaint. Previously identified risk factors should be recorded in the prenatal record. If no new risk factors are found, attention may be focused on the following historical factors:

- time of onset and frequency of contractions,
- status of the membranes,
- presence or absence of bleeding,
- fetal movement,
- history of allergies,
- time, content, and amount of most recent food or fluid ingestion, and
- use of any medication (AAP & ACOG, 1997).

Display 1-2 (cont.)

ASSESSMENTS DURING LABOR AND BIRTH

Maternal Vital Signs

Maternal vital signs should be assessed and recorded at regular intervals, at least every 4 hours. This frequency may be increased, particularly as active labor progresses according to clinical signs and symptoms (AAP & ACOG, 1997)

During oxytocin induction / augmentation, at a minimum, assess blood pressure before every dosage increase (AWHONN, 1993a).

Fetal Heart Rate

The intensity of FHR monitoring used during labor should be based on risk factors.

In the absence of risk factors:

"The standard practice is to evaluate and record the FHR at least every 30 minutes during the active phase of the first stage of labor and at least every 15 minutes during the second stage of labor."

When risk factors are present:

"During the active phase of the first stage of labor: If auscultation is used, the FHR should be evaluated and recorded at least every 15 minutes after a uterine contraction. If continuous electronic monitoring is used, the tracing should be evaluated every 15 minutes."

"During the second stage of labor: With auscultation, the FHR should be evaluated and recorded at least every 5 minutes. When electronic monitoring is used, the FHR should also be evaluated at least every 5 minutes." (ACOG, 1995).

During oxytocin induction/augmentation, at a minimum, assess the FHR before every dosage increase (AWHONN, 1993a).

Uterine Activity/Labor Progress

For women who are at no increased risk for complications, evaluation of the quality of uterine contractions should be sufficient to detect abnormalities in the progress of labor (AAP & ACOG, 1997).

During oxytocin induction / augmentation, at a minimum, assess uterine contractions before every dosage increase (AWHONN, 1993a).

Vaginal examinations should be sufficient to detect abnormalities in the progress of labor (AAP & ACOG, 1992), and include assessment of dilatation and effacement of the cervix, and station of the fetal presenting part (AWHONN, 1993b).

During Regional Analgesia/Anesthesia

Women "who receive epidural analgesia should be monitored in a manner similar to that used for any patient in labor" (ACOG, 1996).

During regional anesthesia for women in labor "vital signs and FHR should be monitored and documented by a qualified individual" (ASA, 1993).

"Maternal vital signs should be monitored at regular intervals by a qualified member of the healthcare team" during epidural anesthesia in labor (AAP & ACOG, 1997).

"When epidural anesthesia/analgesia is initiated, the nurse monitors maternal vital signs and the fetal heart rate based on each patient's status. The fetal heart rate is assessed before and after the procedure, either intermittently or continuously, and as possible during the procedure. Additional monitoring of the patient is provided during epidural anesthesia/analgesia when the patient's condition warrants" (AWHONN 1998).

DISPLAY 1-2 (cont.)

Additional Parameters

Assess character and amount of amniotic fluid: clear, bloody, meconium stained, odor (AWHONN, 1993b)

Assess character and amount of bloody show/vaginal bleeding (AWHONN, 1993b)

Assess maternal affect and response to labor (AWHONN, 1993b)

Assess level of maternal discomfort and effectiveness of pain management/pain relief measures (AWHONN, 1993b)

Assess labor support person/s' abilities (AWHONN, 1993b)

ASSESSMENTS DURING THE IMMEDIATE POSTPARTUM PERIOD

Maternal Assessments

During the period of observation immediately after birth, maternal vital signs and additional signs or events should be monitored and recorded as they occur. Maternal blood pressure and pulse should be assessed and recorded immediately after birth and repeated every 15 minutes for the first hour. These evaluations may be undertaken more frequently if warranted by the woman's condition or findings. The amount of vaginal bleeding should be evaluated often, and the uterine fundus should be identified and massaged and its size and degree of contraction noted (AAP & ACOG, 1997).

Newborn Assessments

Apgar scores should be obtained at 1 minute and 5 minutes after birth and for an extended period until the Apgar score is 7 or greater. During the stabilization period, temperature, heart and respiratory rates, skin color, adequacy of peripheral circulation, type of respiration, level of consciousness, tone, and activity should be monitored and recorded at least once every 30 minutes until the newborn's condition has remained stable for at least 2 hours. (AAP & ACOG, 1997; AWHONN, 1998).

When determining frequency of maternal-fetal assessments during labor, factors such as stage of labor, maternal-fetal risk status, and institutional policies, procedures, and protocols should be taken into consideration (AWHONN, 1993a)

Collaboration between perinatal care providers and review of current published guidelines as outlined here can facilitate development of institutional guidelines for practice.

uterine activity is uninterpretable may indicate that the nurse needs more information and further demonstration about Leopold's maneuvers and correct tocodynamometer placement. Inaccurate notations in the medical record about the fetal heart rate baseline and periodic patterns could be evidence that the nurse needs more practice in fetal heart rate pattern interpretation. Correct interpretation and documentation of nonreassuring fetal heart rate patterns without notations about appropriate nursing interventions suggest that the nurse could benefit from an additional clinical preceptorship and more education about how to respond when the fetal heart rate is nonreassuring. Notations about nonreassuring fetal status accompanied by entries that the physician or CNM is aware and not responding, with no further interventions noted, may indicate that the nurse needs to review the unit chain of command algorithm. A well-documented medical record that is comparable with the electronic monitoring tracing and includes appropriate nursing interventions at frequencies reasonably consistent with institutional policies provides evidence that the nurse has a solid knowledge base about the physiology of fetal heart rate pattern interpretation, labor and birth, and institutional policies and standards of care, and is able to apply that knowledge in clinical practice.

Selected parameters as outlined next can be used to develop a medical record audit tool review nursing care during labor, birth, and the immediate postpartum period. Prior to completion of orientation, at least five randomly selected medical records and EFM strips can be reviewed with the orientee as both a learning exercise and a competence validation process. The person responsible for orientation can use this session to reinforce accuracies in interpretation, documentation, and appropriate nursing interventions. This process can build confidence for nurses new to the specialty and allow a nonthreatening opportunity for the orientee to ask questions and seek clarification as needed. Nurses who need further education and clinical practice experience can be identified before completion of orientation.

When medical record audits are used as a component of annual competence validation for all nurses, nurse members of a unit practice committee are ideal candidates to coordinate the program. At least three random medical records with EFM strips can be selected on an annual basis prior to the nurse's annual performance evaluation. The committee can review the medical record and EFM strips as previously described as a group. A nurse who needs further education and clinical practice experience can be identified and provided close supervision. A follow-up audit should be done that validates competence before this nurse is allowed to be the primary caregiver for a woman in labor. Reviewing at least three randomly selected medical records reflecting different days in the clinical setting for each nurse who is evaluated contributes to overall accuracy of the data collected.

Specific unit quality care issues also can be addressed by medical record audits. The tool should be designed based on individual unit needs. For example, if there is a consistent problem related to incomplete admission assessments, inaccuracies in medical record documentation when compared to the EFM strip, increases in oxytocin when adequate labor is established, or nurse-coached pushing during the second stage when there is evidence of nonreassuring fetal status, the tool can be developed to evaluate these specific practice areas and provide feedback to individual nurses as needed. Heightened awareness of the importance of accurate medical record documentation and the peer review process can be incentives to enhance quality. Audits also can be useful in developing medical record forms that are more user friendly and provide cues or prompts to enter the required data. Areas for noting aspects of nursing care that are often provided but infrequently documented, such as comfort measures during labor and interactions with the woman's support persons, can be added to flow sheets. The sam-

DISPLAY 1-3

Medical Record Audit Tool

Is the admission data complete   Y____ N____
Name of admission nurse_____
Is there a full signature for each RN using the labor flow record? Y____ N____
Names of nurses without signature_____
Are the nurses' notes legible   Y____ N____
Names of nurses with illegible notes_____
Does the EFM FHR baseline match the FHR baseline noted on the labor flow record?
Y_____ N_____
Names of nurses noting inaccurate FHR baselines _____
If there is evidence of a nonreassuring FHR, is this noted on the labor flow record?
Y_____ N_____
Names of nurses not noting nonreassuring FHR on the labor flow record
_____

Are nursing interventions noted on the labor flow record when there is evidence of nonreassuring FHR?
Y_____ N_____
Names of nurses not noting appropriate nursing interventions_____
Is there documentation that the physician/CNM was notified of the nonreassuring FHR?
Y_____ N_____
Names of nurses not documenting physician/CNM notification_____
Is there documentation that the nonreassuring FHR pattern was resolved or if not, is there evidence of continued interventions to establish fetal wellbeing?
Y_____ N_____
Names of nurses not documenting as described_____
Are maternal assessments noted on the labor flow record according to policy?
Y_____ N_____
Names of nurses not noting maternal assessments according to policy
_____

If adequate labor is established, is oxytocin increased?
Y_____ N_____
Names of nurses increasing oxytocin_____
If there is evidence of hyperstimulation, is oxytocin increased?
Y_____ N_____
Names of nurses increasing oxytocin_____
Does contraction frequency on EFM strip match labor flow record documentation?
Y_____ N_____
Names of nurses with inaccurate frequencies_____

Display 1-3 (cont.)

Is the uterine activity monitor (toco or IUPC) adjusted for an accurate baseline?
Y_____ N_____
Names of nurses during periods needing adjustment _____

Are medications administered without evidence of fetal wellbeing?
Y_____ N_____
Names of nurses administering medications without evidence of fetal wellbeing
_____

Does documentation continue during the second stage of labor?
Y_____ N_____
Name of nurse during the second stage _____

Are there maternal VS q 15 minutes for the first hour immediately postpartum?
Y_____ N_____
Name of nurse during the postpartum recovery _____

Are there assessments and VS q 30 minutes for the newborn's first 2 hours of life?
Y_____ N_____
Name of nurse during the newborn transition _____

Is there documentation about discharge (scoring criteria) from OB-PACU care for women with epidurals?
Y_____ N_____
Name of nurse discharging patient to the mother-baby unit _____

Other documentation, assessment, or intervention issues noted _____
_____
_____

Reviewer_____ Date _____

Recommendations _____
_____

Follow-Up _____
_____
_____
_____

ple in Display 1-3 was developed for a labor and delivery unit that was experiencing inconsistencies in quality of nursing documentation during labor and birth. Medical record audits provided evidence of specific practice issues, and feedback helped improve both nursing practice and documentation during labor and birth.

GUIDELINES FOR DESIGNING A MEDICAL RECORD AUDIT TOOL FOR NURSING CARE DURING LABOR, BIRTH, AND THE IMMEDIATE POSTPARTUM PERIOD

Selected medical records of women during labor can be reviewed and compared to the electronic fetal heart rate tracings. Overall accuracy, consistency with established institutional policies and procedures, AWHONN, ACOG, AAP, ASA, ASPAN guidelines, legibility, and clinical practice issues can be evaluated during the intrapartum and immediate postpartum periods using some of the following parameters:

- Are the nurses' notes legible?
- Are the times noted on the Admission Assessment, Labor Progress Chart, and the initial EFM strip consistent within a reasonable time frame?
- Is there documentation of notification of the physician of admission within the time frame outlined in the policies and procedures?
- Is fetal wellbeing established prior to ambulation?
- Does the EFM FHR baseline match the FHR baseline noted on the Labor Progress Chart?
- Does the EFM FHR baseline variability match the FHR baseline variability noted on the Labor Progress Chart?
- If there is evidence of decreased FHR variability, is it noted on the Labor Progress Chart?
- If there is evidence of decreased FHR variability, are appropriate nursing interventions charted on the Labor Progress Chart?
- If there are FHR decelerations on the EFM strip, are they correctly noted on the Labor Progress Chart?
- Are appropriate nursing interventions charted on the Labor Progress Chart, during nonreassuring FHR patterns?
- Is there documentation of physician notification on the Labor Progress Chart during nonreassuring FHR patterns?
- If there are FHR accelerations noted on the Labor Progress Chart are they on the EFM strip?
- Are maternal assessments noted on the Labor Progress Chart according to policy?
- If there is evidence of a nonreassuring FHR pattern, is oxytocin dosage increased?
- If there is evidence of a nonreassuring FHR pattern, is oxytocin dosage decreased or discontinued?
- If there is evidence of uterine hyperstimulation, are appropriate nursing interventions charted on the Labor Progress Chart?
- If there is evidence of adequate labor, is oxytocin dosage increased?
- If there is evidence of uterine hyperstimulation, is oxytocin dosage increased?
- Does the frequency of uterine contractions on the EFM strip match what is noted on the Labor Progress Chart?
- Is the uterine activity monitor (external toco or IUPC) adjusted to maintain an accurate baseline?
- Are oxytocin dosage increases charted when there is an inaccurate uterine baseline tracing or an uninterpretable FHR tracing?
- Are medications given when there is an uninterpretable FHR tracing prior to administration?
- Does documentation continue during the second stage of labor?
- Are women in the second stage of labor encouraged to push with contractions when the FHR is nonreassuring, that is, when variable FHR decelerations are occurring with each contraction?
- If the FHR is nonreassuring during the second stage of labor, is oxytocin discontinued?
- Does the time of birth match the end of the EFM strip?
- If the woman had regional analgesia/anesthesia, is a qualified anesthesia provider involved in the decision to discharge from PACU care?
- If the woman had regional analgesia/anesthesia, is the discharge from PACU care scoring evaluation documented?
- Are maternal assessments documented dur-

ing the immediate postpartum period every 15 minutes for the first hour?
- Are newborn assessments documented during the transition to extrauterine life at least every 30 minutes until the newborn's condition has been stable for 2 hours?

The same framework can be used to develop a medical record audit tool for other aspects of perinatal nursing care.

BENEFITS OF USING MEDICAL RECORD AUDITS TO VALIDATE COMPETENCE

- Medical record audits can be used for both knowledge base evaluation and clinical skills verification.
- Medical record audits are objective and comprehensive while avoiding the observer bias inherent in using skills checklists.
- The process works well when used prior to completion of orientation to reinforce knowledge and clinical skills and can build confidence for nurses new to the speciality.
- The process can be incorporated into the unit's annual competence validation program for all nurses and allows identification of nurses who could benefit from additional education and clinical practice experience.
- Tool development can be useful in ensuring that institutional policies, procedures, protocols, care plans, and clinical pathways are consistent with published guidelines and standards of care from professional organizations.
- The audit process can lead to redesign and enhancements of current medical record forms.
- Feedback can heighten awareness of the importance of accurate documentation on the medical record.
- Results can be used as part of the unit quality improvement process.
- Improvements in documentation and clinical practice can lead to decreased institutional liability.

REFERENCES

American Academy of Pediatrics and American College of Obstetricians and Gynecologists. (1997). Guidelines for perinatal care (4th ed.). Elk Grove Village, IL: Author.

American College of Obstetricians and Gynecologists. (1995). Fetal heart rate patterns: Monitoring, interpretation and management. (Technical Bulletin No. 207), Washington, DC: Author.

American College of Obstetricians and Gynecologists. (1995). Induction of labor. (Technical Bulletin No. 217), Washington, DC: Author.

American College of Obstetricians and Gynecologists. (1996). Obstetric analgesia and anesthesia. (Technical Bulletin No. 225), Washington, DC: Author.

American Society of Anesthesiologists (1993). Guidelines for regional anesthesia in obstetrics. In ASA standards, guidelines and statements (pp. 22–23). Park Ridge, IL: Author.

Association of Women's Health, Obstetric, and Neonatal Nurses. (1993a). Cervical ripening and induction and augmentation of labor. (Practice Resource), Washington, DC: Author.

Association of Women's Health, Obstetric, and Neonatal Nurses. (1993b). Didactic content and clinical skills verification for professional nurse providers of basic, high risk, and critical care intrapartum nursing. Washington, DC: Author.

Association of Women's Health, Obstetric, and Neonatal Nurses. (1998). Standards and guidelines for professional nursing practice in the care of women and newborns (5th ed.). Washington, DC: Author.

Simpson, K. R., & Creehan, P. A. (1996). AWHONN's Perinatal Nursing. Philadelphia: J. B. Lippincott.

CHAPTER 2

Developing a Competence-Based Orientation and Cross-Training Program for Nurses in the Inpatient Setting

Susan D. Guild and Linda Closs Leoni

INTRODUCTION

Most hospitals find themselves at some point along the continuum between a traditional staffing pattern and a totally cross-trained nursing staff. In the traditional department, a nurse works in labor and delivery, postpartum, nursery, or intensive care nursery. In a totally cross-trained department, nurses find themselves working with women and families during three or sometimes four different phases of the childbirth process. Because the majority of hospitals will be somewhere in the middle of this continuum, the goal of this chapter is to describe a comprehensive approach to staff education that includes both orientation and cross-training.

The assumption of this chapter is that a nurse is capable of caring for a variety of patients at different levels of acuity, if the nurse is adequately oriented and provided with ongoing opportunity to maintain and enhance clinical skills. Unlike in the traditional model where patients move through a system coming to the nurse, today's perinatal nurses move to the patient. The perinatal nurse may simultaneously care for an antepartum woman following the placement of a McDonald suture, a woman experiencing an uncomplicated postpartum recovery, and a newborn whose temperature continues to remain unstable. As hospital census and length of stay fluctuate, and managed care and capitation capture a larger share of the healthcare market, perinatal nurse managers no longer have the luxury of staffing distinctly separate units within one department.

A competence-based philosophy of orientation and cross-training provides a flexible, cost-effective means of educating a large number of nurses with a variety of backgrounds, skills, and knowledge (Display 2-1). Competence validation integrates knowledge, psychomotor skills, and the attitudes required for safe practice in a specific role and setting. It is cost-effective when the program is developed around the skills necessary to safely perform the job and implemented individually for each nurse depending on his or her experience and ability to master new skills. Competence is achieved by practicing within established standards of care. Standards are articulated descriptions of the nature of nursing practice, including knowledge and quality of care, that define the accountability of the professional nurse while administering specific care. Standards of care are the foundation of competency. The literature contains many versions of standards of care. Standards of care developed by individual obstetrical departments should be based on recommendations from professional nursing and physician organizations and as much as possible reflect current literature and be research-based.

DISPLAY 2-1

Strong Memorial Hospital Competence-Based Education Philosophy

Strong Memorial Hospital is committed to the utilization of a competence-based education system for the orientation and ongoing education of the nursing staff. Standards of care are authoritative, descriptive statements that define the nature of current nursing practice, knowledge, and quality of patient care that are a means for establishing accountability for care rendered by the professional nurse. Competence-based education derived from these standards facilitates quality patient care through documented competence of nursing staff. Competence-based education emphasizes the learner and the learning process, and recognizes that knowledge and performance are necessary for competence. Competence is the possession of the required knowledge, skills, attitudes, and abilities to function in a given scope of practice. Competence is demonstrated by an individual's performance, and simultaneously integrates the knowledge, skills, and attitudes that are required for minimal safe practice in a designated role and setting (Alspach, 1984). Achieving a successful outcome from competence-based education includes a commitment to the following characteristics (Del Bueno, Barker, & Christmyer, 1981):

1. Assessment of the individual's prior learning
2. Assessment of the individual's learning style
3. Utilization of self-directed learning activities
4. Flexibility and time to achieve expected outcomes
5. Utilization of the teacher/preceptor as a facilitator/resource
6. Emphasis on achievement of performance expectations

A competence-based system helps ensure that the acquisition of beginning level skills is accomplished during orientation, and that intermediate and advanced skills are acquired throughout the individual's career. Maintaining the competence of nursing staff is an ongoing process.

DEVELOPMENT OF A COMPETENCE-BASED ORIENTATION AND CROSS-TRAINING PROGRAM

In the literature, the terms orientation and cross-training may be used interchangeably or to describe separate entities. For clarity in this chapter, **orientation** is defined as the education of new staff to the whole, an entire set of patient care responsibilities, including basic and complex skills and patient care situations. **Cross-Training** is defined as the education of existing staff to an additional set of patient care responsibilities. These new responsibilities may include basic skills for a clinical population they are unfamiliar with, and/or more complex skills and patient care situations within a population they are familiar with. The orientation and cross-training program is divided into a basic program and an advanced program. New nurses complete both parts of the program, while cross-training staff complete those components that are new to their practice. If an orientation and cross-training program is to be successful, input during all phases of development and implementation of the program is necessary from unit managers, advanced practice nurses, staff nurses, and individual nurses who have completed the

DISPLAY 2-2

Creating an Orientation and Cross-Training Program

Develop the structure for the program
Identify content and resources
Design tools to document and evaluate learner progress
Design tools to evaluate program effectiveness
Develop and define roles
Identify lines of communication

---

program. Feedback from all of these individuals must continue as long as the orientation and cross-training programs are in progress. Display 2-2 identifies tasks involved in development, implementation, and evaluation of a successful orientation and cross-training program.

PROGRAM STRUCTURE

Basic Program

The basic program identifies core skills and knowledge required to provide antepartum, intrapartum, postpartum, and neonatal nursing care to a low-risk population (Display 2-3). It forms the basis of orientation for all new staff who must complete all components. Nurses involved in cross-training could quickly demonstrate competence in components that reflect their current clinical expertise by a brief review, followed by sign-off of skills and knowledge. Nurses in orientation might require a more concentrated learning and precepted clinical experience in a component they are not proficient in. Cross-Training nurses will also need more time in a particular clinical area. For example, a newborn nursery nurse cross-training to LDRP care would not have experience in the intrapartum and postpartum components of care. The cross-training program would consist of a brief review and sign-off of the newborn piece and in-depth exposure to intrapartum and postpartum care.

Advanced Program

The advanced program includes high-risk antepartum, intrapartum, postpartum, and special newborn situations (Display 2-4). This portion of the program follows the basic orientation for new staff and forms the basis of cross-training current staff. Current staff review, test out of topics they are experienced in, and receive in-depth information and precepted experience in unfamiliar areas. For example, in the past, postpartum cesarean birth patients were cared for on a self-contained High-Risk Obstetric Unit; today they are cared for on the LDRP unit. Thus, the entire LDRP staff, new and current, will receive education in the care of this population.

PROGRAM CONTENT

Content for each topic includes basic physiology and pathophysiology, an overview of medical interventions, in-depth review of nursing interventions, documentation, and patient education.

Basic Program

Because of limited teaching resources, the wide variety of staff learning needs, great variation in time frames for learning, and commitment to adult learning principles, self-directed learning options were chosen for the basic program. These include a series of videos (Frye, 1992) with study guides and posttests, and collections of readings drawn from a variety of sources (Mattson & Smith, 1993; March of Dimes Perinatal/Neonatal Learning Module Series, 1980–1998; Olds, London & Ladewig, 1996; Simpson & Creehan, 1996). New staff use scheduled time during orientation to view videos, complete the study guides and posttests, and review supplementary readings. Learning is guided by a set of objectives for each area that is included in each person's orientation manual. In essence, each concept section is a detailed

Display 2-3

Basic Program

I. Intrapartum
   A. Admission of the laboring patient
   B. First stage of labor—cervical effacement and dilatation
      (1) early/latent
      (2) active
      (3) transition
   C. Second stage of labor—birth of the newborn
   D. Third stage of labor—delivery of the placenta
   E. Fourth stage of labor—postpartum recovery
   F. Special situations and complications
   G. Medications
II. Postpartum
   A. Admission of the postpartum woman
   B. Physical assessment
   C. Nutrition and hydration
   D. Elimination
   E. Activity and rest
   F. Hygiene and comfort
      (1) breast care—engorgement, sore nipples
      (2) uterine cramping/afterbirth pains
      (3) perineal care—episiotomy/hemorrhoids
      (4) headaches/muscle and joint pains
   G. Special situations and complications
   H. Maternal-newborn-family interaction
   I. Postpartum diagnostic/lab tests/values
   J. Medications and immunizations
   K. Patient and family education
   L. Discharge of the postpartum family
III. Newborn
   A. Admission of the newborn
   B. Physical and gestational age assessment
   C. Nutrition/feeding
   D. Elimination
   E. Hygiene, safety, and security
   F. Special situations and complications
   G. Laboratory values and diagnostic tests
   H. Medications and immunizations

learning plan for review of information on intrapartum, postpartum, or newborn topics; it tells the learner what he or she needs to know to be considered competent. Once review of information and the posttest is completed and a clinical experience is provided, the corresponding skills/learning summary is signed off.

Advanced Program

For the advanced program, learning modules are the central means of education. Each learning module is based on a clinical competence, identifies learning resources, and contains a posttest. Learning resources include textbooks, journal articles, and practice statements/guidelines from

DISPLAY 2-4

Advanced Program

I. Antepartum/Intrapartum
   A. Preterm labor
   B. Cardiac disease
   C. Premature rupture of membranes
   D. Diabetes
   E. Preeclampsia/eclampsia
   F. HELLP Syndrome/DIC
   G. Analgesia/anesthesia
   H. VBAC
   I. Assisted delivery—vacuum, forceps
   J. Cesarean birth
   K. Induction/augmentation of labor
   L. Meconium-stained amniotic fluid
   M. Prolapsed cord
   N. Placenta previa/abruptio
   O. Early postpartum hemorrhage

II. Postpartum
   A. Maternal resuscitation
   B. Uterine atony/subinvolution
   C. Spinal headache
   D. Puerperal infection
   E. Thrombophlebitis
   F. Diabetes
   G. Preeclampsia/eclampsia
   H. HELLP Syndrome/DIC
   I. Postoperative cesarean birth
   J. Postpartum tubal ligation
   K. Maternal substance abuse/Psychosocial complications

III. Newborn
   A. Neonatal resuscitation
   B. Hypothermia/hyperthermia
   C. Hypoglycemia
   D. Polycythemia/anemia
   E. Prematurity/postmaturity
   F. Hyperbilirubinemia
   G. LGA/IDM newborns
   H. SGA/IUGR newborns
   I. Sepsis
   J. Substance withdrawal
   K. HIV

professional organizations, such as Association of Women's Health Obstetrical and Neonatal Nursing (AWHONN) and American College of Obstetrics and Gynecology. The learner reviews the material, takes the posttest, completes a precepted clinical experience, and is signed off on the competence. Whenever possible, readings are condensed into an overview of salient information, rather than requiring the learner to read through all the resources. This has been received very positively by staff struggling with multiple commitments and seeking the most efficient way to obtain essential, up-to-date information. Time is scheduled to complete learning modules, although this is difficult to accomplish if staffing is tight and census is high; in this case, time frames for completion must be flexible.

Learners move at their own pace, but ultimately must independently and satisfactorily demonstrate skill and knowledge to the preceptor and complete a posttest with 90% accuracy. Although each nurse has the option of taking the posttest without reviewing learning options, everyone to this point has elected to complete them. Experience with this program has shown that even seasoned staff benefit from a review of this information.

PROGRAM TOOLS

Development of effective tools is essential to program success. Tools are designed to: (1) evaluate the learner's progress and the program's effectiveness, (2) document staff competence for regulatory agencies, and (3) provide effective lines of communication and organization for preceptor, learner, educator, and manager. Display 2-5 lists documentation tools used during orientation/cross-training. Examples are included in chapter appendices.

Evaluation of Orientation Needs

The unit manager typically reviews the form Evaluation of Orientation Needs (Appendix 2-1) with every new nurse when they are hired. Questions focus on previous experience and knowledge, previous negative work or orientation experiences, experience with precepted orientation, learning style, and barriers to learning. Answers provide the basis for designing an individualized orientation. The tool is useful in planning orientation if the information is communicated between managers, preceptor, and orientation coordinator. The tool has not been used for cross-training.

Orientation/Cross-Training Schedule

The Orientation/Cross-Training Schedule (Appendix 2-2) is a simple tool following a standard calendar format. Each day the preceptor and focus of the clinical experience (labor, mother/baby, antepartum, or nursery) is noted. Although the learner's schedule is always included in the unit scheduling book for overall planning purposes, the calendar's usefulness has evolved in several different ways. In orientation, it is used as a planning tool by the unit orientation coordinator to target the focus of each week's experiences and to identify preceptors. Plans are discussed with the learner and written on the calendar. The calendar is a reference for the learner and a simple means of laying out the orientation plan, and is an alternative to asking a new staff member to refer to a complex unit schedule.

For cross-training the calendar is used slightly differently. Preceptors and learning experiences are usually determined on a daily basis, based on staffing and census. The learner keeps his/her own calendar, recording each day's preceptor and overview of the patient assignment. When the learner meets periodically with the primary preceptor to discuss progress, this calendar is reviewed for consis-

DISPLAY 2-5
Program Tools

Evaluation of Orientation Needs
Orientation/Cross-Training Calendar
Weekly Learning Needs Assessment/Performance Evaluation of Learner
Learner's Evaluation of Preceptor and Orientation/Cross-Training
Intrapartum Study Guide, Posttest, and Skill Competence/Learning Summary
Postpartum Study Guide, Posttest, and Skill Competence/Learning Summary
Newborn Study Guide, Posttest, and Skill Competence/Learning Summary
Advanced Learning Modules

tency of preceptors, balance of assignments, and exposure to appropriate shifts. This tool has proven very useful.

Weekly Learning Needs Assessment/ Performance Evaluation of the Learner

During orientation, time for weekly planning and evaluation is essential. The Weekly Learning Needs Assessment/Performance Evaluation (Appendix 2-3) provides the opportunity for structured feedback and documentation of weekly progress. It is completed by the preceptor and used primarily in the orientation program. The tool contains a section for documenting the learning activities and clinical experiences of the past week, a section for evaluation of the learner's clinical performance and pace of learning, and a section for outlining objectives or experiences for the following week. A new sheet is filled out each week or whenever learner and preceptor meet. At the end of orientation, the learner has an opportunity to comment on the last weekly sheet. All sheets are returned to the unit orientation coordinator and placed in the learner's file. Although time-consuming to complete, the tool is helpful for keeping orientation on track and for early identification of problems.

Evaluation of Preceptor and Orientation/Cross-Training Program

The Evaluation of The Learner's Evaluation and Orientation/Cross-Training Program (Appendix 2-4) provides an organized overview of the learner's perceptions of his or her experience. The tool is divided into sections allowing the learner to comment on the program, primary preceptor, and associate preceptor. In situations where there were multiple preceptors, learners are asked to comment on one or two preceptors they have worked with most consistently. Despite the valuable information this tool has provided on preceptor performance and program effectiveness, it is often difficult to motivate staff to complete and return it at the end of their experience. Time and the task of filling out another form are obstacles to completion.

Study Guides, Posttests and Skill Competency/Learning Summaries

Study guides, posttests, and skill competence/learning summaries for intrapartum care (Appendix S), postpartum care (Appendix U), and newborn care (Appendix T) ensure consistent, organized learning, as well as documentation and evaluation of learner competence. The skill competence/learning summaries use a skills checklist format. Although the summaries are not written in competency form as performance and learning objectives, they go hand-in-hand with the concept sections, which are written in this format. Each summary provides space for documenting that the learner: (1) reviewed necessary information in the concept, either with the preceptor or by using a self-learning option, such as a study guide or video, (2) is able to theoretically apply the concept or learned information to practice, (3) observed/assisted the preceptor in giving care in a particular area, (4) performs the associated skills satisfactorily. Any or all of the columns can be used throughout the learning experience as preceptor and learner feel is appropriate. By the end of orientation/cross-training, the second and fourth columns must be completed or signed off by the preceptor. This indicates the learner knows and integrates appropriate information and performs associated skills satisfactorily in each concept area. Each summary has a section of special situations and complications. Although there may not be an opportunity to be exposed to clinical situations in all of these areas before the end of the learning experience, it is expected that learner and preceptor will at least review the information and skills associated with each of these topics before sign-off is complete.

A study guide and posttest for each core area are central learning resources that document and evaluate learning for that component. Each study guide is a script of the AWHONN cross-training video for that area, with additional unit/hospital specific information added; it provides a means for staff to glean essential information from a fast-paced video packed with facts. Each posttest is drawn from tested questions in recognized test banks. Although study guides currently are not optional, in the future staff can choose to test out of the study guide by successfully passing the posttest for that area. This option is not provided at present, because it was identified from a variety of sources that all nurses could benefit from a review of the basics. Study guides are corrected and returned to staff who keep them for future review. Posttests are not returned, unless they need to be corrected to meet 90% accuracy; in this case, the staff member self-corrects the items and returns the test. To date, most staff have achieved 90% on the first try; all others have achieved it with a second try. There are no special retests and currently no consequences for failure, other than occasionally delaying sign-off of orientation/cross-training. Early in program development, a philosophical agreement was reached by managers that learning would be as positive an experience as possible, that the learner would have the basic, essential information and skills by the end of his or her experience, and that every effort would be made to ensure these two goals. To date, there has been no cause to regret this approach.

Advanced Learning Modules

Learning modules are the foundation of the advanced program. Development of learning modules is ongoing. Modules will eventually replace the special situations sections on the intrapartum, postpartum, and newborn skill competence/learning summaries. Each module identifies the competence, learning options, and posttest. Staff must review the area of competence, complete the learning options as needed, pass the posttest with 90% accuracy, and demonstrate associated skills to a preceptor. Completion of each area of competence is recorded on an individual record sheet, which is kept in the staff members file. It is expected this sheet will eventually replace or supplement the skill/learning summaries.

ORIENTATION TEAM

Advanced Practice Nurses

Advanced practice nurses (APN) provide leadership for orientation and have ultimate accountability for overall program development and implementation. Their role includes developing competencies, learning modules, and tools; identifying, organizing, and coordinating learning activities and resources; evaluating the program; educating staff regarding the program and competence-based approach; and serving as a resource for learners, preceptors, and unit coordinators. This last role may include assisting with individual learning plans, developing an action plan for special learning needs, meeting with learner and preceptor at designated times during the learning experience to assess progress, and coordinating learning activities for each learner as needed.

Nurse Managers

Nurse managers provide and support unit resources for program development and implementation and assist with ongoing program evaluation. This last piece includes reviewing evaluation feedback on preceptors and learners and initiating appropriate follow-up with APN and unit coordinator.

Unit Coordinators

Unit coordinators are clinical nurse leaders who assist with program development and implementation at the unit level by developing an individualized learning plan for each learner, organizing a schedule, identifying and assigning preceptors and learning experiences, meeting with learners periodically to assess progress and address issues, and serving as a resource to preceptors and learners alike. They also provide input into the development of competencies, learning modules, and tools.

Preceptors

The preceptor role has been implemented in a variety of ways. Ideally, preceptors are clinically advanced staff who function as primary preceptors with other experienced staff serving as associate preceptors. All preceptors receive a manual outlining the program and their responsibilities. Many have attended a preceptor workshop. A consistent or primary preceptor is assigned as much as possible. This individual is responsible for meeting with the learner, completing weekly evaluation forms, ensuring that all skills/learning summaries are signed-off, coordinating activities, and communicating with associate preceptors, APN, and/or unit coordinator. All experienced staff serve as associate preceptors, provide learning experiences, assist with completion of the skills/learning summary, and contribute to the learner's evaluation. A learner may have several different preceptors although consistency is provided whenever possible. Preceptors are responsible for identifying when the learner has completed orientation/cross-training.

During periods when there are large numbers of nurses in orientation, unit coordinators or APNs may function as primary preceptors. In this role they meet periodically with learners to assess and document progress, obtain feedback from associate preceptors, and address any concerns.

Two nurses who are cross-training may share an assignment as "buddy preceptors," teaching each other in their areas of expertise. This has worked well with mother/baby assignments of reasonable numbers and acuity when shared by a nursery nurse and a postpartum nurse. The idea of one preceptor working with 2 or 3 learners on 1 shift, each with a small assignment, has been implemented occasionally. Although this is an interesting idea when preceptor resources are few, the assignments of each learner must be similar so learning needs will be similar and group learning will be facilitated.

Learners

Learners are responsible for participating in developing a learning plan, taking advantage of didactic as well as clinical learning experiences, completing orientation and cross-training requirements in a timely fashion, and communicating concerns immediately to the appropriate resource person. Learners are aware of their responsibilities before beginning orientation or cross-training. They are also encouraged to candidly look at their experience on an ongoing basis, to expect a positive experience, and to question and address any negatives. In the past there have been nurses who have completed orientation or cross-training successfully, only to decide they did not like the particular clinical area. In response to this, staff learners have the option of "when to say when," an acceptable choice they can exercise any time during orientation or cross-training. Since this counseling piece has been implemented, a few staff have chosen to leave the department rather than continue in a learning experience they were not enjoying and probably would not be committed to long term.

THE LEARNING PROCESS

How are the people, content, and experiences of orientation and cross-training organized to offer the best learning experience to each person? The ideal described here has sometimes been achieved and sometimes not. In addition to the ideal, lessons learned along the way may help (Display 2-6).

Before beginning orientation or cross-training, each new staff member meets with the unit coordinator and APN. The learner's educational background and experiences are reviewed, and a tentative learning plan is developed. For staff completely new to obstetrics, minimal orientation time is 10–12 weeks. Experienced new staff, who only require a review of information and skills and orientation to hospital/unit specific routines, may complete orientation in 6–8 weeks. No one has completed orientation in under 5 weeks.

For current staff cross-training to additional competencies, time to complete learning experiences increases with the complexity of the topic. For instance, labor nurses cross-training to mother/baby care may complete their experience in 3–4 weeks, whereas nursery nurses require at least 6–8 weeks of experience to begin to feel comfortable with intrapartum care. An effort is made to carefully look at the learner's needs and closely monitor progress, in order to provide sufficient time for each person to cross-train. Time frames can vary widely and experience has shown to expect the unexpected, set flexible time frames, and realize that even when orientation is completed no one feels he or she is completely ready.

Once the orientation/cross-training plan is agreed on, a schedule is developed, preceptors are identified, a tentative end date is set, and orientation materials are reviewed with each learner. Emphasis is placed on consistency of preceptors and coordinating learner and preceptor schedules.

For new staff members, the first day of orientation is spent familiarizing themselves with the unit environment, personnel, and routines and reviewing their orientation plan with the preceptor. After that, the learners are assigned to experiences that gradually increase in complexity. Usually, nurses new to obstetrics are oriented first to care of low-risk mother/baby couplets and then introduced to more complex assignments, such as postoperative cesarean birth or newborns with special care needs. Once the learner attains a solid base of experience in postpartum and newborn care, he or she is introduced to care of the laboring woman with a concentrated exposure to this area over several weeks. Toward the end of orientation, emphasis is placed on integrating skills and knowledge in all three areas and managing larger, more complex, or changing assignments. Throughout orientation, learners meet formally at least every 1–2 weeks with their preceptor to review progress. Issues or concerns that arise at these meetings are brought to the unit coordinator or APN. Reading time is scheduled

DISPLAY 2-6

Lessons Learned

1. Keep lines of communication with administration open and use them. As healthcare delivery systems change, the boundaries and resources for orientation and cross-training will change. Expect that resources will diminish, learning needs will increase, and patient care responsibilities will expand and change. Expect to flex the boundaries of the program and make compromises, but know when you've reached the bottom line and communicate this to administration as soon as possible, so that informed decisions on allocation of resources, contingency plans, and priorities can be determined. No matter how creatively resources are used, orientation and cross-training are still expensive undertakings and require a certain amount of up-front funding to be successful.

2. Develop the essential pieces of the program before it is implemented; this may seem like common sense, but if you are caught in the whirlwind of job responsibilities, you may find yourself trying to implement the beginning pieces of a program, while still developing the remaining pieces. Full attention is needed for development and implementation. Set realistic time frames. Recognize that this is a labor intensive task, even when you use existing tools and resources.

3. In identifying and developing content, keep it simple, stick to the basics, but build in some flexibility and challenges for those who want more. Recognize that the majority will probably be happy just to be proficient in the basics, but that the basics are far more than what they used to be.

4. Keep tools and documentation simple and streamlined, just what is necessary for regulatory agencies.

5. Build adequate time in everyone's schedule to complete responsibilities and keep the process meaningful to those who use it. Identify back-up people or systems. If someone does not have sufficient time to complete his or her part or there is no flexibility or discretion built in for completing a task, that piece and perhaps the whole program will fail.

6. Keep in mind that just as it takes a whole village to raise a child, it really takes a whole unit to educate and support each member in attaining new or expanded knowledge and skills. Involve everyone and keep all staff well-informed about the program. This includes how it is organized, how it changes, and what role each nurse plays. Staff can never have too much information, particularly when they are functioning in multiple roles, such as being learners and preceptors. Celebrate everyone's progress and formally recognize the contributions of preceptors. Build in a means for staff nurse input in program revisions and act on their suggestions in a meaningful way.

7. Provide flexibility in every aspect of the program. After all, this what a competence-based approach is all about!

periodically, giving the learner an opportunity to complete study guides, learning modules, and posttests. Reading is coordinated with clinical experiences. For instance, newborn and postpartum information are reviewed during those clinical experiences, whereas intrapartum reading time is scheduled during labor orientation. The APN is available during these reading days to provide additional resources or answer specific questions on topics of concern. Approximately two-thirds of the way through orientation, the learner meets with a preceptor and the unit coordinator or APN to review written material and skill/learning summaries for completeness. The calendar is evaluated for a balanced exposure to all areas, and any final concerns or gaps in information or experience are identified and plans made to address them. If necessary, a group decision can be made at this time to extend orientation. If an extension of orientation is necessary, the cost versus benefits ratio is carefully weighed by management. Only when the learner and everyone involved in the process is satisfied, is orientation/cross-training considered complete.

During the first month after orientation, the learner remains on the day shift because of the availability of more resources. Learners identify a resource person at the start of each shift; this can be the charge nurse, former preceptor, or leadership person who will be available for questions and support during that shift. These strategies contribute to a smoother transition from orientee to staff member.

For nurses cross-training, time is given to review required information and complete learning modules, study guides, and posttests. The nurse is then scheduled for a concentrated experience in the area to be mastered. For example, nursery staff learning postpartum care will be scheduled for 1–2 weeks on the LDRP unit, with precepted mother/baby assignments every day. Once learning and performance requirements are completed, he or she is signed off as competent to care for that additional patient population. Although there are no set formal meetings with preceptor, APN, or cross-training coordinator, these individuals meet with each learner at least once and then as often as necessary to discuss concerns and plan additional learning experiences. While the process and participants must be flexible and recognize the needs of the department, everyone realizes that varying significantly from this structure compromises learning and delays the cross-training process.

PROGRAM EVALUATION

Although orientation and cross-training are fluid processes that have evolved and will continue to evolve over time, the basic goals remain the same: (1) to prepare each nurse to function at an optimal level by understanding and applying the nursing process to provide quality care to his or her patients and (2) to accomplish this through cost-effective and efficient use of resources. Evaluation of the orientation program is ongoing. Learner feedback through written evaluations has been very positive. Areas that are cited enthusiastically include the amount of communication and organization built into the program and the wide array of in-depth learning options available. Areas cited as needing improvement include more scheduled time for preceptor and learner to: (1) debrief and review patient care situations, (2) discuss progress and resolve issues, and (3) plan future learning experiences. Often this time has been swept away in the demands of patient care or unit operations. In addition to monitoring learner feedback, future plans for program evaluation include examining the following indicators: (1) patient care incidents, complaints, and compliments involving staff during the first 6 months after orientation/cross-training, (2) retention rates of staff during the first 6 months after orientation/cross-training, (3) anecdotal feedback from preceptors, and (4) average cost of orienting/cross-training new staff. Preceptors have also requested a formal program of ongoing support and education.

FUTURE INITIATIVES

The final step in program development is transition to a service-based program. Streamlined, personalized orientation packages will replace the traditional unit-based orientation/cross-training manuals. Modules ranging from the three basic components to those addressing special or complex situations will be stored in a central file. Unit coordinators will pull modules appropriate for nurses based on assessment of their learning needs and the patient population they will care for. Modules will be assembled into an individualized orientation/cross-training notebook. Eventually, learning options and resources will be housed in a staff resource room with TV/VCR, video/audio/reading library, computers with computer-assisted instruction programs, and copies of all learning modules. Nurses could use this room during reading and review days to complete required learning materials. Managers and advanced practice nurses continue to search for new, innovative, and up-to-date learning materials with particular attention to computer-assisted instruction. The preceptor role will be strengthened with formal continuing education programs and direct involvement in program revision. Trends and issues in unit scheduling and shift workload will be examined to identify and address barriers to preceptor consistency and learning time. Tools will be refined to emphasize simplicity and decrease the total number of documentation forms. Ongoing communication between unit groups will provide opportunities to share concerns about orientation/cross-training and collaborate in problem-solving activities. Last, a program of competence-based continuing education will be established for all staff members to strengthen and revitalize learning that occurred during orientation or cross-training.

CONCLUSION

Today's healthcare system requires a flexible staff with a solid knowledge and skill base who are prepared to care for a multifaceted patient population, located in a variety of settings within a rapidly changing environment. Competence-based education provides the vehicle for ensuring that this goal is reached.

ACKNOWLEDGMENTS

The authors wish to acknowledge Deborah A. Stone, RN, MS and Deborah Aylward, RN, BA for their invaluable contributions in initiating CBO/CBE on the Obstetrical Service and the Obstetrical Nursing Leadership, Nursing Staff and Office Staff for their support and contributions to the development and implementation of this program.

REFERENCES

Alspach, J. G. (1984). Designing a competency-based orientation for critical care nurses. Heart & Lung: Journal of Critical Care, 13(6), 655–662.

Del Bueno, D. J., Barker, F., & Christmyer, C. (1981). Implementing a competency-based orientation program. Nurse Educator, 5(3), 16–20.

Frye, B. (1992). AWHONN Cross-Training for Obstetrical Nursing Staff Video Series. Baltimore: Williams & Wilkins.

March of Dimes Perinatal/Neonatal Learning Module Series (1980–1998). White Plains, NY: March of Dimes Birth Defects Foundation.

Mattson, S. & Smith, J. E. (Eds.). (1993). AWHONN Core Curriculum for Maternal-Newborn Nursing. Philadelphia: W.B. Saunders.

Olds, S. B., London, M. L., & Ladewig, P. W. (1996). Maternal-Newborn Nursing: A Family Centered Approach. Menlo Park, CA: Addison-Wesley Nursing.

Simpson, K. R., & Creehan, P. A. (Eds.). (1996). AWHONN's Perinatal Nursing. Philadelphia: Lippincott-Raven.

APPENDIX 2-1. Evaluation of Orientation Needs

University of Rochester - Strong Memorial Hospital
OB/GYN Nursing
Orientation Program

EVALUATION OF ORIENTATION NEEDS

C O N F I D E N T I A L

Instructions: Completed during the hiring process by NM/NL and used as the basis for planning an individualized orientation.

Learner: _____

Start date: _____   Shift: D E N WKND   Status: FT PT UBPD

Years of nursing experience: _____   How recent: _____

Current certifications: _____

Please indicate yes or no to the following:

1. Has previous experience at SMH. _____
   If yes, on what unit(s). _____

2. Has previous experience with LDRP concept. _____

3. Has previous labor and delivery experience. _____
   If yes, high or low risk. _____   # of years _____

4. Has previous nursery experience. _____
   If yes, high or low risk. _____   # of years _____

5. Has previous experience with mother-baby nursing. _____
   If yes, # of years _____

6. Has previous experience working charge. _____

7. Has been oriented in the past by a preceptor. _____

APPENDIX 2-1. Cont.

8. Appears to have a solid knowledge base in nursing care/management of low-risk childbearing family. If not, where are areas of deficit? _____
_____
_____

9. Does this learner have any personal constraints/situations that may impact on orientation (i.e., time, shift, family responsibilities)? _____
_____
_____

10. Does this learner have any past work experiences that he or she views as a negative experience, which may impact on approach to orientation? _____
_____
_____

11. How does this learner learn best (i.e., read material/learn concept first, demonstration/return demonstration)? _____
_____
_____

12. What makes learning difficult for this learner (i.e., "shadowing" by preceptor)?
_____
_____
_____

RECOMMENDATIONS FOR ORIENTATION (i.e., didactic class needs, amount of orientation in each clinical area, etc.): _____
_____
_____
_____
_____

APPENDIX 2-2. Orientation/Cross-Training Schedule

University of Rochester - Strong Memorial Hospital
OB/GYN Nursing
Orientation/Crosstraining Program

ORIENTATION/CROSSTRAINING SCHEDULE

Learner: _____   FT/PT   Preceptor: _____

		Sunday	Monday	Tuesday	Wednesday	Thursday	Friday	Saturday
WEEK 1		Date Shift Preceptor Focus						
WEEK 2		Date Shift Preceptor Focus						
WEEK 3		Date Shift Preceptor Focus						
WEEK 4		Date Shift Preceptor Focus						
WEEK 5		Date Shift Preceptor Focus						
WEEK 6		Date Shift Preceptor Focus						

APPENDIX 2-2. Cont.

UNIVERSITY OF ROCHESTER - STRONG MEMORIAL HOSPITAL
OB/GYN NURSING
ORIENTATION/CROSSTRAINING PROGRAM

ORIENTATION/CROSSTRAINING SCHEDULE

Learner: _____ FT/PT _____ Preceptor: _____

	Sunday	Monday	Tuesday	Wednesday	Thursday	Friday	Saturday
WEEK 7	Date Shift Preceptor Focus						
WEEK 8	Date Shift Preceptor Focus						
WEEK 9	Date Shift Preceptor Focus						
WEEK 10	Date Shift Preceptor Focus						
WEEK 11	Date Shift Preceptor Focus						
WEEK 12	Date Shift Preceptor Focus						

APPENDIX 2-3. Weekly Learning Needs Assessment/Performance Evaluation

University of Rochester - Strong Memorial Hospital
OB/GYN Nursing
Orientation/Crosstraining Program

WEEKLY LEARNING NEEDS ASSESSMENT/EVALUATION OF LEARNER

Instructions: Completed weekly by the preceptor and learner at the end of each week of clinical orientation and returned to the NM/NL for review.

Learner: _____

Primary/Associate Preceptor: _____

Date: _____

At end of week # _____ of clinical orientation

LEARNING ACTIVITIES/CLINICAL EXPERIENCES COMPLETED THIS WEEK (i.e., formal learning activities/reading days/classes attended; information reviewed informally by preceptor; types of clinical experiences provided by assignments; skill competency/learning summaries completed, if any):

_____
_____
_____
_____
_____

PERFORMANCE EVALUATION (this assessment should be based on learner's success in meeting the goals of orientation/crosstraining, the learning objectives for concepts/modules, and performance objectives for skills checklists, which are appropriate for that week and based on the orientee's individualized learning plan):

- The learner's clinical performance this week (circle one):

    1. meets expectations

    2. does not meet expectations

If #2, please indicate reasons:

_____
_____
_____
_____
_____

APPENDIX 2-3. Cont.

- The learner is progressing at the following pace of learning (circle one number on the scale which best describes pace of learning):

slow   average   accelerated

1   2   3   4   5

If other than #3, please explain:
_____
_____
_____
_____

CLINICAL OBJECTIVES FOR THE FOLLOWING WEEK (i.e., what do you hope to accomplish next week in the way of clinical experiences and formal/informal review of information?):

1. _____
2. _____
3. _____
4. _____
5. _____

COMPLETE THIS ADDITIONAL SECTION AT THE END OF THE LAST WEEK OF ORIENTATION/CROSSTRAINING

ORIENTATION EVALUATION SUMMARY (i.e., briefly summarize the learner's performance behaviors, identifying strengths, as well as areas for additional learning):
_____
_____
_____
_____

Learner's comments:
_____
_____
_____
_____

Learner's Signature: _____ Date: _____

Preceptor's Signature: _____ Date: _____

APPENDIX 2-4. Evaluation of Preceptor and Orientation/Cross-Training Program

University of Rochester - Strong Memorial Hospital
OB/GYN Nursing
Orientation/Crosstraining Program

LEARNER'S EVALUATION OF PRECEPTOR AND ORIENTATION/CROSSTRAINING

Instructions: Completed by the learner at the end of orientation/crosstraining and returned to the NM/NL for review.

Learner: _____ Date: _____

PLEASE RATE EACH OF THE LISTED CRITERIA USING THE FOLLOWING SCALE:
1 = STRONGLY AGREE 2 = AGREE 3 = DISAGREE 4 = STRONGLY DISAGREE

<u>ORIENTATION/CROSSTRAINING PROGRAM</u>

- The learning plan was individualized,
  i.e., it recognized my strengths/experience
  and identified my particular learning needs.   1 2 3 4
- I was given the opportunity to participate
  in planning my learning.   1 2 3 4
- The plan remained flexible to accommodate
  changes in my learning needs.   1 2 3 4
- The schedule was organized, manageable and
  appropriate to my learning plan.   1 2 3 4
- I had a clear understanding of the goals
  and plan for my orientation/crosstraining.   1 2 3 4
- Leadership (Nurse Manager, Nurse Leaders,
  Clinical Nurse Specialist) were accessible
  and responsive to my needs and concerns.   1 2 3 4
- Staff on the unit were friendly and
  supportive during my orientation/crosstraining.   1 2 3 4
- My assignments were appropriate and based
  on my capabilities.   1 2 3 4
- There was consistency in the information I
  was given during orientation/crosstraining.   1 2 3 4
- My learning needs in the following areas were
  adequately met:
    . Postpartum-Mother/Baby   1 2 3 4
    . Newborn   1 2 3 4
    . Labor and Delivery   1 2 3 4
    . Unit Operations   1 2 3 4
- My off-shift orientation/crosstraining
  prepared me to function effectively on that shift.   1 2 3 4
- Reading sessions were effective
  in assisting me with my learning.   1 2 3 4

APPENDIX 2-4. Cont.

- The orientation/crosstraining manual was effective in organizing and assisting me with my learning. 1 2 3 4
- Learning materials, ie., videos, readings, study guides, post test, were effective is assisting me with my learning. 1 2 3 4
- Orientation/crosstraining prepared me to effectively organize my care. 1 2 3 4
- Orientation/crosstraining prepared me to problem-solve and function with a beginning independence. 1 2 3 4
- Orientation/crosstraining prepared me to competently perform necessary psychomotor (technical) skills. 1 2 3 4
- Orientation/crosstraining provided me with an adequate knowledge base and helped me apply theory to practice. 1 2 3 4
- My orientation/crosstraining was complete, ie., I have the skills and knowledge to perform effectively. 1 2 3 4

PRIMARY PRECEPTOR: _____

- I had a clear understanding of my primary preceptor's role. 1 2 3 4
- My primary preceptor was accessible and provided adequate supervision. 1 2 3 4
- My primary preceptor encouraged me to act independently. 1 2 3 4
- My primary preceptor was a positive role model. 1 2 3 4
- My primary preceptor was a knowledgeable resource. 1 2 3 4
- My primary preceptor provided clear, frequent, and constructive feedback on my performance. 1 2 3 4
- My primary preceptor was supportive, ie., he/she assisted me in identifying and resolving potential problems or concerns during my orientation/crosstraining. 1 2 3 4
- Weekly meetings with my primary preceptor were positive and productive, ie., my performance/learning needs were appropriately assessed and realistic, short term goals were set. 1 2 3 4

APPENDIX 2-4.   Cont.

If you had more than one associate preceptor and wish to comment on them, please ask for an additional sheet.

ASSOCIATE PRECEPTOR: _____

- I had a clear understanding of my associate preceptor's role.   1 2 3 4
- My associate preceptor was accessible and provided adequate supervision.   1 2 3 4
- My associate preceptor encouraged me to act independently.   1 2 3 4
- My associate preceptor was a positive role model.   1 2 3 4
- My associate preceptor was a knowledgeable resource.   1 2 3 4
- My associate preceptor provided clear, frequent, and constructive feedback on my performance.   1 2 3 4
- My associate preceptor was supportive, ie., he/she assisted me in identifying and resolving potential problems or concerns during my orientation/crosstraining.   1 2 3 4
- Weekly meetings with my associate preceptor were positive and productive, ie., my performance/learning needs were appropriately assessed and realistic short term goals were set.   1 2 3 4

COMMENTS (please let us know what was most/least stressful as well as most/least helpful to you during orientation):

_____
_____
_____
_____

CHAPTER 3

Meeting the Unique Needs of Nurses in Small Rural Hospitals

Bev Deaton, Helen Essenpreis, and Kathleen Rice Simpson

INTRODUCTION

Orientation, continuing education, and competence validation for perinatal care providers present unique challenges in small rural hospitals. Limited financial and personnel resources, a small volume of patients, and geographic isolation from other perinatal centers are some of the contributing factors. Countless rural communities rely on quality care during the childbirth process. Women are reluctant to travel far distances from family and support persons and leave their familiar healthcare providers during this intimate family experience. Creativity and flexibility are the hallmark of many rural community hospitals. These healthcare providers are experienced in doing their best with limited resources. Although there are challenges, it is possible to provide excellent services and employ competent quality caregivers. The innovative strategies discussed in this chapter have been developed by perinatal healthcare providers in small rural hospitals; however, many of their ideas can be adapted for use in any perinatal center.

PROFESSIONAL ORGANIZATIONS AND REGULATORY AGENCIES

Perinatal nurses in all practice settings are responsible for the care of women and newborns in a safe and therapeutic environment. This level of care requires specialized knowledge and skills as outlined by the Association of Obstetric, Gynecologic, and Neonatal Nurses (AWHONN) in *Didactic Content and Clinical Skills Verification for Professional Nurse Providers of Basic, High-Risk and Critical Care Intrapartum Nursing* (1993) and *Standards and Guidelines for Professional Nursing Practice in the Care of Women and Newborns* (1998). In addition, most perinatal services are licensed through their state agencies such as the Department of Health and are directly affected by the requirements set by their state as well as other regulatory agencies such as the Joint Commission on Accreditation of Healthcare Organizations (JCAHO). Each of these agencies mandates competence for perinatal care providers. It is important to review the state Department of Health regulations when developing competence validation programs. There may be areas of clinical practice that mandate specific programs and documentation. For example, in the State of Illinois Administrative Code (1987), three areas for perinatal nurses are mentioned individually: "perinatal nurses must be knowledgeable and skilled in electronic fetal monitoring, aspects of infection control, and neonatal resuscitation."

The JCAHO (1997) standards for Human Resources Planning provide clear guidelines as follows:

HR.3 The leaders ensure that the competence of all staff members is assessed, maintained, demonstrated, and improved continually.

HR.3.1 The hospital encourages and supports self-development and learning for all staff.

HR.4 An orientation process provides initial job training and information and assesses the staff's ability to fulfill specified responsibilities.

HR.4.1 The hospital orients and educates staff about their responsibilities related to patient care.

HR.4.2 Ongoing inservice and other education and training maintain staff and improve staff competence.

HR.4.3 The hospital regularly collects aggregate data on competence patterns and trends to identify and respond to the staff's learning needs.

Thus perinatal services must provide documentation of some type of systematic process to assure the public that professional care providers are competent. Typically this process involves orientation, continuing education, and periodic competence validation.

Although state agencies and accrediting bodies require competence validation in general terms, various professional nursing organizations have published guidelines and content outlines in greater detail for the recommended educational needs for perinatal nursing that provide the framework for developing a comprehensive program. Every perinatal unit should maintain current issues of these publications and have them readily available as resources. Ideally, nurses belong to their professional nursing organization and have their own copy of the professional guidelines and standards. Because perinatal nursing crosses many speciality practice areas such as neonatal nursing, perioperative nursing, and perinanesthesia nursing, other professional organizations publish guidelines and standards of care that are applicable. The National Association of Neonatal Nurses (NANN), Association of Operating Room Nurses (AORN), American Society of Perinanesthesia Nurses (ASPAN), and the American Association of Critical Care Nurses (AACN) are examples of professional nursing organizations that contribute to perinatal nursing practice.

There are fewer opportunities for clinical experiences and limited financial and personnel resources in most small rural hospitals; however, the nurse responsible for orientation, continuing education, and competence validation must find a way to meet these professional criteria. Many times this person is also the nurse manager with all of the responsibilities that are associated with an administrative role. Few small rural hospitals have the resources for a budgeted position for perinatal educator or clinical nurse specialist. This chapter presents ideas for maximizing existing resources and developing innovative programs using both internal and external resources that have proven successful for nurses in small rural hospitals.

CHALLENGES

Typically, nurses in small rural hospitals care for women who are at low risk for complications of pregnancy, labor, and birth and for healthy full-term newborns. However, pregnancy, labor, and birth are dynamic processes. Unforeseen events can and do arise. Although nurses in the community hospitals may not be required to care for a pregnant woman who needs invasive hemodynamic monitoring or for a preterm newborn, they must have the requisite knowledge and clinical skills to assess women and newborns with complications, identify patients who should be transferred to a tertiary referral center, and provide care until stabilization and transport can be accomplished safely. Unlike nurses in larger perinatal centers, this must be accomplished for the most part without continuous in-house physician coverage. In many ways, the nurse practicing in a small rural hospital must be able to practice more autonomously, have keener assessment skills, be able to recognize signs of impending complications quicker, and plan further ahead because the ability to call for a resident physician or in-house attending physician does not exist. The nearest primary healthcare provider may be 30 minutes away. They must have an understanding of the limitations of their resources and clinical setting and work within these limitations to provide the highest quality of perinatal care possible.

To develop a continuing education and competence validation program or evaluate, expand, and/or improve an existing program several factors must be considered. Institutional philosophy/mission is an important factor. How does the institution view continuing education for staff? What priority do they place on quality patient care? The role of the department of nursing is also critical. Ideally, the institutional philosophy is consistent with that of the department of nursing. Is research-based practice encouraged and supported? Does this support include financial resources for continuing education for nurses? A nursing philosophy that is grounded in quality patient care delivery must include financial support for nursing continuing education programs that provide opportunities for nurses to keep up with the latest research and clinical practice in their speciality field. There is less money available than in the past for nursing education in most institution budgets. No longer can nurses expect to have several paid days off per year to attend continuing education programs. Funds for travel to out-of-town conferences have also decreased dramatically in most institutions. However, there remains a joint responsibility between professional nurses and the employing institution to ensure that nurses have current knowledge in the speciality area of practice. Fortunately, there are innovative methods to develop a quality continuing education program that can be less costly than the traditional approach. Forming partnerships with local nursing school colleagues, using educational offerings from vendors, participating in home study programs, and developing a library of resources including videotapes, computer programs, and learning modules that nurses can access during fluctuations in census are examples of low cost–high yield ways to get current information about clinical practice and research to perinatal nursing staff. Suggestions for implementing these non-traditional methods will be discussed in detail in this chapter and throughout this text. Suggested resources for home study, videotape series, computer-assisted instructional programs, and learning modules are provided in the text appendices.

ORIENTATION

Today most perinatal units in the rural setting "cross-train" nurses. Limited staffing due to the small volume of births does not permit employing nurses with clinical skills exclusive to the Labor and Delivery, Nursery, or Postpartum units. Perinatal nurses in rural hospitals must be competent in antepartum, intrapartum, postpartum, and newborn nursing care. Thus the orientation program must be extensive to cover all aspects of care for childbearing women and their newborns. As more institutions have adopted a mother-baby model of care, it is unusual to hire an experienced perinatal nurse who does not have at least a knowledge of postpartum and newborn care or labor and birth care. There are still many institutions that have separate labor-delivery-recovery units and mother-baby units so it is possible to hire a new employee with experience in perinatal nursing but who will need cross-training to be able to meet the needs of the unit.

Core Competence Development

Development of perinatal unit core competencies is the essential first step in designing the orientation program. There are multiple resources available to provide a framework for this process. Program content may be developed within the institution or may be purchased and adapted for the institution. AWHONN's *Didactic Content and Clinical Skills Verification for Professional Nurse Providers of Basic, High-Risk and Critical Care Intrapartum Nursing* (1993) and *Standards and Guidelines for Professional Nursing Practice in the Care of Women and Newborns* (1998) are excellent references for unit competence development. Selected competencies as appropriate to the individual perinatal unit can be adopted from these resources.

Evaluation of expected nursing skills for each unit guides the decision-making process for selecting competencies to be included. An example of a perinatal core competence tool that is based on these AWHONN publications is included in Appendix B. The Rural Wisconsin Health Cooperative's (1995) program covers competence criteria for all areas of perinatal nursing practice, is available for purchase, and can be used for both initial orientation and ongoing competence validation. For perinatal centers that do not have the financial or personnel resources to develop and maintain a quality orientation and competence validation program, purchasing this type of existing program can help fill the void.

Instead of developing an orientation manual in-house, use of learning modules that include comprehensive coverage of perinatal content areas is an excellent alternative. *Intrapartum Management Modules* (Martin, 1996) for labor-delivery-recovery content and *Family-Centered Maternal-Newborn Care* (Phillips, 1996) for mother-baby content are useful texts because they provide the needed information and include self-assessment components that the new nurse can complete during the orientation process. Similar resources with self-assessment components are the *AWHONN Compendium on Postpartum Care* (AWHONN, 1996) and *Physical Assessment of the Newborn: A Comprehensive Approach to the Art of Physical Examination* (Tappero & Honeyfield, 1996). *Fetal Monitoring and Assessment* (Tucker, 1996) is an excellent resource for nurses new to fetal monitoring and is small enough to be carried in the pocket for frequent referral during orientation. For units that have a manual with the focus on care of low-risk mothers and newborns, use of learning modules specific to common complications of pregnancy can provide information targeted to this type of nursing care. The March of Dimes nursing modules are excellent low-cost comprehensive resources that cover a variety of perinatal nursing topics. March of Dimes nursing modules such as *Preterm Labor: Prevention and Nursing Management* (Freda & Patterson, 1994), *Multiple Gestation* (Drukker, 1997), *Hypertension During Pregnancy* (Poole, 1997), and *Obstetrical Complications for the Perinatal Nurse* (White & Poole, 1996) can be used as adjunct references to the orientation manual for low-risk perinatal units. (See Appendix T for a complete listing of March of Dimes Nursing Modules).

Selection of Preceptors

Most perinatal units have a formal preceptor program, which includes additional education for this group about the special role of the preceptor and recognition of this contribution to the unit. The preceptor is assigned to coordinate orientation for the new nurse employee and acts as a clinical role model. Usually the preceptor works side by side with the new employee for a number of weeks and is the person responsible for validating competence at the completion of the orientation program. Other perinatal units have found that a less formal approach using multiple clinical experts and senior staff members works well, with each person validating the clinical skills observed during the time spent with the new employee. As with any method of orientation, there are advantages and disadvantages to both systems. The formal preceptor program provides consistency and ideally involves a nurse preceptor who has volunteered for this role, and thus is motivated to be helpful and nurturing. A potential disadvantage to the formal preceptor system is the limited interaction with other staff members until orientation is completed. The less formal approach allows the new nurse to work with many of those she or he will be working with after orientation and to get a sense of similarities and differences in individual practice styles. The new nurse is also exposed to a potentially larger group of nurses who can provide reassurance and encouragement, which ideally builds confidence and collegial relationships. One disadvantage to having multiple preceptors during orientation is the potential frustration of having one clinical expert show the new nurse his or her method of clinical interventions and then having another clinical expert demonstrate a different but equally acceptable approach.

Nurturing and providing recognition for the contribution to the unit for nurses who agree to act as clinical role models is essential no matter which method of preceptorship is used. The preceptor must be a clinical expert and have a clear understanding of the expected clinical skills, a familiarity with the perinatal core competence tool, and the ability to encourage the new employee to complete orientation within the expected time frame.

Length of Orientation

Although there is merit in developing a time frame for acquiring requisite knowledge and mastering expected clinical skills, orientation to the perinatal unit must be individualized to meet the needs of each new employee. Experienced and inexperienced nurses have very different levels of knowledge and skill. The type of clinical experience is also a contributing factor in setting a realistic time for completion of orientation. Nurses who are not experienced in working in the rural hospital setting without the clinical resources and immediate back-up that are found in larger institutions may need assistance in developing autonomy and the ability to predict well in advance when the primary healthcare provider will be needed to come to the institution. Before completion of orientation in the rural hospital setting, the preceptor must feel comfortable that the new nurse will be able to accurately assess women and newborns and competently handle common perinatal emergencies until the primary healthcare provider can arrive.

The time frame for completion of orientation therefore must be dynamic and flexible with additional clinical preceptorship available if needed. Completion of the perinatal core competence tool is one of the last steps. Ideally, a discussion with the new employee and the preceptor provides the framework for determining areas where improvement is needed and clinical skills that have been mastered. The nurse manager participates in the final decision that the nurse has met criteria for completion of orientation. Some units use a "buddy system" or identify a resource person for the nurse who has recently completed orientation. This works well because there is always a person available to answer questions and provide support when the new nurse encounters the inevitable situation that was not covered during orientation. This practice also encourages mentoring and nurturing, which can provide the foundation for long-term professional relationships. One of the more rewarding aspects of participating in the orientation of a new nurse is observing that person's professional growth and stimulating his or her enthusiasm for perinatal nursing specialty.

Examples of Orientation Programs in Hospitals in the Rural Setting

St. Francis Hospital in Litchfield, Illinois has a formal preceptorship program that teams the new employee with a preceptor for the period of time needed to ensure initial competence in the clinical setting. The Maternity Department averages 400 births annually and maintains 3 staff nurses on 12-hour shifts. The preceptor has been provided education about adult-learning skills and is knowledgeable in all aspects of the functions of the department. The preceptor and new employee meet weekly, or as indicated, with the nurse manager to review progress/issues and discuss goals for the coming week(s). Activities for each day of orientation are flexible, depending on the activity of the department. Because the department may not have an active labor patient on a specific day, the preceptor must consider all expected competencies rather than focus on specific clinical skills in isolation. In this type of setting, it is unrealistic to plan to complete a list of expected clinical skills in a rigid order of progression. Opportunities for learning are seized as they present themselves.

During the first days of orientation the preceptor does not function as part of the department staffing. After this initial period, the preceptor and new employee function as one of the three staff members for the day, taking the most appropriate assignment of learning. To ensure that all aspects of clinical practice and unit policies are covered during orientation, a checklist is used. If actual patient care for a specific area of competence is not covered during orientation due to lack of clinical opportunity, the procedures and expected nursing interventions are reviewed carefully and a discussion is held during which the new employee demonstrates understanding of the requisite knowledge and clinical skills. This is a frequent occurrence during orientation in the rural hospital setting. For example, the new employee must have knowledge and clinical skills related to the care of women in labor with complications such as pregnancy-induced hypertension or placenta previa. However, during orientation, this clinical situation may not occur. It is critically important to cover this material during orientation to ensure that the new nurse will be able to handle this clinical situation when it does occur in the future. One way to validate that the new nurse has an understanding of common complications of pregnancy that may not present during orientation is the completion of learning modules (Drukker, 1997; Freda & Patterson, 1994; Martin, 1996; Phillips, 1996; Poole, 1997; White & Poole, 1996). The learning module approach provides written documentation that the material was covered and the nurse successfully completed the self-assessment for common pregnancy complications. Orientation generally lasts 6 weeks depending on the needs of the new employee and includes a period of time on the shift the new employee will be working.

St. Joseph's Hospital in Breese, Illinois with an average of 600 births per year uses a combination of senior staff nurses rather than a formal preceptor. The new employee is assigned to work with that nurse for the day. Nurses feel that one of the advantages of assigning the new employee to different nurses is that the new nurse is exposed to a variety of skills and perspectives and can adopt the best practice of each nurse. It is important to consider that although there are many ways to provide quality care and thus variety is acceptable and even beneficial, the new nurse may not have the knowledge and skill to discriminate from practices that are not the best approach or are not current. Thus for this type of program to be successful, it is critical that the nurse role-model be a clinical expert.

The orientation content includes the organization's mission, governance, policies and procedures, departmental/service policies and procedures, review of job description, performance expectations, plant and safety management programs and the individual's safety role, infection control program and the individual's role in the prevention of infection, and the quality assurance/continuous quality improvement programs. Each nurse is expected to complete the Neonatal Resuscitation Program (NRP) co-developed by the American Heart Association and the American Academy of Pediatrics (1994). This program must be completed by the end of the orientation program. The NRP program is essential in rural institutions because an emergency situation can occur during times when pediatric coverage may not be in-house. NRP is a self-study program with six lessons, including initial steps in stabilizing the newborn, use of hospital resuscitation equipment, cardiac compressions, endotracheal intubation, and administration of emergency medications. After completion of the six lessons, a test and skills demonstration is completed to validate competence. It is recommended that the course be repeated every 2 years. Some organizations have found it beneficial to repeat the course annually due to the infrequency of using the resuscitation skills. Having in-house educators for this program facilitates giving the classes as frequently as needed.

Use of the self-study modules by Martin (1996) as well as the *Perinatal Continuing Education Program Modules* developed by the Southern New Jersey Perinatal Cooperative (1992) are also a part of orientation. The modules contain pre- and posttests for each chapter. Although many of the modules are primarily didactic content, several are skill activities and require demonstration of that skill, such as the performance of Leopold Maneuvers.

Most rural hospitals do not have a surgery staff in-house 24 hours a day. In the event of an emergent cesarean birth, perinatal staff may be called upon to start the functions of the scrub nurse and circulating nurse. Orientation to the operating room (OR) can involve a one-day course presented by the Operating Room/Recovery Room staff reviewing principles of perioperative and perianesthesia nursing. After the day of orientation, the obstetrical nurse then rotates into the Operating Room to observe cases and the activities of nurses in the scrub and circulator role. A critical component of this program is the continued validation of competence. The perinatal nurse works with the OR nurse to do a mock emergency cesarean birth setup on a quarterly basis.

CONTINUING EDUCATION

Fetal monitoring continuing education is a top priority in most departments. The traditional approach to fetal monitoring continuing education is a formal full-day workshop. If there is no one at the institution with the knowledge and skill to present this type of workshop, outside sources are available. One approach is to partner with the local nursing school and invite the perinatal nursing faculty to be a guest speaker. Those most likely to accept an invitation are nursing school faculty that use the institution as their clinical site for student nurses. As an alternative choice, the fetal monitoring equipment sales representative can arrange for a company-sponsored speaker at no charge to the institution. If funds are available, the AWHONN (1997) *Fetal Heart Monitoring Principles and Practices* workshop is a quality program. This program offers both didactic content and hands-on clinical skills. Regional faculty members can be found by calling the AWHONN national office. Some institutions elect to sponsor a formal fetal monitoring workshop every other year. During years when a workshop is not offered EFM continuing education can be provided through non-traditional quality fetal monitoring education programs such as use of a videotape series, computer-assisted instructional programs, or strip of the month clubs (see Appendix J). The Perifax Program offered through Strong Memorial Hospital in Rochester, New York is an innovative program that provides fetal monitoring case studies on a monthly basis. This program can be purchased for all staff on a yearly basis and is an ideal alternative for small rural hospitals without the resources of a perinatal educator. A committee of senior perinatal staff nurses can collect interesting fetal monitoring strips and compile case studies with portions of the FHR strip and patient history. Nurses can be asked to interpret the FHR and select appropriate nursing interventions. One institution uses a "nurse presenter of the month" who posts a FHR strip for 2 weeks to allow all staff to review and complete the review form. After the forms are completed and returned to this nurse, correct answers are posted and a discussion is held at the monthly staff meeting. This is a great learning process for the nurse who developed the fetal monitoring case study, as well as for the other staff who complete the process.

Other perinatal topics can be presented using the same nontraditional approaches. Many companies that sell services and products to the institution have clinical educators that will provide continuing education for nurses. For example, one of the infant formula companies presented a newborn abduction education program at no charge. Although some companies do not provide this type of service, they will usually agree to provide small education grants to support an outside speaker on a perinatal nursing topic. Recently Johnson and Johnson Consumer Products worked with AWHONN to develop the *Compendium of Postpartum Care*. This is an excellent comprehensive resource that includes a self-study module and it is free to AWHONN members. The National Certification Corporation for the Obstetric, Gynecologic and Neonatal Nursing Specialties (NCC) has developed self-study modules on various perinatal nursing topics that can be purchased for a nominal fee by calling 312-951-0207. Other self-study modules covering a wide variety of perinatal nursing topics are available through the March of Dimes at a very low price (see Appendix Q). As more nurses are comfortable using computers, use of interactive computer programs has become an additional method of quality continuing education. Many nurses enjoy using these programs because they are interactive and different from reading a traditional nursing text (Simpson, 1993). Videotape series have been developed by AWHONN, Williams & Wilkins, Mosby, and Lippincott-Raven on many perinatal nursing topics. The advantage to using learning modules, CAIs, and videotape series is that they can be loaned to nurses for use at home.

Journal club participation is another method to encourage staff nurses to keep abreast of new developments and current research. Monthly meetings to discuss interesting articles and educational resources, position statements, and committee opinions from professional organizations can stimulate practice changes. Many journals such as the *Journal of Obstetric, Gynecologic and Neonatal Nursing, the Journal of Nurse Midwifery, Journal of Perinatal and Neonatal Nursing, The American Journal of Maternal-Child Nursing,* and *Neonatal Network* offer continuing education credit for selected articles.

Attendance at outside educational programs may not be possible for all staff nurses, especially if they must cover their own expenses. However, those staff who are sponsored by the hospital to attend a conference should then present the new material to the other staff members. Nurses who attend conferences that are not sponsored by the hospital also can be encouraged to present a summary of the conference content. Although funds are limited to cover tuition and travel costs, payment for the time spent attending the conference is one way to support the nurse financially.

Perinatal outreach educators can be valuable resources. In most states, rural hospitals are part of a larger Perinatal Network. In Illinois, each level I and level II hospital is directly linked to a level III Perinatal Center. Outreach education is a required component of the program. These programs are free or at a very reduced cost and generally offer continuing education credits. Public health department staff can be invited to present information about services and programs such as the hepatitis vaccine initiative, mother-baby homecare, sexually transmitted disease prevention, and genetic issues.

Use of expert care providers from other departments in the institution is an avenue that is many times overlooked. Use the hospital directory to get ideas about possible speakers and topics. Physician colleagues can be invited to present inservices on perinatal topics or to conduct case study reviews. Anesthesia care providers are available to provide education on types of anesthesia, medications used, effects and adverse reactions, and nursing care of women receiving anesthesia/analgesia. At St. Francis Hospital, where epidural anesthesia is provided for women in labor, attendance at the annual inservice covering these topics is mandatory. An excellent reference for a staff education program for post anesthesia care of childbearing women was developed by a cooperative group of clinical nurse specialists and nurse managers in the state of Washington (O'Brien-Abel, et al., 1994). The article provides a clear outline for the educational module as well as a sample checklist and can easily be adapted to the individual setting. Pharmacists can offer educational programs on medications for perinatal patients such as cervical ripening agents, oxytocin for labor induction and augmentation, antihypertensives and heparin therapy. Social workers have information about programs such as Medicaid, the women and infants supplemental food and nutrition program, and community resources that is beneficial to nursing staff. A registered dietician may agree to present an inservice on prenatal nutrition or managing diabetes during pregnancy. The security department can be invited to present information about infant abduction and personal safety. Pastoral care services may be available to share information about how to handle perinatal loss. There are multiple untapped resources within any institution.

PERIODIC COMPETENCE VALIDATION

A quality orientation program for new nurse employees is the foundation for periodic competence validation and follow-up with experienced perinatal nurses. The challenge is to develop a program with meaning that is truly an opportunity to ensure that experienced staff nurses have maintained expected perinatal competencies. The perinatal core competence checklist can be used as a framework to validate competence on an annual basis (see Appendix B). Multiple methods such as evaluation of self-assessment components of learning modules, videotape series and CAIs, medical record audits, peer review, and patient feedback tools can be used (see the text appendices).

PROGRAM EVALUATION

The continuing quality-improvement process provides an excellent framework for program evaluation. Meeting the standards of care while maintaining an outcome focus will offer a needs assessment for the department. Using the previous focus from JCAHO of high-risk, low-volume or problem-prone areas still offers valid targets for education and competence validation. The current JCAHO (1997) standards require data collection, program evaluation, and documentation of these activities. At St. Francis Hospital, staff nurses assist with program reviews and concurrent chart audits as part of the department's improvement process. Employee performance evaluations should also focus on learning needs assessment. Using this process as an annual mechanism for professional growth and development rather than as a punitive measure is essential to the continued progress of a perinatal unit. St. Joseph's Hospital incorporates a skills validation checklist. The checklist is used throughout the year as key skills are identified and competence is validated. Staff members are assessed for skills and aspects of clinical judgment that could potentially place the patient at risk if not performed at the level of expected competence. The validation process is completed by senior (level III) nurses as they review and observe the level I and level II nurses. The level I designation means the employee is dependent on others to meet practice specifications as during orientation. Level II designation is characterized by independence in practice and ability to perform it without supervision. The level III practitioner has mastered the competencies and can fulfill the resource and consultative role within the department. The skills validation checklist must remain on the unit and be accessible to the persons making assignments for the shift. A workable solution is the placement of binders at the central station identified for the competence validation checklists. Sections for each employee contain a summary sheet that reflects the staff member's performance level as well as the completion of required institutional programs. This system provides the nurse manager with a reference for the annual performance evaluation as well as the opportunity to work with employees in setting performance goals for the next year.

SUMMARY

Validation of staff competence is an ongoing challenge nurse managers in small rural hospitals face daily. Few have perinatal educators to coordinate a competence validation program. Maintaining a focus on quality outcomes while complying with guidelines and standards from multiple professional organizations and regulatory agencies works well. To meet these demands, the nurse responsible for competence validation must seek innovative educational opportunities within the institution and in the community and use the extensive excellent resources that have been developed by experts in the perinatal nursing specialty. There is no reason to "reinvent the wheel." Although institutions have responsibilities for certain aspects of this educational process, individual nurses are also responsible (AWHONN, 1993). Perinatal nurses must actively seek opportunities for professional knowledge enhancement to meet the needs of childbearing families. Research-based practice is a joint responsibility and a critical component of quality perinatal nursing care.

REFERENCES

American Academy of Pediatrics & American College of Obstetricians and Gynecologists. (1997). <u>Guidelines for perinatal care</u>. Washington, DC: Author.

American Heart Association & American Academy of Pediatrics. (1994). <u>Neonatal resuscitation program</u>. Elk Grove Village, IL: Author.

Association of Women's Health, Obstetric and Neonatal Nurses. (1993). <u>Didactic content and clinical skills verification for professional nurse providers of basic, high-risk and critical-care intrapartum nursing</u>. Washington, DC: Author.

Association of Women's Health, Obstetric, and Neonatal Nurses. (1998). <u>Standards and guidelines for professional nursing practice in the care of women and newborns</u>. Washington, DC: Author.

Drukker, J. (1997). Multiple gestation. March of Dimes Nursing Module. March of Dimes Birth Defects Foundation, White Plains, NY.

Feinstein, N., & McCartney, P. (1997). AWHONN's Fetal heart monitoring principles and practices. Dubuque, IA: Kendall/Hunt Publishing Co.

Freda, M. C., & Patterson, E. T. (1994). Preterm labor: Prevention and nursing management. March of Dimes Nursing Module, March of Dimes Birth Defects Foundation, White Plains, NY.

Johnson & Johnson Consumer Products. (1996). Compendium of postpartum care. Skillman, NY: Author.

Joint Commission on Accreditation of Healthcare Organizations. (1997). Accreditation manual for hospitals, Standards. 1. Oakbrook Terrace, IL: Author.

Martin, E. J. (1996). Intrapartum management modules (2nd ed.). Baltimore: Williams & Wilkins.

National Certification Corporation for the Obstetric, Gynecologic and Neonatal Nursing Specialities (NCC). (1995). Certification program. Chicago: Author.

Northrop, C. E., & Kelly, M. E. (1987). Legal issues in nursing. St. Louis, MO: C.V. Mosby.

O'Brien-Abel, N., Reinke, C., Warner, P., & Nelson, C. (1994). Obstetrical postanesthesia nursing: A staff education program. The Journal of Perinatal & Neonatal Nursing, 8(3), 17–32.

Phillips, C. (1996). Family-Centered Maternal-Newborn Care, St. Louis: Mosby.

Poole, J. H. (1997). Hypertension during pregnancy. March of Dimes Nursing Module. March of Dimes Birth Defects Foundation, White Plains, NY.

Rural Wisconsin Health Cooperative. (1995). Competency based orientation program: Maternity department. Sauk City, WI: Author.

Simpson, K. R. (1993). Meeting the challenge of the 1990's: Strategies to provide quality perinatal services in an era of decreasing reimbursement. The Journal of Perinatal and Neonatal Nursing, 7(2), 1–9.

Simpson, K. R. & Creehan, P. A. (Eds.). (1996). AWHONN's perinatal nursing. Philadelphia: Lippincott-Raven.

Southern New Jersey Perinatal Cooperative. (1992). Perinatal continuing education program modules. Pennsauken, NJ: Author.

State of Illinois. (1987). Illinois administrative code. Springfield, IL: Author.

Tappero, E. P., & Honeyfield, M. E. (1996). Physical assessment of the newborn: A comprehensive approach to the art of physical assessment (2nd ed.). Petaluma, CA: NICU INK.

Tucker, S. M. (1996). Fetal Monitoring and Assessment (3rd ed.). St. Louis: Mosby.

White, D., & Poole, J. H. (1996). Obstetrical emergencies for the perinatal nurse. March of Dimes Nursing Module. March of Dimes Birth Defects Foundation, White Plains, NY.

CHAPTER 4

Challenges of Perinatal Outreach: Identifying and Meeting Educational Needs of Nurses in Network Hospitals

Mary Neuman and Susan Weekly

INTRODUCTION

Perinatal outreach programs play a critical role in the delivery of quality perinatal services in their network area. Perinatal educators, nurses, and physicians provide a vital link between small rural community hospitals and the specialty knowledge, technologies, and providers that may only be available in tertiary care centers. The availability of perinatal outreach programs that provide consultation and referral services, educational support, and assistance with the development of evidence-based protocols and practice guidelines contributes greatly to the ability of small rural hospitals to care for childbearing women and their families in their own communities.

Even with the existence of comprehensive perinatal outreach programs, there are ongoing issues and special challenges for small rural hospitals that support specialty care services. Administrators of small rural hospitals and community leaders may elect to eliminate speciality services such as perinatal care that benefit small populations in favor of speciality services that potentially benefit more patients in the community such as orthopedics, geriatrics, cardiology, rehabilitation, and pediatrics. These clinical areas are easily integrated with existing medical-surgical and family practice care models. Perinatal services require a major financial and human resource commitment. Allocation of physical space, purchase of high-tech equipment, and commitment for education to attain and maintain competence of perinatal care providers in a hospital that expects under 250 births annually may not be feasible. Thus, small hospitals in rural communities face a dilemma when providing full-scope specialty services. Perinatal services in many institutions do not generate a profit. However, there are data showing that a positive childbearing experience may result in return business for hospitals for future healthcare needs of the entire family. If women in the community are forced to travel distances to receive perinatal care, they may be more comfortable with the tertiary care center where they gave birth when other healthcare needs arise. Community support and utilization of services in small hospitals are crucial for their financial survival. The decision to continue to provide specialty care that is not profitable is difficult for any hospital but is especially complex in smaller rural hospitals that have limited financial and personnel resources and less flexibility in absorbing the costs of nonreimbursed care.

Common concerns that must be addressed by a smaller hospital providing perinatal care are both logistical and financial. Financial resources for costly equipment such as electronic fetal monitors and birthing beds and for education to attain and maintain competence of the nursing staff may be limited. Even if financial resources are adequate, the ability to maintain competence in perinatal nursing for nurses who work in a hospital where births occur infrequently is a challenge. The opportunity for perinatal nurses to care for childbearing women in this setting may arise only once or twice a month. When nursing competence in caring for childbearing women and newborns is difficult to achieve, maintain, and validate, liability risk management and compliance with JCAHO standards for performance expectations become problematic.

The basic nursing education for many nurses who work in rural community hospitals provides limited perinatal clinical nursing experience. This is due, in part, to the fact that nurses who work in the rural area were also educated in that same community where clinical experiences in obstetrics were either not available or rare. In some cases there may have been an opportunity to observe only one labor and birth or perhaps view a videotape of a labor and birth. Fetal monitoring is not a component of most basic nursing school curriculums. Hours of lecture and clinical practice in specialty nursing areas such as perinatal nursing have been decreased or eliminated in many nursing schools. The lack of formal education and clinical practice in perinatal nursing before graduation provides unique challenges for perinatal units in rural settings because these graduates often go directly to their community hospital to practice.

Small community hospitals that do continue to provide perinatal care must design a program that ensures that care provided is consistent with current guidelines and that standards of care and competent nurses are available when necessary. A designated nurse coordinator for perinatal services is one component of a quality perinatal program. This nurse can ensure that clinical practice is current and can act as a champion for the perinatal specialty. Most small rural hospitals do not have positions for perinatal educators or clinical nurse specialists. Traditionally, in addition to nursing staff education, nurses in these roles are also responsible for the development of perinatal policies, procedures, and evidence-based protocols or practice guidelines that are consistent with guidelines and standards of care. The ability of perinatal care providers in small rural hospitals to consult with the tertiary care center through perinatal outreach programs when developing these types of practice guidelines is essential. Nevertheless, it remains challenging to offer appropriate healthcare provider education and to facilitate a practice environment that will allow them to provide safe and effective care to pregnant women and newborns.

This chapter describes Nebraska Methodist Hospital (NMH) Perinatal Center's formal education program currently used in rural community hospitals, and provides suggestions for implementation by perinatal outreach educators.

THE MISSION OF NEBRASKA METHODIST PERINATAL OUTREACH PROGRAM

The Nebraska Methodist Perinatal Outreach Program is part of a tertiary perinatal center averaging 3000 births annually. The program's mission is to improve quality of perinatal care in participating rural community hospitals. In 1984, the program started when perinatologists established a remote fetal monitoring consultation service in three rural hospitals in Iowa and Nebraska. Soon after, a part-time perinatal nurse outreach coordinator and a full-time nurse educator were added to the outreach team. Currently, there are over 30 rural community hospitals in Nebraska, Iowa, northern Kansas, and northwest Missouri that are enrolled in the program. Annual birth volumes in participating hospitals vary as follows: 45% of hospitals (24–99 births), 35% (100–250), and 20% (250–900). Locations range from a 30-minute drive to as much as a 5-hour drive, with an average driving time from Nebraska Methodist Hospital (NMH) of 2–3 hours. In addition to the clinical consultation service, the other major program component is continuing education for the healthcare providers, which serves as a framework for promoting evidence-based clinical care by competent clinicians.

CONCEPTUAL FRAMEWORK FOR EDUCATIONAL ASSESSMENT

A first step in providing education to outreach hospitals is to identify the learning needs of the healthcare providers. An excellent conceptual framework (Jones and Modica, 1989) that can be used for rural community staff learning needs assessment including assessment objectives, target groups, assessment category, and method is depicted in Display 4-1.

Ideally, several methods are used for needs assessment for any target population. Both informal and formal methods are helpful. Informal methods used by NMH include information gathered during telephone calls from providers at the outreach hospitals, educational presentations, remote fetal monitoring fax transmissions, and patient transfers. Formal methods are written questionnaires and chart reviews/quality indicators (QI) data. Information from all sources help to construct a more comprehensive and reliable assessment of each unit's specific learning needs.

DISTINGUISHING EDUCATIONAL WANTS FROM EDUCATIONAL NEEDS

One of the major difficulties encountered by the perinatal outreach staff when conducting an educational assessment was how to identify the knowledge level of the rural community nurses. For several years, the process involved asking the nursing contact person at each rural hospital to complete a questionnaire indicating educational programs that were of interest. One of the major problems with using questionnaires and surveys asking for programs of interest to

DISPLAY 4-1

Conceptual Framework for Assessment

Assessment Objective

Target Groups	Assessment Category	Method
Individual	Knowledge	Informal
Agency	Equipment and services	Discussions
Region	Psychomotor skills	Grand rounds
	Care practices	Transport
		Conferences
		Formal
		Questionnaire or survey
		Interview
		Chart review
		Written examination
		Observation

For example: Objective —> Target population —> Assessment categories —> Methods
Conceptual framework for assessment

identify educational needs is that they assess individuals' interests or "wants" rather than "actual" learning needs (Farley & Fay, 1988; Puetz & Jazwiec, 1991). Several authors have discussed the importance of distinguishing between educational wants versus actual educational needs (Farley & Fay, 1988; Puetz & Jazwiec, 1991; Kristjanson & Scanlon, 1989; Maloney & Kane, 1995; Timms, 1995). A "felt" need is a conscious desire or interest that is best known by the individual, whereas a "real" need is a gap in knowledge, attitude, or skills measured according to some objective criteria (Monette, 1977). Individuals may or may not be aware of their real educational needs.

By 1992, strong relationships between the outreach staff and the staff in the participating hospitals had developed that allowed the outreach staff to make accurate observations about real education needs. Many requested programs involved new technologies or complex clinical issues. However, most likely the rural hospital making the request would not keep patients or perform the procedures about which they requested information. It became apparent that a significant difference existed between what the contact people identified as "wants" or "felt needs" versus a "real" educational need. Although felt needs should not be ignored, it was important to find a system to assess actual needs and to plan appropriate educational opportunities.

Due to the limitations of a traditional questionnaire, an assessment model that would more accurately identify "actual" learning needs was necessary. By addressing "actual" learning needs, education could be provided to promote competence of the nursing staff in providing perinatal care. Therefore, a competence model of assessment was the most appropriate for meeting the goal. In addition, a competence model for assessment is consistent with the following Joint Commission on Accreditation of Healthcare Organizations (JACHO) standards: (a) HR.3: The leaders ensure that the competence of all staff members is assessed, maintained, demonstrated, and improved continually and (b) HR-4.3: The hospital regularly collects aggregate data on competence patterns and trends to identify and respond to the staff's learning needs (1996).

COMPETENCE MODEL

Competence models assess learning needs of individuals in relation to some standard of performance or competence (Puetz & Jazwiec, 1991). They are designed by first deciding what capabilities or expertise are necessary for practice in a specific area. More specifically, they identified the dimensions of competent performance which include the successful integration of technical, interpersonal, and critical thinking skills. Competence statements must be specific and measurable. They should clearly describe what is expected including both knowledge and clinical skills. Current level of competence is determined by how accurately the expected competence statements describe the nurses' knowledge and clinical skills. Learning needs are defined by identifying gaps between expected competence and current demonstrated competence.

THE PERFORMANCE-BASED DEVELOPMENT SYSTEM (PBDS)

In 1986, Nebraska Methodist Hospital purchased the Performance Based Development System (PBDS) for use in the orientation of newly employed nurses (Del Bueno, Weeks, & Brown-Stuart, 1987). PBDS, a competency-based performance assessment, was developed in 1985 by nine acute care hospitals in conjunction with Baxter Management Services (Del Bueno, 1990). Dorothy Del Bueno, RN, PhD acted as Chief Consultant for Development. This system currently has modules to assess clinical competence in the following areas: obstetrics, medical-surgical, intensive care, and neonatal intensive care. An assessment for managerial competence is also available.

PBDS uses a critical pathway concept in determining individual development needs. The concept is based on a reliable assessment through objective measurement. Objective measurement includes methods and tools that evaluate three dimensions of competent performance including (a) critical thinking, (b) interpersonal relations, and (c) technical skills. The theoretic framework is illustrated in Figure 4-1, where three overlapping circles in a square

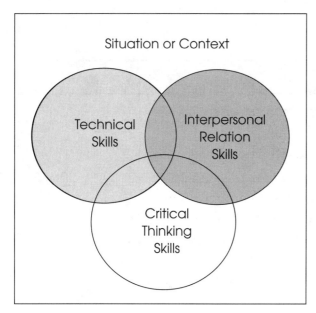

Figure 4-1. Dimensions of competent performance.

represent the interrelated skill dimensions inherent in any role. The square represents the clinical environment, such as the hospital, unit, or shift. Measurement of these three dimensions of competent performance is accomplished through the use of various exercises including video simulations, prioritization activities, audiotapes, games, and criterion checklists.

These methods allow an evaluation of a nurse's current performance ability relative to desired performance. Desired performance is evaluated by the use of criterion-based model answers. Model answers for each exercise include both acceptable and unacceptable responses agreed upon by a group of clinical experts. Analysis of the gaps in performance allows an identification of steps needed to close these gaps. If a lack of knowledge or the inability to perform a skill is identified, an individualized learning plan can be developed to address the learner's needs.

THREE DIMENSIONS OF COMPETENT PERFORMANCE

Critical Thinking Skills

Objective measurement of critical thinking or clinical judgment is difficult. The various dimensions of critical thinking that are necessary for competent nursing practice are outlined in Display 4-2: critical thinking dimensions (Del Bueno, Weeks, & Brown-Stewart, 1987). These dimensions are assessed by a variety of simulation methods including clinical video vignettes, prioritization exercises, problem-solving algorithms, and care planning exercises.

Clinical Vignettes

Clinical vignettes are 2- to 5-minute video simulations for each patient situation. Each simulation presents a patient portrayed by an actress who follows a structured script. The patient is experiencing a specific perinatal problem. The nurses are evaluated on their ability to recognize specific clinical problems and to identify interventions for these problems along with an acceptable rationale for each intervention listed. For example:

(a) In a video simulation of placental abruption, the actress complains of symptoms of abruption, such as constant abdominal pain and vaginal bleeding; other cues presented are vital signs, a rigid uterus, and an electronic fetal monitoring strip depicting uterine irritability.

(b) In a video simulation of intraamniotic infection, the actress describes symptoms of fever, chills, general malaise, and diarrhea, and the FHR pattern is tachycardia with decreased FHR baseline variability.

Top Priority

Top Priority uses a game approach in which event cards present various clinical situations. The nurse must prioritize each card as an urgent priority (must do) or as something that must be done but can be delayed. For example, the nurse may be given several cards representing patient situations such as:

(a) a newly admitted pregnant woman who needs a speculum exam to rule out ruptured membranes,

(b) a woman in labor with hyperstimulation related to oxytocin administration and a nonreassuring fetal heart rate, or

(c) a woman in labor reporting increasing perineal pressure.

The nurse evaluates the clinical situations presented on the cards and identifies which is most urgent with rationale.

Display 4-2

Critical Thinking Dimensions

Clinical Decision Making
- Ability to identify a priority risk to a patient's health.
- Ability to describe nursing interventions to correct or minimize identified risks.
- Ability to identify nursing interventions that may prevent potential risks.
- Ability to defend decisions using scientific knowledge principles or proven practice.
- Ability to make decisions related to urgent risks with a predetermined time limit.

Priority Setting/Revising
- Ability to differentiate the priority of both independent and dependent nursing activities required by a specific patient.
- Ability to determine the relative priority of specific uncontrolled events that occur in clinical units.
- Ability to describe or demonstrate interventions that will correct or minimize harm from specific uncontrolled events.

Problem Solving/Troubleshooting
- Ability to identify malfunction problems of specific invasive monitoring devices.
- Ability to describe/demonstrate nursing actions to be taken in response to malfunction problems.
- Ability to determine variables causing specific interpersonal problems and subsequent outcomes.

Care Planning
- Ability to develop or revise a nursing care plan for a specific patient based on a primary and secondary data base.
- Ability to develop a discharge plan to manage actual and potential health risks for a specific patient.

Source: Del Bueno, Weeks, & Brown-Stewart (1987).

What If

"What if" exercises present clinical situations that require a response as to what the nurse would do or say in a certain situation. These exercises are particularly helpful for future reference if this clinical situation presents at a later date. For example the nurse may be asked:

(a) "What if" a physician requests that a patient be admitted for elective induction of labor and there are insufficient nursing staff resources available to provide safe care for that patient?

(b) "What if" a woman in labor with a nonreassuring fetal heart rate expresses a desire to ambulate despite explanations about concerns for fetal status?

(c) "What if" a pregnant woman in preterm labor presents with a prolapsed umbilical cord?

(d) "What if" a women in labor attempting a vaginal birth after cesarean birth reports sharp pain in the lower abdomen?

(e) "What if" the physician begins closing the skin during cesarean birth and final instrument and needle counts are not correct?

Problem-Solving Algorithm

The Problem-Solving Algorithm is an exercise used to differentiate reassuring situations from dangerous or potentially dangerous situations. The nurse is then asked to describe or demonstrate appropriate nursing interventions for these clinical situations. The nurse's ability to recognize reassuring versus nonreassuring fetal monitoring patterns along with effective nursing interventions for nonreassuring patterns can be assessed using this method. Appropriate nursing interventions can be evaluated for each step. For example, it is not enough to correctly interpret the FHR and initiate intrauterine resuscitation interventions. The nurse must also know what to do and who to call if the FHR does not return to a reassuring pattern. The ability to follow through a course of a complex problem-solving algorithm is required, especially in the rural hospital where the perinatal nurse may be the only nurse available with expertise in caring for pregnant women.

Care Planning Activities

Care planning activities include assessment of the ability of the nurse to prioritize a patient assignment and to develop and/or revise a plan of care. The nurse is given a typical patient census list with diagnoses and conditions. The nurse must be able to correctly decide patient acuity and make appropriate patient care assignments based on that decision.

Interpersonal Relationship Skills

Interpersonal relationship simulations use audiotaped conversations between two nurses, a nurse and a patient, or a nurse and a physician. The nurse is assessed based on ability to analyze interpersonal strategies and to identify ineffective and effective communication strategies. Some examples are:

(a) A nurse receives a report from the nurse on the previous shift that a physician has ordered magnesium sulfate prophylaxis for a woman in labor with pregnancy-induced hypertension 2 hours ago, but the nurse hasn't started the intravenous infusion,
(b) The visitor policy limits one person at the bedside for birth and the woman in labor requests that her mother and sister also be present in addition to the father of the baby.
(c) A physician is notified of a nonreassuring FHR pattern and asked to come to the hospital to evaluate the patient, but refuses to do so.
(d) A physician requests that the nurse bring a vacuum extractor in the room for birth and the nurse knows this physician does not have privileges for operative vaginal births.
(e) The father of the baby is obviously intoxicated and becomes verbally abusive to the woman in labor.

Technical Skills

Technical skills involve checklists to evaluate the nurse's ability to perform specific technical skills either by simulation or with an actual patient (Display 4-3). Technical skills requiring assessment are selected based on unit expected competence statements, how often the skills are used, and the potential for risk of adverse patient outcomes if competence was not ensured (Del Bueno, Weeks, & Brown-Stewart, 1987).

DEVELOPMENT OF THE UNIT-BASED ASSESSMENT MODEL

We felt that the PBDS program would provide the appropriate philosophy, tools, and components to more accurately assess the actual learning needs of nurses in the rural hospitals in a time-efficient manner. In 1992, the designated "perinatal" nurse from each perinatal outreach participating hospital was invited to a focus group to gather data for development of a unit-based assessment program that could evaluate learning needs of the nursing staff at his or her hospital. A 2-day workshop was held with 16 hospitals represented.

The philosophy and components of the PBDS program were explained. Each component was administered to the focus group members. Their responses served to validate the model answers that the perinatal outreach team educators had developed as applicable for their institution. An evaluation of the maximum time that would be allowed for completion of the assessment was discussed by the group. It was decided that a 4-hour evaluation session would be the most realistic for staffing and for monetary compensation to the

DISPLAY 4-3

FUNDAL CHECK

CRITICAL ELEMENTS

	Met	Not Met
1. Assures patient privacy by closing curtain and pulling sheet.	☐	☐
2. Raises nightgown over abdomen.	☐	☐
3. Explains procedure.	☐	☐
4. Positions patient comfortably on back.	☐	☐
5. Places one hand over symphysis.	☐	☐
6. Palpates fundus for firmness.	☐	☐
7. Massages fundus with cupped hand or fingertips, if fundus is boggy.	☐	☐
8. Measures fundal height in fingerbreadths below or above the umbilicus.	☐	☐
9. Documents	☐	☐
a. Fundal height.	☐	☐
b. Fundal firm or boggy.	☐	☐

_____ Passed _____ Needs to repeat

Validated by_____ Date_____

---

staff. Members of the focus group also decided that it would be optional to divide the staff into groups of 10 or fewer, with enough sessions to evaluate all of the staff. An institutional assessment form was given to determine facility accommodations and needs of each community hospital. (See Display 4-4.) Group members were informed that the program would be piloted in two to three sites to assist in the resolution of unanticipated operational issues. After the pilot phase, the program was offered to all interested sites at a charge to the outreach hospital based on the number of nurses who participated.

Critical thinking, interpersonal skills, and technical skills were evaluated; however, the program required modification in order to complete the assessment in a 4-hour time period. As originally designed, the assessment of critical thinking alone can take anywhere from 6 to 18 hours based upon how many dimensions are assessed and the number of clinical areas evaluated (Del Bueno, Weeks, & Brown-Stuart, 1987).

After a review of all the possible tools and exercises that are available for PBDS obstetric assessment, the program was modified to include the components that were appropriate for a 4-hour perinatal unit-based assessment. See Display 4-5 for an outline of the components used, along with explanations of the assessment purpose for each component. New exercises were developed to assess breastfeeding, pharmacology, labor progress, and electronic fetal monitoring. Care planning exercises were omitted and the total number of situations/questions

DISPLAY 4-4

Institutional Assessment

1. Anticipated number of your staff to be assessed. _____
2. Is there meeting room space available at your hospital? _____
3. Do you have a VCR available? _____
4. Would you be able to send your staff to a nearby hospital for assessment if necessary to best utilize the facilitator's time? _____
5. Would a fee per person be workable? _____
6. Is your staff currently allowed to do the following?

   Place scalp electrodes. Yes _____ No _____
   Place intrauterine pressure catheters. Yes _____ No _____
   Perform cervical checks. Yes _____ No _____
   Perform gestational age assessments. Yes _____ No _____

   If you answered no to any of the above, please describe if the staff is not trained or the physicians do not want them to perform the skills. If you would like assistance in these areas, please explain.
7. Please describe your staff's strengths as a unit.
8. Please describe your staff's weaknesses as a unit.
9. How do you feel this assessment program will help your staff?
10. Was there anything missing from this assessment program?
11. Are there any specific needs, problems, or concerns we should be aware of before bringing this assessment program to your staff? Please be specific.
12. Additional comments or suggestions?

---

in some of the components was reduced to meet the 4-hour time limitation. For example, the ten situations presented in the "What If" exercise were reduced to four. The only component where the total number of situations was not reduced was clinical videotapes, because this was a major component of clinical judgment and was most likely to provide data about how the nurse may perform in an actual clinical situation.

IMPLEMENTATION OF THE UNIT-BASED ASSESSMENT

In 1993, the program was trialed at three community hospitals. The number of nurses in each group were 6, 10, and 29. The larger group was at a level II hospital where nurses practiced in a mother/baby (MB) or labor/birth/recovery (LDR) care model. They were divided into separate groups for MB and LDR with videos and other exercises specific for their area of clinical practice. In smaller hospitals using the labor/birth/recovery/postpartum (LDRP) model and where LPNs are used, exercises were geared for each role.

Further refinement of the tools used for evaluation was completed. The results for each component were obtained based on the analysis of the total number of acceptable answers divided by the total number of participants. A process was developed to report the results in an objective manner that detailed the unit strengths as well as their educational needs. The

DISPLAY 4-5

Outline of Components Used for Unit-Based Assessment for Obstetrics

PBDS Component	Assessment Purpose

1. Clinical Judgment Skills
   a. (Videotapes 11-12)
      Problem diagnoses:
      -Prolapsed cord
      -Precipitous labor
      -Preeclampsia
      -Uterine hyperstimulation from pitocin
      -Preterm labor
      -Nonreassuring fetal heart rate pattern
      -Placental abruption
      -Postpartum urinary retention
      -Postpartum hemorrhage
      -Neonatal hypoglycemia
      -Neonatal cardiorespiratory arrest
      -Neonatal sepsis
	Assesses ability to identify patient problems, describe appropriate interventions, and rationale for those interventions.

b. -Fetal monitoring case studies
      2 NSTs
      3 labor strips
	Assesses the ability to interpret fetal monitoring strips based upon the patients history including risk factors. Assesses ability to identify appropriate nursing interventions.

c. -Event cards
      23 cards total with nursery, postpartum, antepartum, labor, birth, and Delivery Recovery events
      Example: Your patient with PIH complains of a severe headache and refuses pain medication
Priority determination: Must Do
	Assesses ability to identify priority situations from situations that must be addressed but not immediately.

d. What If Exercise (4 situations) Example: A labor patient with spontaneous rupture of membranes states her fluid was green-colored. She refuses fetal monitoring and an IV.	Assesses ability to identify acceptable interventions for priority events requiring immediate action.
e. Fetal monitoring algorithm (11 strips with patient history)	Assesses ability to recognize reassuring versus nonreassuring fetal monitoring patterns along with effective nursing interventions for nonreassuring patterns.

DISPLAY 4-5 (cont.)

f. Graphing and Interpreting labor curves (2 cases)	Assesses ability to graph labor curve and appropriately interpret.
g. Breastfeeding -Multiple choice questions	Assesses basic knowledge about breastfeeding.
h. Pharmacology -Questions (multiple choice, true-false and matching)	Assesses knowledge of common medication used in obstetrics.
2. Interpersonal (4 audiotaped simulations) -2 nurse-patient interactions -1 nurse-MD interaction -1 nurse-nurse interaction IPR example: A mother receives inconsistent information regarding breastfeeding.	Assesses ability to identify ineffective and effective interpersonal/communication strategies.
3. Technical Skills -Fundal check -Bulb syringe infant -Newborn lavage -Deep tendon reflexes -Application of scalp electrode -Cervical models	Uses criterion checklists to assess the ability to perform specific technical skills.
4. Miscellaneous Stages and phase of labor (short answer)	Assesses ability to identify/define stages and phases of labor.

---

results were reported in percentages so that both the perinatal outreach educator, the perinatal contact nurse, and the nursing staff could discuss how to prioritize the learning needs. The outreach educator provided recommendations about areas that might be the most important to address first. Learning options to address the educational needs were also included in the report. A copy of the report was sent to the perinatal contact nurse. (See Appendix 4-1 for a sample report.) The program was then offered to community hospitals participating in the perinatal outreach program that had been represented in the focus group. All but two have used the program.

ASSESSMENT FORMAT

The participants were informed of this activity by their supervisor and scheduled for a morning or afternoon session. Although the nurses on the perinatal outreach team were known to the participants, anxiety was a universal emotion for session participants. An informational letter has since been drafted that details the philosophy, purpose, and mechanism in an effort to relieve unnecessary anxiety prior to the assessment session.

Before the assessment is formally started, the nurse participants are assured that individual performance assessment data would not be reported and they would be asked only to designate RN or

LPN and area of clinical practice specialty. No names are used and the answer sheets remain the property of Nebraska Methodist Hospital. The purpose of the assessment is to evaluate the competence of the group of nurses as a whole rather than as individuals. (See Display 4-6 for description of the format followed for the 4-hour assessment session.)

EVALUATION

In 1995, representatives from hospitals that participated in the unit-based assessment program in 1993 and 1994 were asked to complete an evaluation about their experience with the program. All those participating indicated that they felt that both the assessment process and the data reported were helpful. Although most perinatal contact nurses indicated they were not surprised at the results, there were some who were surprised at specific areas of learning needs that they had taken for granted.

At one hospital it was noted that nurses were unable to identify a prolapsed cord and that they did not know to push the presenting part off the cord. Although this information was shocking to the unit nurse manager, it gave an opportunity for education and competence validation before a potential adverse outcome occurred.

The evaluation also included a grid that reflected learning needs. (See Display 4-7 for a sample.) This allowed the perinatal outreach team and nurses in participating hospitals to see progress and identify follow-up learning needs. Assistance for follow-up educational opportunities was offered in the form of self-studies, protocols to discuss in unit meetings, case studies the perinatal unit manager could present, and formal presentations by the outreach team at the participating community hospital.

MODIFICATION FOR USE BY OTHER HOSPITALS

For hospitals that would like to use this type of program but do not have access to the PBDS system, a similar program can be designed by developing exercises to evaluate critical thinking, interpersonal relationship, and technical skills. It is important to incorporate all components and to trial the components to ensure that they are clear, accurate, and effectively evaluate the desired areas. The first step is the development of expected perinatal unit competence statements (see Appendix B). An excellent reference for designing and critiquing competence statements for nursing performance evaluation has been written by Gurvis and Grey (1995). Although it is time-saving to purchase video- and audiotapes and other available learning activity resources, it is not necessary to do so if there are limited financial resources for education and competence validation. The professionally produced videotapes in the critical thinking component can be replaced by written

Display 4-6

Format for Unit-Based Assessment

Group activities (1.5 hours)
  Introductions
    philosophy
    purpose
    anonymity of performance
    explanation of materials
  Video vignettes
    time limited to 5–7 minutes of writing for each problem
  Audiotapes
    time limited to 5 minutes of writing for each problem
  Break
Self-Paced Materials (2.5 hours)
  (Divide room into workstations)
  Fetal monitoring exercises
  Breastfeeding
  Pharmacology
  Top Priority
  What If
  Labor curve
  Stages and phase of labor
  Technical skills

Display 4-7

Recommended Learning Options

The recommended learning options included in your assessment report follow. Please check the appropriate corresponding comments.

	Done	Planned	Need Resources	Need A Program
Self-Studies				
Fetal Monitoring				
Breastfeeding Self-Study				
Pharmacology of the Alpha and Beta Receptors (includes Terbutaline)				
Presentations				
Fetal Monitoring Case Studies (If you'd like to present some, or, we could send you some to use.)				
Labor Curve (reviewing terminology and abnormals)				
Pitocin Augmentation and Induction				
Reflex and Clonus Assessment				
Determining Care of the At-Risk Obstetric Patient Through the Use of Video Simulation (We could use either the same or different videos than those used at the assessment with the problems we used in the assessment. We show each situation, have staff write answers, and then discuss as a group. We could focus on nursing interventions and rationale as well as nursing diagnosis.)				
Fetal Monitoring Interpretation and Nursing Management				
Breastfeeding				
Nursing Assessment of the Postpartum Woman (Hematoma and postpartum hemorrhage could be focused on.)				
Pregnancy Induced Hypertension.				
Labor and Delivery Complications (Talk could focus on your assessed needs: nursing interventions and rationale for these complications such as prolapsed cord, PIH, abruption, etc.)				
Videos				
Newborn Thermoregulation				
Fetal Monitoring Interpretation				
Printed Material				
$MgSO_4$, Information Sheet				
Others				
Interpersonal Relations (audiotapes, roleplaying).				
Priority Setting (discussion of situations presented for the assessment, other situations also could be developed.)				
Discussion in staff meetings regarding dealing with physicians; how to negotiate.				

perinatal case studies that include clinical signs and symptoms, laboratory data, and electronic fetal monitoring strips. Interpersonal relationship exercises can be developed and easily audio-recorded. Top priority games, what if exercises, problem-solving algorithms, and care planning activities can be developed in a reasonable timeframe.

CONCLUSION

Although this program is very labor-intensive, the information has been most helpful in planning educational programs that are appropriate and individualized for each participating outreach hospital. Identification of strengths and weaknesses of the clinical skills and knowledge levels of an aggregate group of nurses representing unit competence are critical to guide the planning of targeted education programs for each hospital. Perinatal outreach programs include a number of participating hospitals. The opportunity to have the perinatal outreach education team on-site is limited, thus the programs that are provided must be appropriate and accurately reflect each participating hospital's needs. Objective data gathered in a systematic approach through a program described in this chapter is one way to make sure this occurs.

Having a formal program not only helps facilitate appropriate education for participating outreach hospitals, it also allows the tertiary hospital to allocate their resources most efficiently. Teamwork between the outreach providers and the participants improves perinatal care delivery in small rural community hospitals.

REFERENCES

Del Bueno, D. J. (1990). Experience, education and nurses' ability to make clinical judgements. Nursing and Health Care, 11(6), 290–294.

Del Bueno, D. J., Weeks, L., & Brown-Stewart, P. (1987). Clinical assessment centers: A cost-effective alternative for competency development. Nursing Economics, 5(1), 21–26.

Farley, J. K., & Fay, P. (1988). A system for assessing the learning needs of registered nurses. Journal of Continuing Education in Nursing, 19(1), 13–16.

Gurvis, J. P., & Grey, M. T. (1995). The anatomy of a competency. Journal of Nursing Staff Development, 11(5), 247–252.

Joint Commission on Accreditation of Health Care Organizations (1996). Comprehensive Accreditation Manual for Hospitals: The Official Handbook. OakBrook Terrace, IL.

Jones, D. B., & Modica, M. M. (1989). Assessment strategies for the outreach educator. Journal of Perinatal and Neonatal Nursing, 2(3), 1–10.

Kristjanson, L. J., & Scanlan, J. M. (1989). Assessment of continuing nursing education needs: A literature review. The Journal of Continuing Education in Nursing, 20(3), 118–123.

Laurent, C. L. & Johnston, C. R. (1995). Implementing the performance based development system (PBDS) at Naval Medical Center San Diego. Journal of Nursing Staff Development, 11(3), 156–159.

Maloney, P., & Kane, J. W. (1995). An innovative solution to assessing staff learning needs. The Journal of Continuing Education in Nursing, 26(2), 67–72.

Monette, M. L. (1977). The concept of educational need: An analysis of selected literature. Adult Education, 27(2), 116–127.

Puetz, B. E., & Jazwiec, R. M. (1991). Learning needs assessment. Concepts and process. Journal of Nursing Staff Development, 7(2), 91–94.

Timms, J. (1995). Needs assessment surveys in gerontological nursing: Are we really assessing continuing education needs and priorities? The Journal of Continuing Education in Nursing, 26(2), 84–88.

APPENDIX 4-1. Unit-Based Educational Assessment—Obstetrics

UNIT-BASED EDUCATIONAL ASSESSMENT—PERINATAL
CRITICAL THINKING ASSESSMENT

Clinical Video Vignettes

Strengths

A total of eight nurses completed this exercise. The majority (75% or more) were able to identify 9 of the 11 problems presented as follows:

    100% were able to identify preterm labor, PIH, and neonatal respiratory arrest.

    100% of nurses were able to identify nonreassuring FHR patterns (50% labeled it as nonreassuring, and 50% said late decelerations).

    88% were able to identify uterine hyperstimulation, distended bladder, and neonatal hypoglycemia,

    75% were able to identify precipitous labor and abruptio placenta.

Nurses were able to identify the majority of the critical nursing interventions for nonreassuring FHR patterns, uterine hyperstimulation, and neonatal respiratory arrest.

- 88% appropriately identified the need to feed the hypoglycemic infant some D5/W.
- 88% identified the need to empty the bladder of the postpartum woman.

Educational Needs Identified

- Only 62% identified postpartum hemorrhage.
- Only 50% of nurses identified a prolapsed cord and none specified they would do a vaginal exam in order to assess for prolapsed cord and attempt to push the presenting part off of the cord.
- 62% omitted stating they would prepare for a precipitous birth and 50% did not specify that they would notify the MD of a precipitous labor.
- 75% omitted turning the woman in preterm labor to her side and to increase IV fluids.
- 50% or more omitted the following interventions for PIH: lateral position, assessment of maternal vital signs, and deep tendon reflexes.
- 75% omitted assessing maternal vital signs for a suspected abruption and 38% omitted increasing IV fluids and assessing the FHR.
- 62% omitted checking the fundus for a distended bladder.
- 50% or more omitted the following interventions for a postpartum hemorrhage: assess bladder, pad count, and massage uterus.
- 88% omitted continuing to assess the hypoglycemic baby for further signs of hypoglycemia.
- 25% omitted potentially increasing IV fluids for nonreassuring FHR and for uterine hyperstimulation.

Overall, the participants did not identify specific rationale for most of the critical nursing interventions. The majority were unable to list nursing diagnoses for the majority of problems.

NOTE: A common finding throughout the videos, as well as the fetal monitoring exercises, was the repeated omission of IV hydration and positioning as critical nursing interventions for several of the problems presented. Participants are able to identify problems, but need to increase their knowledge of nursing interventions along with rationale for those interventions.

Fetal Monitoring

Strengths

- 87% of participants were able to interpret NSTs as reactive versus nonreactive (this result does not include the nurse who does not work in L&D and one LPN).
- The nurse who said she does not work in L&D was able to correctly interpret NSTs.
- 75% to 100% of all participants were able to correctly identify fetal monitoring strips as reassuring versus nonreassuring in seven of the ten strips illustrated.
- 100% were able to identify decreased variability on three of the three strips that showed decreased variability. (The non-L&D nurse and one LPN were not included in the result.)

APPENDIX 4-1. Cont.

- 87% identified hypertonic contractions, i.e., uterine hyperstimulation (excludes LPN and non-L&D nurse.)
- Both the LPN and non-L&D nurse took the appropriate action for hypertonic contractions (LPN said to notify RN; non-L&D nurse identified hyperstimulation and said to contact L&D RN but did not say to discontinue pitocin.)
- All of the participants were able to identify the seriousness of a prolonged deceleration even though they did not know the correct terminology.

Educational Needs Assessed

- Participants were unable to identify subtle late decelerations in two different strips. Only 38% of participants identified subtle late decelerations in both strips. (The LPN and non-L&D person were excluded from these statistics.) Some of the participants identified them as early decelerations, one said variable with a late component, and others did not specify type of decelerations. Because late decelerations were not identified, the correct interventions were not listed.
- 40 to 50% were unable to identify variable decelerations and the need for a position change.
- Only one participant identified baseline tachycardia and no one listed the intervention of assessing the maternal temperature for baseline tachycardia.
- 70% omitted discontinuing pitocin for uterine hyperstimulation, and 60% omitted administering oxygen via face mask and potentially increasing IV fluids.
- 70% did not identify marked variability although the majority *did* list the appropriate interventions.
- 70% were unable to label accelerations, however, 80% *did* know that the strip was reassuring.
- The majority of participants (60–70%) did not list all of the appropriate interventions for decreased variability. Actions omitted included: possible application of scalp electrode for further assessment, maternal repositioning, oxygen via face mask, potentially increasing IV fluids, and discontinuing pitocin. Most staff did say they would try to stimulate the baby.
- 100% omitted the need to perform a vaginal exam and ask the woman to stop pushing for a prolonged deceleration. Also omitted by at least 50% of the participants was potentially increasing IV fluids, assessing maternal blood pressure for hypotension, administering oxygen via face mask, and notifying MD.
- There was inconsistency in the terminology to describe variability (often the word "poor" was used to describe decreased variability.)

NOTE: Regarding the LPN and non-L&D staff member. The majority of the time, both of these individuals were able to identify when strips were nonreassuring and stated they would notify the OB nurse. The only exception to this was the subtle late decelerations: they did not identify these as nonreassuring.

Breastfeeding

Overall, the participants demonstrated *excellent* knowledge of breastfeeding. Eight of the ten participants had attended the breastfeeding inservice presented in April. There was a definite improvement in the knowledge level on this assessment compared to the assessment completed prior to the April workshop. The results show a knowledge deficit in the following areas:

Early initiation of breastfeeding—25% of those who attended the workshop continued to feel that early initiation of breastfeeding is not associated with longer duration of nursing.

Breastpumping for NICU—50% of those who attended the workshop still did not know how long the woman should pump each breast. 50% of all participants showed a lack of knowledge about the advantages of double breastpumping.

Breastfeeding frequency—75% of those who attended the workshop continue to incorrectly believe that breastfeeding babies 0–6 weeks of age should be nursing every 3–4 hours.

Sore nipples—25% of all participants are unaware of the causes of sore nipples.

Flat or inverted nipples—50% or more of all participants omitted the use of an electric breast pump for treatment and 40% omitted the use of breast shells. 30% of all participants still selected a nipple shield as treatment (20% of those who selected the shield had not attended the workshop.)

APPENDIX 4-1. Cont.

Hazards of nipple shields—50% of total did not know that a shield can result in newborn dehydration (20% of the total had not attended the workshop.)

Pharmacology

Of all the exercises completed, pharmacology was the one with which the majority of the participants had the most difficulty. The following educational needs were identified:

Oxytocin—70% unable to identify side effects.

MgSO4—60% unable to identify action of MgSO4; 70% unable to identify toxicity level of MgSO4.

Aspirin—50% unable to identify medication that does not contain aspirin.

Ritodrine (Yutopar)—90% unable to identify side effects.

Terbutaline (Brethine)—90% unable to identify primary nursing assessment.

Cervical Dilation

The nurses are able to appropriately identify cervical dilatation and effacement.

Labor Curve

Approximately 50% of the nurses who completed this exercise were able to properly graph both dilation and descent on the labor curves. Several participants did not properly graph descent. Slightly over 50% were able to identify the multiparous woman's labor curve as normal. However, only 43% were able to identify the nulliparous woman's labor curve as normal. No one identified a longer than average mean for the active phase of the nulliparous woman; 43% identified it as a prolonged latent or early phase of labor.

Priority Setting

Almost all of the nurses (80%) were able to prioritize correctly the majority of the time. The one situation that was *under*-prioritized by 70% of the staff was the newborn with an *axillary* temperature of 97.2. The one situation that was consistently *over*-prioritized by 60% of the staff was the hyperemesis patient putting food in the trash. Forty percent of the nurses did not identify a woman after a vaginal birth complaining of rectal pressure in the immediate postpartum period as a priority (possible hematoma).

Overall, the majority of the nurses were able to identify the key interventions to five situations that may arise on the perinatal unit. Most responses indicated attention directed toward addressing the patient's identified needs and interventions to promote maternal and fetal wellbeing. Participants were inconsistent as to how they would handle the patient's mother who wants to visit her laboring daughter (daughter doesn't want mother in room). Although all of the participants respected the daughter's wishes, how to relay this to the mother was not always addressed consistently.

INTERPERSONAL SKILLS ASSESSMENT

Strengths

A majority of the time, nurses' responses promoted direct communication with involved people and attempted to reach a win-win outcome.

Educational Needs Identified

Participants could use more practice with responses to include:

- Acknowledging the frustration of the breastfeeding woman (example: "It must be frustrating that the nurses are giving you different instructions about pumping your breasts.")
- Taking positive steps to correct a departmental problem (example: inconsistent breastfeeding practices).
- Acting as a patient advocate by providing information needed for the woman in order to make an informed decision; then supporting and facilitating client's decision (example: breastfeeding baby during the night).
- Negotiating for a better outcome in situations where the nurse disagrees with MD decision.

TECHNICAL SKILLS ASSESSMENT

Fundal Check

All of the nurses demonstrated the proper procedure for a fundal check.

APPENDIX 4-1. Cont.

Bulb Syringe
Almost all of the nurses demonstrated the proper procedure for use of the bulb syringe. A few did not position the baby on its side and did not suction out both mouth and nose. Several nurses were unaware that the mouth should usually be suctioned before the nose.

Newborn Lavage
All participants were able to properly demonstrate correct placement of a nasogastric feeding tube, verification of tube placement, aspiration of stomach contents, and removal of the tube.

Deep Tendon Reflexes
Nine nurses were evaluated. Seventy percent assessed properly for clonus. All nurses knew at least one reflex and 70% assessed more than one. Several nurses need to apply more pressure with the reflex hammer to be certain to elicit the appropriate reflex.

LEARNING OPTIONS

Self-Studies
- Fetal Monitoring
- Breastfeeding Self-Study
- Pharmacology of the Alpha and Beta Receptors (includes Terbutaline)

Presentations
- Fetal Monitoring Case Studies (if you'd like to present some, or we could send you some to use)
- Labor Curve (reviewing terminology and abnormals)
- Pitocin Augmentation and Induction
- Reflex and Clonus Assessment
- Determining Care of the At-Risk Pregnant Patient Through the Use of Video Simulation (we could use either the same or different videos than those used at the assessment with the problems we used in the assessment. We show each situation, have staff write answers, and then discuss as a group. We could focus on nursing interventions and rationale as well as nursing diagnosis.)
- Fetal Monitoring Interpretation and Nursing Management
- Breastfeeding
- Nursing Assessment of the postpartum woman (the focus could be on hematoma and postpartum hemorrhage)
- Pregnancy-Induced Hypertension
- Labor and Birth complications (talk could focus on your assessed needs: nursing interventions and rationale for these complications such as prolapsed cord, PIH, abruption, etc.)

Videos
- Newborn Thermoregulation
- Fetal Monitoring Interpretation

Printed Material
- MgSO4 information sheet

Others
- Interpersonal Relations (audiotapes, role-playing).
- Priority setting (discussion of situations presented for the assessment, other situations also could be developed)
- Discussion in nursing staff meetings about working collaboratively with physicians; how to negotiate.

APPENDIX 4-1. Cont.

Summary

The nurses are able to identify problems for childbearing women and appropriately prioritize patient situations.

We expect to find that learning needs and addressing those identified for nurses at your hospital will enhance their ability to provide appropriate nursing interventions.

Recommendations

The best initial learning options are:

1. Complete the fetal monitoring self-study.
2. Videotaped simulations of OB problems (used in the assessment) along with a discussion of interventions and rationale.
3. Fetal monitoring case studies.

    Strips could be used to address your educational needs, including pitocin. Cases can be presented by your staff or by us.

    Options #2 and #3 can be supplemented by written handouts.

CHAPTER 5

The Perinatal Education Consortium: A Regional Approach to Nursing Education and Collaboration

Nancy O'Brien-Abel, Judy Schroeder, Mary Burroughs, and Julie Wehmeyer

INTRODUCTION

Orientation to the perinatal nursing speciality typically consists of self-study, formal classroom instruction, and a clinical preceptorship. Orientation programs are implemented on an as-needed basis in most hospitals, that is, when nurses are hired to fill vacancies that may occur periodically. In small hospitals it is possible to have only one nurse in orientation at any one time. Classroom instruction for one nurse is not feasible or desirable, yet important content must be covered during the orientation period. Some hospitals have designed self-study components of orientation to meet the education needs of orientees such as computer-assisted instructional programs, self-assessment learning modules, and videotape series. Although these educational resources provide valuable information, limitations of this approach include the inability to interact with other nurses new to the speciality and to ask questions and seek clarification from a "live" educator and clinical expert.

This chapter discusses the development and implementation of a perinatal education consortium (PEC). Nurse educators and administrators in hospitals in the northwest region of Washington state collaborated to plan, implement, and evaluate a basic orientation program for newly hired and cross-trained perinatal nurses (see Appendix 5-1). Roles and responsibilities for nurses who coordinate the program in participating hospitals are clearly defined and outlined (see Appendix 5-2). This program of shared resources and expertise is financially advantageous and has contributed to quality perinatal nursing orientation, continuing education, and competence validation in participating hospitals.

This collaboration has also been beneficial for clinical practice. During formal and informal meetings, information beyond perinatal education programs is shared among participants. There are opportunities to discuss emerging practice trends, new standards and guidelines, and clinical practice protocols. Thus, not only is time saved developing educational programs, but sharing practice protocols, policies, and procedures can also eliminate duplication in research and writing these essential unit resources. Professional relationships that otherwise may not have developed have proven to be an additional valuable outcome of the consortium.

THE PERINATAL EDUCATION CONSORTIUM

The Northwest Regional Perinatal Outreach Program at the University of Washington in Seattle, consisting of 30 participating hospitals, was founded nearly 20 years ago. Nurse managers from these hospitals meet as a group three to four times annually to discuss common concerns about referrals, consultation, clinical practice, and education. A consistent theme in the discussions over the years has been the challenges of providing comprehensive nursing orientation programs to small groups of nurses or individual nurses hired on an as-needed basis.

In 1991, five perinatal and neonatal clinical nurse specialists from several of the outreach hospitals met to consider collaborating on nursing orientation. Together they developed a survey to explore interest in a collaborative didactic education program for perinatal and neonatal nurses. The survey was mailed to perinatal and neonatal nurse managers, educators, and clinical nurse specialists in 45 hospitals in western Washington. Questions included interest in forming a consortium, length and description of their current orientation program, average number of staff nurses oriented annually, and estimated cost of orientation per staff nurse. Response to the survey was overwhelming. Representatives from 41 of the 45 hospitals surveyed indicated interest in joining the consortium. However, this number of hospitals, located throughout a large geographic area, seemed unmanageable. Had it been known that there would be this much interest, the initial survey would have been limited to a more local group of hospitals in the northwestern area of the state. Like many other states, Washington is divided into regions for the coordination and provision of perinatal care. To expedite coordination and development of the PEC, membership was limited to hospitals participating in the outreach program. These hospitals are located in Seattle and its outlying areas. Presently 16 outreach hospitals, the Northwest Perinatal Outreach Program at the University of Washington, and Children's Hospital Medical Center form the North Puget Sound PEC. For the most part the hospitals that are full members of the PEC are major medical centers with level II and level III status, although there are several level I members. Because few level I hospitals have perinatal clinical nurse specialists or educators, the ability to meet the criteria for full membership is difficult (see Appendix 5-3); however, for a nominal fee per nurse, these hospitals can send orientees to the orientation program. Thus, the 14 other hospitals in the Northwest Regional Outreach Program do participate in the PEC.

A full program description is provided in Appendix 5-1. Core content was developed by the group and includes key clinical topics in the perinatal and neonatal nursing specialities. Content for each day is devoted to a subspecialty area such as labor and birth, postpartum care and infant feeding, perinatal complications, newborn stabilization and resuscitation, and care of newborns in the special care nursery. Thus, program attendance can be tailored to meet the clinical practice model at each hospital. For example, if nurses are expected to provide care to women during the antepartum, intrapartum, and postpartum period, as well as to the healthy full-term newborn and newborns requiring special care nursery admission, completion of the entire 8-day program would be beneficial. Nurses who care for women only during labor and birth or who only provide mother-baby care can attend the appropriate days based on content. The PEC education program is provided twice annually, usually in the spring and the fall. Sites are rotated among member hospitals and are set more than a year in advance to ensure room accommodations. Some years, the course is offered 4 days each week over a 2-week period. In other years the course has been offered 2 days per week over a 4-week period. Members of the advisory committee meet semiannually to set dates and sites. Knowing dates well in advance allows for scheduling and planning. Some hospitals attempt to limit hiring of new nurses to near the time of the next PED education program.

MEMBERSHIP RESPONSIBILITIES AND BENEFITS

Each member hospital is required to select one representative to actively participate on the PEC advisory committee. This representative selects one job, also known as a major service (Appendix 5-2) that contributes to the production of the PEC education program. Major services are reassigned annually. Any costs incurred in providing the services, with the exception of printing course materials, are assumed by member hospitals. In addition each hospital must provide an educator to teach a minimum of 4 hours of instruction per program. Typically this instruction is provided by members of the PEC advisory committee and other perinatal-neonatal clinical educators and clinical nurse specialists from the member hospitals.

To make commitment to the PEC formal, member hospitals sign a letter of understanding stating each hospital's willingness to participate for 1 year as a member of the consortium (Appendix 5-3). This letter serves as a contract outlining the consortium benefits, definition of major services to be provided for each education program, membership requirements, organizational structure, and financial arrangements. The agreement is reviewed annually or may be terminated by the member hospital on 90-day written notice to the PEC board of directors.

PEC sets a community standard for perinatal and neonatal nursing education. Using the expertise of the most highly qualified perinatal and neonatal nurse educators and clinical nurse specialists in the region, PEC provides nursing education superior to any program that an individual hospital could offer. Nurses employed at member hospitals can enroll in any or all of the 8-day lecture series at no charge. Continuing nursing education credits are provided to program attendees at the conclusion of each day of the program.

ORGANIZATIONAL STRUCTURE

The PEC's organizational structure is modeled closely after a critical care consortium developed in the Seattle area (Jacobsen, 1990). The foundation of the PEC is the advisory committee, which consists of one representative from each member hospital. The advisory committee meets a minimum of twice annually to evaluate the most recent consortium education program, discuss concerns, and make recommendations to the board of directors. The board of directors consists of five members of the advisory committee and includes the president, vice president, secretary, treasurer, and continuing education application and credit coordinator. They are elected by members of the advisory committee and serve 2-year terms designed in a way so that the entire board does not go out of office in any one year. The board of directors manages the financial status of the PEC, monitors contract compliance by member hospitals, and implements changes based on the education program evaluations and recommendations from the advisory committee.

FINANCES

Revenue is generated by charging nurses from nonmember hospitals $40 per day or $300 for the entire 8-day program. In addition, vendors who exhibit products pay a fee. Hospitals who recently joined the PEC and did not participate in the early development of the program pay a one-time fee of $500. This combined revenue is used to cover the costs of course materials (our primary direct expense) and costs associated with the semiannual advisory committee and board of directors meetings. Nonprofit status has been obtained. Initial expenses for nonprofit status included a business license and attorney fees for development of the articles of incorporation and bylaws. State-required reports are submitted annually, with a minimum filing fee.

PROGRAM EVALUATION

Participants have consistently described the PEC education program as clinically focused, challenging, helpful, exciting, innovative, and a great way to meet other nurses from around the region. Suggestions for improvements have been easily incorporated into the program. Many of the attendees are nurses new to the perinatal and neonatal nursing specialty, thus although they may have feedback about presentation style, their ability to accurately assess instructors for omissions in critical content or inaccurate information is limited. To maintain high quality education, one advisory committee member serves as a facilitator each day of the program (see Appendix 5-4). This facilitator shares his or her expert evaluation with the advisory committee at the conclusion of the 8-day program.

The PEC education program is also evaluated by the advisory committee at the semiannual meeting. Representatives from member hospitals agree that the benefits of the PEC are enormous. Pooling expertise saves time and financial resources. Collaboration on education overlaps frequently to collaboration on clinical practice issues. Quality perinatal and neonatal nursing education contributes to quality perinatal and neonatal clinical practice. Nurses who provide care to childbearing women and newborns in the member hospitals have a solid foundation in speciality clinical knowledge.

CONCLUSION

The success of this excellent program is particularly remarkable given that the many participating hospitals represent different health systems and financial networks. The nursing leaders who had the initial vision and the commitment to make the PEC program a reality are to be commended. Collaboration between perinatal nurses across healthcare systems is becoming less common as competition for perinatal services in a geographic area may be intense. Sharing expertise and pooling human and financial resources must be the hallmark of contemporary nursing practice. Traditional methods for orientation and continuing education are no longer working in some institutions. Classroom orientation for one or two nurses is prohibitive, but the new nurse must have the opportunity to learn the essentials of perinatal and neonatal nursing. Development of a program based on this model is possible in any community when nurses are willing to work together and forget "the way we've always done it" when considering nursing education. Collaboration between perinatal nurses can only enhance clinical practice in the nursing care of childbearing women and newborns.

REFERENCES

Jacobsen, C., Malan, S., Perkins, T. & Slatten, R. (1990). A regional approach to entry-level critical care education. Journal of Critical Care: AACN, 17(5), 385–393.

Nelson, C., Edwards, J., O'Brien-Abel, N., Blanchard, K., Kearns, S., & Wehmeyer, J. (1995). Development and implementation of a perinatal education consortium. Journal of Obstetric, Gynecologic, and Neonatal Nursing, 24(8), 708–712.

APPENDIX 5-1. Perinatal Education Consortium Lecture Series for Basic Labor and Birth, Mother-Baby, & Special Care Nursery Nursing

COURSE AGENDA

DAY 1
LABOR AND BIRTH

Labor Process/Pelvic Anatomy	3 hours, 45 minutes
Diabetes	1 hour, 30 minutes
Preterm Labor/PROM	1 hour, 45 minutes

DAY 2
LABOR AND BIRTH

Hypertension in Pregnancy	1 hour, 30 minutes
Bleeding during Pregnancy	1 hour, 15 minutes
Placental Pathology	30 minutes
Fetal Monitoring	2 hours, 30 minutes
Legal Issues	1 hour

DAY 3
LABOR AND BIRTH

Nonpharmacologic Pain Relief	1 hour, 15 minutes
Pharmacologic Pain Relief	1 hour
Birthing Complications	1 hour
Induction/Augmentation of Labor	1 hour, 15 minutes
Cesarean Birth and PACU Care	1 hour
ECG Interpretation for OB Care	1 hour, 30 minutes

DAY 4
POSTPARTUM CARE AND INFANT FEEDING

Postpartum Assessment and Care	1 hour, 30 minutes
Postpartum Complications	1 hour, 15 minutes
Post-Discharge Mother-Baby Follow-Up Care	1 hour, 15 minutes
Infant Feeding	2 hours

DAY 5
PERINATAL CHALLENGES

Adolescent Pregnancy and Parenting	1 hour, 30 minutes
Contraception	2 hours
Maternal Infections (HIV, HSV, BV, Hepatitis, GBS)	2 hours
Perinatal Grief and Loss	1 hour, 30 minutes

DAY 6
THE NEWBORN

Newborn Transition and Stabilization	1 hour, 15 minutes
Gestational Age Assessment	45 minutes
Newborn Physical Assessment	1 hour, 30 minutes
Newborn Behavioral Assessment	1 hour
Common Newborn Complications	1 hour, 30 minutes
Asphyxia in the Newborn	1 hour, 15 minutes

DAY 7
THE NEWBORN

Fetal Development	1 hour
Newborn Cardiac Anomalies	45 minutes
Newborn Surgical Emergencies	45 minutes
Respiratory Complications	1 hour, 30 minutes
HBV, HS, HIV in the Newborn	1 hour, 30 minutes
Neonatal Sepsis	1 hour, 30 minutes

DAY 8
SPECIAL CARE NURSERY

Newborn Stabilization and Transport	45 minutes
Prematurity Clinical Issues	3 hours, 15 minutes
Parenting in the NICU	30 minutes
Discharge Preparations	15 minutes
Breastfeeding the Preterm Infant	2 hours

APPENDIX 5-2.

NORTH PUGET SOUND PERINATAL EDUCATION CONSORTIUM

Major Service Job Description

MAJOR SERVICE: President,
    Member, Board of Directors
FUNCTIONS:

1. Acts as resource to member hospital representatives regarding Consortium activities, rules, procedures, and major job descriptions.

2. Oversees functioning of Consortium and provide consultation as needed to assure Consortium comes off smoothly.

3. Presides over PEC Board and Advisory Committee meetings. Provide agenda to Secretary 3-4 weeks prior to Board and Advisory meetings.

4. Receives feedback from Evaluation Coordinator and the Content Committee regarding individual speaker performance. Counsel or arrange mentorship, as needed, to improve speaker performance.

5. Calls for elections of Board of Directors officers every other year. Call for major service redistribution annually.

6. Oversees update of PEC job descriptions annually or as needed.

7. President elected by Advisory Committee for a two-year term.

NORTH PUGET SOUND PERINATAL EDUCATION CONSORTIUM

Major Service Job Description

MAJOR SERVICE: Vice President
    Member, Board of Directors
FUNCTIONS:

1. Acts on behalf of President if President is unable to fulfill duties on a temporary or permanent basis (e.g., illness, extended absence, position change).

2. Assumes additional major service as able.

3. Attends Board and Advisory Committee meetings and presides over these meetings as necessary in President's absence.

4. Vice President elected by Advisory Committee for a two-year term.

APPENDIX 5-2. Cont.

NORTH PUGET SOUND PERINATAL EDUCATION CONSORTIUM

Major Service Job Description

MAJOR SERVICE: Secretary
  Member, Board of Directors

FUNCTIONS:

1. Takes minutes at all Advisory Committee and Board meetings. Types and disseminates to Board of Directors and Advisory Committee members.

2. Maintains a current mailing list for the Advisory Committee.

3. Receives agenda from Board President 3 weeks prior to Board of Directors and Advisory Committee meetings. Types and distributes at least 2 weeks prior to meeting(s).

4. Maintains records for consortium activities and correspondence.

5. Maintains the file of Letters of Understanding from each member hospital and sends out renewal letters every year in October to assure receipt by January 1st.

6. Provides new members with job description packet.

7. Secretary elected by Advisory Committee for a two-year term.

APPENDIX 5-2. Cont.

NORTH PUGET SOUND PERINATAL EDUCATION CONSORTIUM

Major Service Job Description

MAJOR SERVICE: Treasurer
  Member, Board of Directors

FUNCTIONS:

1. Establishes / maintains a checking account to handle all monetary transactions.

2. Establishes nonprofit status and maintains a business license from the State of Washington.

3. Receives all checks for payment of tuition and reimbursement from vendors. Maintains separate tracking mechanisms for reporting purposes. Notifies registrar of late fees received.

4. Provides a written Treasurer report at each Advisory Committee meeting and as requested by the Board.

5. Provides a written annual report.

6. Submits required Business and Occupation Tax forms to state agency according to required timeline.

7. Completes and submits appropriate forms to non-member hospitals, providing tax number for their accounting purposes.

8. Pays any PEC bills pending approval of Board of Directors.

9. Treasurer elected by Advisory Committee for a two-year term.

Appendix 5-2. Cont.

NORTH PUGET SOUND PERINATAL EDUCATION CONSORTIUM

Major Service Job Description

MAJOR SERVICE: CEARP Coordinator
Member, Board of Directors

FUNCTIONS:

1. Completes CEARP application to the Washington State Nurses Association which is accredited as an approver of continuing education in nursing by the American Nurses' Association's Board on Accreditation. Individual days within the course will be given CEARP credits to benefit participants attending selected days.

2. Requests speakers to complete the "Offering Approval Documentation Form" for each new talk they give or whenever they make content changes.

3. Prepares CEARP certificates. Places certificates in a separate envelope for each day. Distributes the envelopes of certificates to the Site Coordinator prior to the beginning of the course.

4. At conclusion of the course, requests originals of attendance sign-in sheets for course. (Site Coordinator will forward originals and retain copy for back-up.)

5. At conclusion of the course, requests copy of evaluation summary.

6. Maintains on file a copy of the CEARP application and syllabus for each Consortium offering.

7. Prepares report for Advisory Committee meeting.

8. Elected by Advisory Committee for a two-year term.

Appendix 5-2. Cont.

NORTH PUGET SOUND PERINATAL EDUCATION CONSORTIUM

Major Service Job Description

MAJOR SERVICE: Content Coordinators

FUNCTIONS:

1. Provides maternal and neonatal expertise in evaluating course content.

2. Meets after each PEC program and as needed to review evaluations and make changes in course content.

3. Updates course content and course/topic objectives.

4. Communicates revisions of course content to Course, CEARP and Syllabus Coordinators.

5. Calls on other Advisory Committee members for expertise as needed.

6. Coordinates with Course Coordinator for speaker arrangements.

7. Reviews CEARP applications from speakers to ensure consistency with objectives, as needed.

8. Prepares report of hours of instruction provided by member hospitals.

9. Reallocated as a major service annually (Jan-Dec).

Appendix 5-2. Cont.

NORTH PUGET SOUND PERINATAL EDUCATION CONSORTIUM

Major Service Job Description

MAJOR SERVICE: Site Coordinator

FUNCTIONS:

1. Reserves room for duration of course, classroom style preferred.

2. Arranges for the following to be set up and available in the classroom each day:
   a. slide projector
   b. overhead projector
   c. pointer
   d. lavaliere microphone
   e. stationary microphone
   f. extra blank overheads
   g. colored pens
   h. VCR or film projector

3. Requests members to sign up to act as facilitators for the next Consortium.

4. Confirms facilitator for each day. Conducts facilitator orientation approximately one week before course at PEC site. Stores syllabi, registration and evaluation materials for daily distribution.

5. Every morning checks in with daily facilitator. Provides facilitator with reference list, including number of on-site contact person for use throughout the day for troubleshooting, (e.g., AV problems, environmental concerns, aid to speakers). Provides facilitator with syllabi, sign in sheets and evaluations. Reminder notes of the particulars of your site are also helpful.

6. Collects sign-in sheets at the end of the day. Makes two copies and forwards originals to CEARP Coordinator. Forwards one copy to Registration Coordinator for tally of attendees, and retains one copy.

7. Sends evaluations to the Evaluation Coordinator.

8. Sends collected late registration fees to Treasurer.

9. Prepares report for the Advisory Committee meeting.

10. Service as Site Coordinator is required only once in a calendar year. If PEC is offered twice in a year, two hospitals may chose Site Coordinator as a major service.

11. Reallocated as a major service annually (Jan-Dec).

Appendix 5-2. Cont.

NORTH PUGET SOUND PERINATAL EDUCATION CONSORTIUM

Major Service Job Description

MAJOR SERVICE: Registration Coordinator

FUNCTIONS:

1. Coordinates closing date of registration with Syllabus, Advertising, Site and Course Coordinators.

2. Coordinates with registration provider to verify brochure information, phone numbers, correct information for confirmation letters including map, and late registration information.

3. Coordinates with registration provider to get daily roster of registrants prior to beginning of classes to Site Coordinator.

4. Coordinates with registration provider for data after classes completed: name and number attended by day and hospital; name and number of no shows by hospital; total attended by day; number of late registrants by hospital; record of late fee and non-Consortium tuition payments.

5. Maintains record of registrants for review by the Board. This report will be available at Advisory Committee meeting.

6. Prepares copies of report for Advisory Committee meeting.

7. Tracks payment of late registration fees and follow up.

8. Reallocated as a major service annually (Jan-Dec).

APPENDIX 5-2. Cont.

NORTH PUGET SOUND PERINATAL EDUCATION CONSORTIUM

Major Service Job Description

MAJOR SERVICE: Advertising Coordinator

FUNCTIONS:

1. Confers with Course, Syllabus and Registration Coordinators to establish registration deadline.

2. Distributes brochure two months prior to the beginning of each course. Maintains mailing list in collaboration with the NW Regional Care Program office and/or secretary of PEC.

3. Brochure should include:

    a. title
    b. sponsored by: *North Puget Sound Perinatal Education Consortium and the NW Regional Perinatal Care Program*
    c. dates
    d. course description
    e. course content
    f. member hospitals and representatives
    g. registration fees
    h. registration deadline
    i. refund policy
    j. faculty
    k. CEARP credits (verify with CEARP Coordinator)
    l. contact person with phone number (Registration Coordinator)
    m. registration form -- include role (RN____   LPN___   Other____)

4. Prepares report for Advisory Committee meeting.

5. Reallocated as a major service annually (Jan-Dec).

APPENDIX 5-2. Cont.

NORTH PUGET SOUND PERINATAL EDUCATION CONSORTIUM

Major Service Job Description

MAJOR SERVICE: Syllabus Coordinator

FUNCTIONS:

1. In collaboration with Registration, Advertising, Site and Course Coordinators, sets deadline for the submission of course materials and close of registration. Material not received by the deadline will become the responsibility of the speaker to duplicate. If no new material is received, material from prior PEC sessions will be placed in syllabus.

2. Obtains agenda, including schedule and faculty list, from Course Coordinator or content committee. Copies first page on assorted colored paper to distinguish individual days.

3. Syllabi should be copied single-sided, not exceeding 4 pages per hour lecture, no articles. Each day's syllabus should be stapled together as packet.

4. Delivers syllabi to facilitator's orientation meeting.

5. Prepares an invoice for all duplicating costs and forwards it to Treasurer.

6. Makes sufficient syllabi for pre-registered attendees, plus 20 for potential late registrants. In the Spring makes one extra copy for each member hospital.

7. Prepares report for Advisory Committee meeting.

8. At Advisory Committee meeting following the Spring Consortium, distributes additional copies of syllabi.

9. Reallocated as a major service annually (Jan-Dec).

APPENDIX 5-2. Cont.

NORTH PUGET SOUND PERINATAL EDUCATION CONSORTIUM
Major Service Job Description

MAJOR SERVICE: Course Coordinator

FUNCTIONS:

1. Confers with Site, Advertising, Syllabus and Registration Coordinators regarding chronology of deadlines, including brochure.

2. Obtains course schedule from Content Committee chair one month before brochure is due out. Forwards to Advertising Coordinator.

3. Contacts and confirms speakers by phone for the course if not done by Content Committee. Once commitment is made, speakers will be responsible to replace themselves and contact Course Coordinator.

4. When all speakers are verbally confirmed, types schedule with speakers included and forwards to Advertising, Syllabus, Site and Evaluation Coordinators, including speaker phone list. (May be delegated to Content Committee).

5. Sends confirmation letter to all speakers at least one month prior to deadline required for syllabus printing. Letter should include:

    Date and time of presentation(s); map of facility and parking (as needed); handout guidelines (4 pages/hour of presentation, no articles, include objectives); name and mailing address of Syllabus Coordinator; name of Site Coordinator to communicate special AV needs; name and address of CEARP Coordinator to send completed CEARP forms (include sample CEARP forms).

6. Sends copy of course agenda to all Advisory Committee members who have not already received one.

7. Notifies CEARP Coordinator immediately if there are changes or speaker substitutions that alter number of applicable credit hours.

8. Prepares report for Advisory Committee meeting.

9. Reallocated as a major service annually (Jan-Dec).

APPENDIX 5-2. Cont.

NORTH PUGET SOUND PERINATAL EDUCATION CONSORTIUM

Major Service Job Description

MAJOR SERVICE: Evaluation Coordinator

FUNCTIONS:

1. Prepares evaluations in consultation with CEARP Coordinator. Places evaluations in a separate envelope for each day. Distributes the envelopes of evaluations to Site Coordinator prior to the start of the course.

2. At end of Consortium, receives evaluations back from Site Coordinator.

3. Collates results of evaluations by speaker and prepares master list of speakers and their rating for review by Board prior to the Advisory Committee meeting.

4. Distributes brief speaker evaluation to each speaker, through hospital representative at Advisory Committee meeting.

5. Collates overall course evaluations and prepares written summary to distribute at the Advisory Committee meeting.

6. Reallocated as a major service annually (Jan-Dec).

APPENDIX 5-3.

NORTH PUGET SOUND PERINATAL EDUCATION CONSORTIUM

1998 PEC Membership Agreement -Letter of Understanding

THE NEED FOR A CONSORTIUM

Providing extensive perinatal education to prepare staff to work in labor and birth, mother-baby, and special care nursery units is not only costly, but consumes many hours of preparation and teaching time. In light of the current cost containment activities affecting all health care facilities, an effort to share perinatal education resources, including educators, materials and support services, is seen as desirable. In cooperation with the Northwest Regional Perinatal Outreach Program, several clinical nurse specialists from area institutions met in spring 1991 to discuss the feasibility of developing a consortium for perinatal education. The concept of shared educational resources for perinatal education is even more efficacious at the present time with the decreasing resources to meet the educational demand of preparing nurses to work in this rapidly changing specialty.

THE PERINATAL EDUCATION CONSORTIUM (PEC) PROVIDES FOR:

1) A broad availability and sharing of expertise of perinatal educators and clinical nurse specialists
2) A reduction of duplicate efforts in perinatal courses and offerings
3) A community standard for perinatal education
4) Reduced costs to member hospitals for perinatal education
5) Access to quality perinatal education for the nursing community
6) CEARP credits for participants

MEMBERSHIP

Membership shall be for a term of one (1) year beginning January 1, 1998, and may be renewed every year by each member of the Consortium. A Consortium hospital electing to discontinue its membership shall provide not less than 90 days' prior written notice of its intent not to renew its membership.

Membership in the Consortium requires that the hospital is willing and able to provide all of the following:
1) A minimum of one major service per year;
2) Instruction for a minimum of four (4) hours of content for each program (consideration will be given to availability of instructors at each hospital). In the unusual event that a member hospital cannot provide any speaking hours, member hospital will provide a facilitator for two days during each program. When a member hospital's agreed upon speaker, major service and/or facilitator person(s) is/are no longer available, the member hospital maintains responsibility for fulfilling these requirements;
3) Active participation on the Consortium Advisory Committee; and
4) Rotational service on Board of Directors.

Participants from member hospitals will not be charged a fee to attend the Consortium. Hospitals joining the Consortium after January 1, 1993, will be charged a one-time fee of $500.

DEFINITION OF MAJOR SERVICES (See attached complete major service description)

1) **Site Coordinator:** Two site coordinators per year. Arranges conference room, provides audio-visual equipment and assists vendors and exhibitors. Oversees site facilitator on daily basis.
2) **Advertisement Coordinator:** Develops and mails brochures to PEC members and area hospitals.
3) **Registration Coordinator:** Collects registrations, and maintains an updated list of participants. Forwards non-member registration monies to the treasurer. Sends confirmation letter with all necessary information (maps, locations, lists of texts, etc.) to all participants.

APPENDIX 5-3. Cont.

4) **Course Coordinator:** Confirms speakers and distributes course information (objectives, course schedules) to speakers and Advisory Committee. Generally oversees flow of program.
5) **Syllabus Coordinator:** Collects teaching materials from instructors and prepares syllabi for participants. Printing costs will be reimbursed by the Consortium.
6) **Content Coordinators:** Reviews each speaker's content outline to make sure it covers consortium objectives. Updates consortium objectives as needed. Alters course content to reflect current community needs.
7) **Evaluation Coordinator:** Prepares evaluation, collates program and instructor evaluations. Sends feedback to speakers and Board of Directors.
8) **CEARP Coordinator:** Member, Board of Directors. Prepares CEARP application and maintains application materials on file. Issues certificates of completion and maintains related records.
9) **Secretary:** Member, Board of Directors. Records, types and distributes materials for Advisory Committee and Board of Directors. Distributes annual contracts to members. Maintains records, including contracts.
10) **Treasurer:** Member, Board of Directors. Deposits all registration monies and pays all approved expenses from the nonprofit account. Provides semi-annual budget reports to Advisory Committee. Maintains nonprofit organization status.
11) **Vice President:** Member, Board of Directors. Fills President role in absence of President
12) **President:** Member, Board of Directors. Presides over Advisory Committee and Board of Directors, Oversees functions of entire Consortium.

Major services will be rotated among the Consortium members as determined by the Board of Directors. Costs incurred providing major services are assumed by the hospital except syllabus reproduction.

STRUCTURE

ADVISORY COMMITTEE:

1) Consists of one representative from each member hospital
2) Meets a minimum of two times per year
3) Assesses needs and determines frequency of programs
4) Provides input regarding functioning of the Consortium and community needs

BOARD OF DIRECTORS:

1) Consists of a representative from four hospitals and the Northwest Regional Perinatal Care Program on a rotating basis for two year terms
2) Develops budget, fee structure, and manages financial status of the Consortium. Authorizes treasurer to make disbursements to member hospitals, if applicable
3) Recommends frequency of program based on needs of member hospitals
4) Implements program changes based on evaluations
5) Monitors and ensures compliance with membership requirements
6) Facilitates changes in the Consortium's Letter of Understanding
7) Receives and evaluates applications for membership in the Consortium
8) Sets policy regarding membership
9) Meets once a year and as needed

FINANCIAL STRUCTURE

The North Puget Sound Perinatal Education Consortium is a nonprofit corporation with a bank account into which all Consortium monies are deposited. In addition, the Board of Directors will, on an annual basis, develop a proposed operating budget for the Consortium activities.

For each program offering, a number of spaces may be opened for community enrollment depending on availability of space. Employees of non-member hospitals may enroll in these spaces for a fee determined by the Board. A fee discount for individual non-member institutions may be implemented by the Board in exchange for needed

APPENDIX 5-3. Cont.

instructional services. If income from community participants is sufficient, expenses for all syllabus reproduction will be paid from this account. Any course income received in excess of the amount needed to cover course expenses will be designated for use in the production of future courses.

TERM OF AGREEMENT

This agreement shall become effective on January 1, 1998 and shall continue until December 31, 1998. A Consortium hospital electing to not renew its membership shall provide not less than 90 days' prior written notice of its intent not to renew membership.

The following hospital agrees to participate as a member of the North Puget Sound Perinatal Education Consortium from January 1, 1998 through December 31, 1998. In recognition of the human and monetary resource benefits, we are willing to provide to the Consortium the following:
1) Mandatory participation on the Advisory Committee;
2) At least one major service per year;
3) Educator(s) to provide 4 hours of instruction per program; and
4) Rotational service on the Board of Directors.
5) In the unusual event that compliance with item number 3) above is not possible, the member hospital will provide a facilitator for two days during each program.

Hospital Name: _____

Address: _____

_____

_____   _____
Nursing Executive Officer/Hospital Administrator   Date

_____
Title

Please return to: Secretary

Deadline for completed membership agreement - December 31, 1997

APPENDIX 5-4.

NORTH PUGET SOUND PERINATAL EDUCATION CONSORTIUM

Facilitator Responsibilities:

1. Attends facilitator orientation meeting 1-2 weeks prior to start of PEC. Facilitators come from membership of Advisory Committee. Members are expected to facilitate at least once each year.

2. Arrives early, well before registrants. Reviews facilitator notes.

3. Sets-up attendance sheets for participants to sign (must sign in each day). Maintains separate, ongoing list of late registrants and walk-ins. (Collects one-time late registration fee, payable by check to PEC. Gives receipt to participant. Participant will need to show receipt each day).

4. Distributes materials to all pre-registered attendees first. If, at the time of morning announcements there are additional syllabi, distributes them on a first come-first serve basis to late registrants and walk-ins. Otherwise, attendees may share materials with peers and obtain own copy from the hospital Advisory Committee member.

5. Makes announcements as needed and introduces speakers.

6. Keeps speakers on time. Starts each lecture on time as scheduled (even if all participants are not back from break).

7. Calls site contact person for any crisis!

8. At end of day, collects evaluations and distributes CEARP certificates. Prepares a facilitator evaluation for that day. Returns evaluations and attendance sheets to Site Coordinator.

APPENDIX 5-4. Cont.

Acknowledgments

Esther Anderson-Crook, MN, RNC
Perinatal Clinical Nurse Specialist
Group Health Cooperative, Redmond

Chris Ashbey, RNC, BSN
Perinatal Manager
Affiliated Health Services, Mount Vernon

Undrea Bostic, MN, RN
Perinatal Staff Nurse
University of Washington Medical Center, Seattle

Bonnie Bowie, MSN, MBA, RN
Director, Family Childbirth Center
Providence Medical Center, Seattle

Liz Graf-Brennen, MSN, RN
Neonatal Clinical Nurse Specialist
Swedish Medical Center, Seattle

Ann Keppler, MN, RN
Maternal-Child Clinical Nurse Specialist
Evergreen Hospital Medical Center, Kirkland

Terrie Lockridge, MS, RNC
Neonatal Clinical Nurse Specialist
Northwest Regional Perinatal Outreach Program
Children's Hospital and Regional Medical Center, Seattle

Denise Mahboub, MSN, RN
Perinatal Staff, Family Birth Center
Highline Community Hospital, Seattle

David Neal, RNC
Clinical Educator
St. Joseph Hospital, Bellingham

Carole White, MN, RNC, ARNP
Neonatal Nurse Practitioner
Providence General Medical Center, Everett

Nancy Wilk, MS, RNC, ARNP
Director, Prenatal Care Center
Island Hospital, Anacortes

Sue Williams-Judge, MN, RN
Perinatal Clinical Nurse Specialist
Stevens Hospital, Edmonds

CHAPTER 6

Competence Assessment for Nurses Providing Mother-Baby Home Care

Lenore Williams

INTRODUCTION

In 1982, Professional Nurse Associates, Inc. (PNA), a private nursing practice, was established to provide high-quality nursing care to women and childbearing families. The first clinical area developed was a home care program for women and newborns discharged following brief postpartum hospitalization. Comprehensive short-stay maternity programs combining a brief hospitalization with nursing follow-up in the home are reported to be safe, cost-effective, and satisfying for women and families (Braveman, Egerter, Pearl, Marci, & Miller, 1995; Brooten et. al., 1994; Carty & Bradley, 1990; Evans, 1995; Hurt, 1994; Lemmer, 1989; Norr & Nacion, 1987; Norr, Nacion, & Abrahamson, 1989; Soskolne, Schumacjer, Fyock, Young, & Schork, 1996. Nursing literature contains many examples of home care programs developed to address the needs of postpartum families (Arnold & Bakewell-Sachs, 1991; Evans, 1991; Evans, 1995; Gillerman & Beckman, 1991; Lynch, Kordish, & Williams, 1996; Stern, 1991; Williams & Cooper, 1993; Williams & Cooper, 1996).

The basic philosophical tenets guiding the practice of nurses providing care to women, newborns, and families in their home is highlighted in Display 6-1. Postpartum care provided in the home is family-centered and logistically more simple, and brings the care to mothers and newborns rather than asking them to travel to outpatient facilities early in the postpartum period. Home visits provide nursing care on a one-to-one basis based on individual needs, decrease exposure to hospital-acquired infections, and provide a natural opportunity to support parent-infant interaction and family adaptation. Home visits also provide opportunities for primary health promotion for every family member. The

DISPLAY 6-1

Philosophy

Postpartum care is an essential component of maternity care traditionally managed by nurses.

The concept of family-centered care is central to decision making.

Care is provided to the mother, newborn, and family.

The focus of care is the recovery of the mother, adaptation of the newborn physically and within the family unit, family adjustment, and general health.

The home is the preferred environment for post-birth recovery.

83

overall goals of the postpartum home visit program are to: (1) provide skilled postpartum home nursing care; (2) validate the need for postpartum home nursing care through use of nursing diagnoses; and (3) evaluate cost-effectiveness, readmission rates, and patient satisfaction.

DEFINING POSTPARTUM HOME NURSING CARE

The challenge to define skilled postpartum home nursing care is vital in order to sell the product. Reimbursement for this care depends on whether a visit is "skilled" and "medically necessary." Skilled care must be tangible and defined in terms that are quantifiable and understandable to buyers. Because home care replaces a portion of care traditionally provided in the hospital, skills required to provide care in the home are adapted from community health and maternity nursing literature (Carr & Walton, 1992; Dahlberg & Loloroutis, 1994; Eidelman, Hoffman, & Kaitz, 1993; Goodwin, 1994; Johnson & Johnson & Association of Women's Health, Obstetric, and Neonatal Nurses, 1996; Kish, 1993; Lowdermilk, 1995; Williams & Cooper, 1993), research (Brooten, 1994; Olds & Kitzman, 1993), and guidelines developed by professional organizations (American Academy of Pediatrics & American College of Obstetricians and Gynecologists, 1997; American Academy of Pediatrics, Committee on Practice, 1995; American Nurses Association, 1996; Association of Women's Health, Obstetric, and Neonatal Nurses, 1994). Appendix 6-1 provides an example of performance criteria and how they can be integrated into a competence checklist.

COMPETENCE-BASED ORIENTATION

After meeting a minimum set of hiring requirements, new nurses attend a didactic program that includes reviewing agency policies and procedures and a 4-hour class focused on postpartum and newborn assessment and care. The overall objective of orientation is that the registered nurse would be competent to complete a home visit including the appropriate assessment, interventions, and evaluation of care provided to women, newborns, and families. The expected outcomes for the nurse who has completed orientation are identified in Display 6-2.

Following the didactic program, orientation is divided into two segments. The length of the first segment varies depending on previous experience and the ability of the orientee to master new skills. Orientees are paired with a preceptor who evaluates them during 4–6 home visits, after which they collaboratively identify learning needs and develop a plan for additional learning opportunities. At all times the goal is to facilitate a nurturing, mentoring exchange between the orientee and preceptor. During this portion of orientation, the orientee and preceptor complete a skills checklist (Appendix 6-1). The orientee begins to master a comprehensive documentation system including the Postpartum Home Care Record and agency-specific referral forms, maternal, newborn, and family care plans; and client progress reports. An orientation manual is provided to all orientees that takes them through a home visit step by step using the documentation system as a basis. This manual includes a description of a complete assessment and interventions for the care of mother, newborn, and family as well as sugges-

DISPLAY 6-2

Orientation Outcomes

Demonstrate competence interacting with and performing assessments of mothers, newborns, and families.

Identify nursing diagnoses according to the North American Nursing Diagnosis Association (1994) with 90% proficiency.

Implement appropriate interventions related to nursing diagnoses.

Communicate and collaborate with other members of the healthcare team.

Complete all documentation.

tions for eliciting information necessary to identify problems and complete documentation. Throughout the manual, the idea of an interactive-therapeutic approach to the nurse-patient relationship is emphasized. Learning is supplemented with videos on newborn and postpartum assessment, lab drawing techniques, and breastfeeding. Time is spent learning how the concepts of case management are implemented in the agency. Orientees also meet with a certified lactation consultant to increase their knowledge of breastfeeding in order to effectively assist mothers with common breastfeeding problems and recognize situations where referrals to this resource would be appropriate. Until it is established that the orientee has reached a level of practice which is both safe and competent, the orientee does not make home visits alone. Once the orientee is making visits alone, a clinical nurse specialist is always available should questions arise about specific clinical situations.

The second part of the orientation is a mentoring period of 3 months. During this time, the nurse is making home visits independently while supervisory staff serve as resources. A supervisor or clinical specialist reviews the nurses' charts and patient evaluations regarding the care they received and is available to answer any questions the nurse may have about actual clinical situations in the home or agency policies and procedures. Opportunities for continuing education in the form of seminars outside the agency are provided based on individual needs.

CONCLUSION

The transition of postpartum care from hospital to home continues to have implications for providers and families. For providers, it has necessitated refining the existing model of maternity care by creating and validating the role of perinatal home care specialist. For families, it has meant progressing from being mere consumers of health care to being their own case managers. Despite media efforts and state and federal legislation promoting hospitalization as the preferred environment for recovery of mother and newborn, for most women and families there is no place like home. As we move forward in perinatal nursing care, it is the responsibility of the profession to engineer a model of care that meets the health-care needs of the family. We need to move beyond the immediacy of the post-birth period and begin to define and contribute to true family health. Recognizing the importance of the fourth trimester and the contribution nurses can make to the outcomes of perinatal care during this period will ensure that we build healthy communities, one healthy family at a time. To accomplish this expertise of home care nurses is essential.

REFERENCES

American Academy of Pediatrics and American College of Obstetricians and Gynecologists. (1997). Guidelines for perinatal care (4th ed.). Elk Grove Village, IL: Author.

American Academy of Pediatrics, Committee on Fetus and Newborn. (1995). Hospital stay for healthy term newborns. Pediatrics, 96(4), 788–789.

American Nurses Association. (1996). Position statement of home care for mother, infant, and family following birth. Washington, DC: Author.

Arnold, L. S., & Bakewell-Sachs, S. (1991). Models of perinatal home follow-up. Journal of Perinatal and Neonatal Nursing, 5(1), 18–26.

Association of Women's Health, Obstetric, and Neonatal Nurses. (1994). Didactic content and clinical skills verification for professional nurse providers of perinatal home care. Washington, DC: Author.

Braveman, P., Egerter, S., Pearl, M., Marchi, K., & Miller, C. (1995). Problems associated with early discharge of newborn infants— Early discharge of newborns and mothers: A critical review of the literature. Pediatrics, 96(4), 716–726.

Brooten, D., Roncoli, M., Finkler, S., Arnold, L., Cohen, A., & Mennuti, M. (1994). A randomized trial of early hospital discharge and home follow-up of women having cesarean birth. Obstetrics & Gynecology, 84(5), 832–838.

Carty, E., & Bradley, C. (1990). A randomized, controlled evaluation of early postpartum hospital discharge. Birth, 17(4), 199–204.

Dahlberg, N. L., & Koloroutis, M. (1994). Hospital based perinatal home-care program. Journal of Obstetric, Gynecologic, and Neonatal Nursing, 23(8), 682–686.

Eidelman, A. I., Hoffman, N. W., & Kaitz, M. (1993). Cognitive deficits in women after childbirth. Obstetrics & Gynecology, 81(5), 764–767.

Evans, C. (1991). Description of a home follow-up program for childbearing families. Journal of Obstetric, Gynecologic, and Neonatal Nursing, 20(2), 113–118.

Evans, C. J. (1995). Postpartum home care in the United States. Journal of Obstetric, Gynecologic, and Neonatal Nursing, 24(2), 180–186.

Gillerman, H., & Beckham, M. (1991). The postpartum early discharge dilemma: An innovative solution. Journal of Perinatal and Neonatal Nursing, 5(1), 9–17.

Goodwin, L. (1994). Essential program components for perinatal home care. Journal of Obstetrics, Gynecologic, and Neonatal Nursing, 23(8), 667–674.

Hurt, H. (1994). Early discharge for newborns—when is it safe? Contemporary Pediatrics, 11(8), 68–88.

Johnson & Johnson Consumer Products, Inc. and Association of Women's Health, Obstetric, and Neonatal Nurses. (1996). Compendium of postpartum care. Skillman, NJ: Author.

Kish, C. (1993). Home care. In Bobak, I., & Jensen, M. Maternity & gynecologic care: The nurse and the family. St. Louis: Mosby.

Lemmer, C. (1989). Early discharge: Outcomes of primiparas and their infants. Journal of Obstetric, Gynecologic, and Neonatal Nursing, 16(4), 230–236.

Lowdermilk, D. L. (1995). Home care. In Bobak, I. M., Lowdermilk, D. L., and Jensen, M. D. Maternity nursing (4th ed.). St. Louis: Mosby-Year Book.

Lynch, A., Kordish, R., & Williams, L. (1996). Maternal-child nursing: Postpartum home care. In Rice, R. (Ed.). Home health nursing practice: Concepts and applications (2nd ed.). St Louis: Mosby.

Norr, K., & Nacion, K. (1987). Outcomes of postpartum early discharge 1960–1986. A comparative review. Birth, 14(3), 135–141.

Norr, K., Nacion, K., & Abrahamson, R. (1989). Early discharge with home follow-up: Impacts on low-income mothers and infants. Journal of Obstetric, Gynecologic, and Neonatal Nursing, 18(2) 133–141.

North American Nursing Diagnosis Association. (1994). NANDA nursing diagnoses: Definitions and classifications 1995–1996. Philadelphia: Author.

Olds, D., & Kitzman, H. (1993). Home visiting: Review of research on home visiting for pregnant women and parents of young children. The Future of Children, 3(3), 53–92.

Soskolne, E., Schumacjer, R., Fyock, C., Young, M., & Schork, A. (1996). The effects of early discharge and other factors on readmission rates of newborns. Arch Pediatrics Adolescent Medicine, 150(4), 373–379.

Stern, T. (1991). An early discharge program. An entrepreneurial nursing practice becomes a hospital-affiliated agency. Journal of Perinatal and Neonatal Nursing, 5(1), 1–8.

Williams, L., & Cooper, M. (1993). Nurse-managed postpartum home care. Journal of Obstetric, Gynecologic, and Neonatal Nursing, 22(1), 25–31.

Williams, L., Cooper, M. (1996). A new paradigm for postpartum care. Journal of Obstetric, Gynecologic, and Neonatal Nursing, 25(9), 745–749.

APPENDIX 6-1.

Postpartum Home Care Competence Checklist

Name:_____

Maternal Care	Demonstrates Competence (Date/Initial)	Comments
Physical Assessment		
<u>Previous Health History</u>: Reviews and identifies pertinent data		
<u>Vital Signs (T,P,R,BP)</u>: Measures accurately		
Identifies deviations, prescribes appropriate interventions, notifies primary provider of abnormal findings		
<u>Breasts</u>: Examines for lumps, reddened or painful areas		
Describes as soft, filling, engorged, nodular		
Demonstrates breast exam or evaluates breast self exam		
Explains breast care and engorgement management for non-nursing mother		
<u>Breastfeeding Mothers</u>: Identifies nipple variations and condition		
Recommends appropriate interventions to resolve nipple variations or conditions		
Discusses lactation physiology		
Discusses nipple and breast care and engorgement management		
Demonstrates appropriate use of lactation aids (pump, shells, lact-aid)		
Identifies deviations, prescribes appropriate interventions, notifies primary provider of abnormal findings		
<u>Abdomen</u>: Palpates for diastasis recti and recommends appropriate exercises if identified		
Determines condition of incision if present		
Instructs mother on incision care		
Identifies deviations, prescribes appropriate interventions, notifies primary provider of abnormal findings		
<u>Reproductive Tract</u>: Describes normal uterine involution		
Palpates uterus for height, consistency, position, tenderness		
Identifies lochia type, amount, odor and any presence of clots		

Copyright 1996 by Professional Nurse Associates, Inc.

APPENDIX 6-1. Cont.

Maternal Care	Demonstrates Competence (Date/Initial)	Comments
Instructs mother on uterine palpation and lochial progression, danger signs of subinvolution and excessive lochia, signs of endometritis		
Determines condition of perineum using the REEDA scale (Redness, Ecchymosis, Edema, Discharge, Approximation)		
Identifies vulvar hematomas/varicosities		
Instructs mother on appropriate perineal care		
Identifies deviations, prescribes appropriate interventions, notifies primary provider of abnormal findings		
<u>Elimination:</u>		
Determines return to normal voiding pattern		
Identifies signs of bladder distention, urinary tract infections (urgency, frequency, dysuria, CVA tenderness)		
Instructs mother on clean catch urine sample		
Determines return to normal bowel habits		
Identifies constipation, diarrhea, hemorrhoids		
Discusses proper diet and appropriate use of laxatives or stool softeners		
Identifies deviations, prescribes appropriate interventions, notifies primary provider of abnormal findings		
<u>Lower Extremities:</u>		
Determines presence of thrombophlebitis (redness, pain, warmth, swelling)		
Performs Homan's sign		
Evaluates presence and location of edema		
Identifies presence and location of varicosities		
Identifies deviations, prescribes appropriate interventions, notifies primary provider of abnormal findings		
<u>Pain:</u>		
Identifies location and level of discomfort		
Determines use and effectiveness of comfort measures and analgesics		
Identifies deviations, prescribes appropriate interventions, notifies primary provider of abnormal findings		
Activities of Daily Living		
<u>Nutrition:</u>		
Determines adequate fluids and dietary intake for both lactating and non-lactating women		
Identifies use of vitamin or iron supplements		

Copyright 1996 by Professional Nurse Associates, Inc.

APPENDIX 6-1. Cont.

Maternal Care	Demonstrates Competence (Date/Initial)	Comments
Activity:		
Describes activity/sleep pattern, presence of fatigue		
Recommends appropriate exercises and timetable, activity level		
Determines level of self-care ability		
Identifies deviations, prescribes appropriate interventions, notifies primary provider of abnormal findings		
Psychological Assessment		
General:		
Determines emotional status, feelings about body image, and level of self-confidence		
Reviews birth experience and identifies any "missing pieces"		
Determines the postpartum timetable phase		
Addresses concerns expressed by the mother		
Specific:		
Evaluates for the presence of postpartum depression		
Counsels mother and supports appropriate person about signs and symptoms of postpartum depression and action steps		
Evaluates grief process and provides appropriate counseling, if there is a perinatal loss		
Determines level of attachment and social support		
Identifies deviations, prescribes appropriate interventions, notifies primary provider of abnormal findings		
Sexuality:		
Explains return of the menstrual cycle, decreased libido, and relationship adjustments in the initial postpartum period		
Discusses normal variations in the lactating woman such as vaginal dryness and breasts leaking during orgasm		
Counsels about birth control options: types, effectiveness, side effects, appropriate choice		
Discusses comfort and lack of lochia as parameters for appropriate time to resume intercourse		
Advises methods other than sexual intercourse to display affection		

Copyright 1996 by Professional Nurse Associates, Inc.

APPENDIX 6-1. Cont.

Infant Care	Demonstrates Competency (Date/Initial)	Comments
Physical Assessment		
Previous Health History:		
Reviews perinatal history to identify pertinent risks		
Vital Signs and Measurements:		
Measures T,P,R accurately		
Measures weight, length, head and chest circumference and compares from baseline data		
Identifies deviations, prescribes appropriate interventions, notifies primary provider of abnormal findings		
Head:		
Palpates fontanels and suture lines		
Denotes presence of molding, caput, cephalhematoma		
Observes face for symmetry		
Checks neck for folds, range of motion, masses		
Checks eyes for symmetry, normal conjunctiva, sclera and eyelids, pupils equal and reactive to light (PERL)		
Checks ears for, shape, size, position, auditory response		
Determines position and patency of nose, normal bridge, presence of discharge		
Observes mouth for normal palate, mucous membranes, tongue, lips		
Chest:		
Auscultates lungs for clear and equal breath sounds bilaterally		
Inspects for normal shape, breast, nipples		
Palpates for intact clavicles		
Cardiovascular:		
Auscultates heart to determine normal rate and rhythm and detect murmurs		
Compares femoral pulses for strength and equality		
Abdomen:		
Palpates abdomen for general condition, liver location		
Observes cord condition - drying, moist, drainage, signs of infection		
Detaches cord clamp if appropriate		
Instructs parents on cord care, normal drying process		
Genitalia:		
Determines normal male and female genitalia		

Copyright 1996 by Professional Nurse Associates, Inc.

APPENDIX 6-1. Cont.

Infant Care	Demonstrates Competency (Date/Initial)	Comments
Instructs on proper care of female genitalia		
Discusses vaginal discharge and pseudomenses		
Recognizes normal healing of circumcision		
Instructs on proper care of intact and circumcised penis		
Skeletal:		
Observes for symmetry of extremities		
Checks for presence of hip clicks		
Observes back for proper alignment, presence of pilonidal cyst or dimple		
Elimination (24 hour assessment):		
Determines color, consistency, and number of stools		
Determines color, amount, number of urines		
Instructs on normal bowel and urine elimination patterns for breast or formula fed infants		
Neuromuscular:		
Determines muscle tone as normal, hypotonic, hypertonic		
Elicits moro, grasp, Babinski reflexes for presence and symmetry		
Skin:		
Observes skin for condition, color, turgor		
Determines presence and level of jaundice as appropriate for days of age		
Explains jaundice etiology, cephalo-caudal progression, when to notify provider		
Examines for presence of rashes, lesions, birthmarks		
Identifies deviations, prescribes appropriate interventions, notifies primary provider of abnormal findings		
Nutrition Assessment		
General:		
Determines presence of root, suck, swallow, gag reflexes		
Describes type and use of pacifier		
Describes amount, frequency, type of emesis		
Observes response to hunger cues, maternal-infant feeding interaction		
Correlates feeding pattern and weight trend		
Instructs on burping techniques		
Breastfeeding:		
Assesses for latch, position, correct suck, audible swallow		

Copyright 1996 by Professional Nurse Associates, Inc.

APPENDIX 6-1. Cont.

Infant Care	Demonstrates Competency (Date/Initial)	Comments
Determines frequency/length of feedings		
Identifies problems and uses correct information or devices to solve them		
Instructs on hydration adequacy using elimination parameters		
Reinforces breastfeeding success		
Formula feeding:		
Determines frequency/amount of feedings		
Identifies proper mixing of formula and use of bottles		
Calculates appropriate ounces per pound of body weight per day		
Identifies deviations, prescribes appropriate interventions, notifies primary provider of abnormal findings		
Behavioral Assessment		
Identifies 24 hour behavior pattern and appropriate sleep/awake states		
Identifies abnormal cry and behavior patterns		
Instructs on sleep/awake states, consoling measures, self-comforting abilities		
Additional Skills		
Clinical		
Collects and transports specimens correctly		
Maternal venipuncture for ordered lab tests		
Clean catch urine		
Vaginal or wound culture		
Infant/newborn metabolic screens		
Hematocrit and hemoglobin		
Bilirubin		
Cord culture		
Explains purpose, procedure, and significance of results to family		
Establishes home phototherapy per protocol		
Demonstrates proper technique for wound care		
Interpersonal		
Communication:		
Demonstrates appropriate interview skills		
Uses direct questioning and open ended statements		
Identifies cultural variations and overcomes barriers		
Has an interactive-therapeutic approach		
Able to obtain sensitive information		

Copyright 1996 by Professional Nurse Associates, Inc.

APPENDIX 6-1. Cont.

Infant Care	Demonstrates Competency (Date/Initial)	Comments
Teaching:		
Uses principles of adult learning		
Gives clear, concise instructions		
Uses written materials appropriately		
General		
Reports information to appropriate member(s) of the health care team		
Refers to appropriate community resources		
Acts as a patient advocate		
Initiates appropriate nursing interventions		
Employs follow-up management as indicated		
Documents nursing care accurately		
Health Promotion Activities		
Parenting		
Describes the process of parent/infant attachment		
Assists family to recognize infant cues and respond appropriately and recognize infant capabilities		
Evaluates infant care-taking abilities and provides appropriate instructions for any deficits identified (may be covered during physical exam)		
Evaluates environmental safety, sleeping arrangements		
Discusses appropriate discipline measures		
Evaluates knowledge of growth and development		
Family Adaptation		
Assesses for adaptation of mother and family members to new roles		
Observes for integration of infant into family unit		
Assesses for sibling adjustment and discusses solutions if problematic		
Determines influence and support of extended family members related to infant care		
Assesses for coping abilities		
Evaluates infant care-taking abilities and provides appropriate instructions for any deficits identified (may be covered during physical exam)		
Bathing/skin/nail care		
Diapering		
Cord care		
Intact or circumcised penis care		
Female genitalia care		
Clothing		

Copyright 1996 by Professional Nurse Associates, Inc.

APPENDIX 6-1. Cont.

Infant Care	Demonstrates Competency (Date/Initial)	Comments
Feeding		
Use of thermometer		
Use of bulb syringe		
Normal elimination patterns		
Signs and symptoms of illness		
Sensory stimulation		
Consoling techniques		
Follow-up care/immunization schedule		
Evaluates environmental safety, sleeping arrangements		
Discusses appropriate discipline measures		
Evaluates knowledge of growth and development		
Family Adaptation		
Assesses for adaptation of mother and family members to new roles		
Observes for integration of infant into family unit		
Assesses for sibling adjustment and discusses solutions if problematic		
Determines influence and support of extended family members related to infant care		
Assesses for coping abilities		
Identification of needs		
Information seeking		
Reorganization of lifestyle		
Mobilization of resources		
Situation adaptation		
Instructs on coping strategies, stress management techniques		
Determines if mother is in a safe relationship and if there is any physical or emotional harm occurring. If present, provides counseling and referral sources.		
Determines if financial needs are present and refers to appropriate community resources		
Discusses issues related to returning to work outside the home		
Provides written information on danger signs, when and where to call for help for both mother and infant		
Identifies follow-up care for mother and refers to community support/educational resources as indicated		

Copyright 1996 by Professional Nurse Associates, Inc.

APPENDIX 6-1. Cont.

Preceptor

Comments:

Initials	Signature

I have demonstrated the competencies for postpartum home care.

Signature:_____

Copyright 1996 by Professional Nurse Associates, Inc.

CHAPTER 7

Competence-Based Orientation and Education: A Working Perinatal Model

Bette-Jo Moore

INTRODUCTION

Identification of the Need for a Comprehensive Orientation Program

In May 1992, changes in healthcare delivery to childbearing women and newborns forced administrators and clinical experts at HealthEast St. John's Hospital Perinatal Services to evaluate their current system of providing nursing education and validating nursing staff competence. St. John's Hospital had just opened a new Single Room Maternity Care Center (SRMCC) with a much higher census than their previous traditional labor and birth unit. Many nurses were not only new to St. John's Hospital, but also new to intrapartum care. The physical layout of the previous unit had allowed nurses to always be in close proximity, which made it easier to mentor new nurses and for new nurses to ask questions and seek clarification from experienced nurses when complex clinical issues arose. The new unit was spread out over a larger area with multiple small "pods," which made this type of communication and collaboration between nurses more difficult.

Managers and preceptors were concerned that the lack of a formal system for nursing orientation and competence validation and the inability to work closely side-by-side with experienced nurses as they had in the previous unit would contribute to the possibility that new nurses would miss learning key clinical concepts. There was a concern that this knowledge deficit would not become evident until there was an adverse maternal-fetal outcome. The group came to a consensus that a new more formal process was needed to validate competence for nurses who worked in the SRMCC. They agreed that the present system was outdated and did not meet their needs.

DEVELOPMENT OF THE COMPETENCE-BASED ORIENTATION AND EDUCATION PROGRAM

A task force was formed to evaluate perinatal nursing orientation, continuing education, and competence validation at St. John's Hospital. After careful consideration and much discussion, task force members decided that a Competence-Based Orientation/ Education (CBO/E) program was the best approach. The program that was developed followed the six characteristics that Dorothy Del Bueno (1980) described: emphases on **outcome** or **achievement** of performance expectations, use of **self-directed** learning activities, **flexibility** and **time** allowed for achievement of outcomes, use of the teacher as a **facilitator** and resource, assessment of **previous knowledge** and learning, and assessment of **learning styles.**

The task force evaluated various CBO/E models looking for a program that could be easily integrated into existing education programs at

HealthEast St. John's Hospital. Unfortunately, the task force was unable to find a program that fully met the identified needs. The decision was then made to design a new CBO/E program to meet the specific needs of the SRMCC at HealthEast St. John's. Based on that premise and the following goals, the HealthEast Perinatal CBO/E model was conceived.

The goals established for the CBO/E task force were to develop a program that included:
- A process to assess individual nurse's current competence and learning needs.
- An orientation program that clearly defined expectations of the orientee to complete orientation for their specific position.
- Clearly defined resources available to assist the orientee to meet those expectations.
- Descriptions of what the preceptor was expected to teach and/or to validate during orientation.
- Descriptions of expectations for successful return demonstrations for validation.
- Descriptions of what was expected to maintain competence and to advance to higher competence levels in Perinatal Services.

Initially the group collected all of the tools and resources that had previously been developed over the past years to identify pieces that could be used in the new program. A formal orientation program was initiated and new competence validation forms were developed. (See Display 7-1 for definitions used in the program.) By September 1993, the task force had made great progress in standardizing the orientation process and in documenting/tracking competence validation for SRMCC nurses. The task force was very excited about what they had developed and how helpful it had been, and thus wanted to share it with others across the HealthEast system. The task force hosted a systemwide perinatal preceptor meeting to introduce the CBO/E program and the labor and birth orientation packets (with validation tools and resources that they had identified or developed). After this meeting, the other three labor and birth units that are part of the HealthEast system decided to use the resources St. John's had developed.

Special Care Nursery (SCN) preceptors decided that they needed a similar program because

DISPLAY 7-1

HealthEast Definitions for Competence-Based Orientation:

Competence	The noun for the skills and knowledge required to perform the position responsibilities.
Assessment	Evaluation/determination of present competence.
Competence-Based	Objective validation of identified key areas of competence. Validation is not required for all position areas of competence. The focus is on those areas of competence that are crucial, high risk, problem prone, or seldom done.
Orientation	The initial training and experience needed to enable a new staff person to function independently in the new role.
Education	The ongoing need for training and experience to maintain and develop new skills to meet the expectations of the position.
Validation	The objective process of ensuring that a staff member can competently perform a skill.

SCN nurses often worked individually and independently as well. In November 1993, the HealthEast SCN CBO/E task force was established. Building on the experiences from the SRMCC task force, the SCN task force continued to improve and refine the process. The task force identified that there were many characteristics of clinical competence that needed validation, but that some types of competence validation processes were difficult to accomplish in the clinical area. They also identified the need for a method of supporting existing competence that was not threatening for experienced nurses.

In response to those needs, the first "HealthEast Perinatal Skills Day" was held in May 1994. That year nearly one fifth of the nursing staff participated and earned 120 continuing education units. By 1996 more than one third of the nursing staff participated and more than 360 continuing education units were awarded in only 9 hours. The now Annual Perinatal Skills Day is a collection of 20–25 small/short sessions that focus on "hands on" experience, demonstration, informational/discussion groups, and many mock scenarios. The nurse attendees choose the sessions that are most applicable for their needs. Internal and external experts share their knowledge on the various competencies. The presenters/validators have been very creative as they seek to make the settings as realistic as possible. Effective scenarios have included mock code pinks where the NRP resuscitation process is reenacted by the participants; labor and birth emergency scenarios; and even the use of a live model for speculum exams.

In August 1994, during our accreditation visit, one of the Joint Commission on Accreditation of Healthcare Organizations (JCAHO) surveyors asked how nursing competence validation was accomplished in Perinatal Services at HealthEast. When the new CBO/E orientation folder and first learning modules were explained, one JACHO surveyor indicated that this program was exactly the type and quality that JCAHO expects but rarely finds. It was gratifying to learn that the group efforts had been rewarded by the CBO/E program meeting JCAHO Standards.

The SRMCC preceptors felt the tools and resources that had been developed were very helpful. However, there were a few more issues to be addressed. There was a need to create some competence statements that considered the cultural differences between the facilities and there were some competence statements that could be standardized across all four facilities. This additional work expanded the CBO/E program overall. In October 1994, the HealthEast-wide Labor & Delivery Task Force was established to form a collaborative group between all four institutions.

During 1995 and 1996 there was further development and full implementation of the program for all existing nurses in addition to nurses who were newly hired. There was a lengthy debate to determine whether to "grandmother in" current nurses based on the assumption that long-term nurses were competent. The decision to include all nurses in the competence validation program proved to be a wise choice. It provided learning opportunities that had not been anticipated. After going through the process even experienced nurses now have a common understanding of what is expected of them, what they can expect of others, and how they can help new nurses develop the level of expected competence.

In August 1996, after reviewing multiple models, HealthEast chose to use the Perinatal model as a building block for developing a systemwide CBO/E program, for all employees including unlicensed assistive personnel (UAPs). During the implementation of the systemwide program the same benefits have been experienced for both clinical and nonclinical staff (see Display 7-2). It is felt that these benefits ultimately lead to financial savings, although data are being gathered to evaluate the exact amount of financial benefits. The key disadvantages of the CBO/E program have included meeting the challenge of change; up-front development costs; and, as with any competence validation program, the inability to be absolutely sure that an individual nurse is and always will be 100% competent, regardless of the validation system in place. We concluded that the benefits of developing a CBO/E program outweighed the challenges.

DISPLAY 7-2

Program Benefits

The key benefits HealthEast has experienced due to implementation of the CBO/E program have been

- clear expectations of competence needed to recruit new staff
- clarity for the preceptor, preceptee, and manager of their roles and expected time lines
- consistency in orientation processes
- ability to individualize orientation to meet specific needs
- decreased unproductive time in unnecessary learning experiences
- increased orientee's self-confidence and decreased anxiety associated with new position experiences
- development of learning resources that support orientation and ongoing education for nursing staff
- increased staff retention
- identification of unit educational needs
- encouragement for nurses to take responsibility for their own educational needs
- problem-area identification such as staff not getting experiences to maintain skills
- increased staff confidence that they are maintaining expected level of competence
- ease in objectively identifying why an individual does not meet expectations, which may lead to disciplining, retraining, reassigning, or relieving
- ease in justifying an extension of orientation and identify goals to be met

KEY POINTS ABOUT COMPETENCE-BASED ORIENTATION AND EDUCATION

The CBO/E philosophy is that every employee is expected to perform at a certain level of competence following orientation. However, learning is a process that should continue along the continuum of beginner, advanced/experienced, and expert. There are three domains within most categories of competence: technical, critical thinking, and interpersonal. Traditionally the primary focus has been on technical competence, because it is the easiest to describe in objective terms. Yet, most personnel issues arise from the critical thinking (problem solving and prioritizing) and interpersonal areas.

The primary methods used for assessing competence are self-assessment, written tests, oral quizzing, return demonstration of competence (simulated or actual outside of the work setting), mock scenarios (including multiple areas of competence), observation of care given and/or clinical tasks performed in the actual work setting, case studies or exemplars (reflection stories), peer review, discussion groups or presentations, and quality improvement indicators that reflect individual performance. When validating competence, it is best to use a variety of methods and allow options when possible.

HEALTHEAST PERINATAL NURSING ORIENTATION PROCESS

During the interview process the preemployment competence inventory is used. The inventory highlights key areas of competence that are desired for the position. Examples include circulating for cesarean births or caring for infants on ventilators. The inventory is used by the manager when interviewing prospective nurses to assess baseline competence and as a springboard for interview questions about experience.

After the new nurse is hired, she or he meets with the Clinical Nurse Specialist (CNS) to receive the orientation folder and schedule. During that meeting the CNS explains the CBO/E program and answers questions. The new nurse is asked to complete the self-assessment form with areas of competence listed on the HealthEast General RN/LPN Competence Checklist, the Mother-Baby Competence Checklist, and position-specific competence checklists (such as Labor and Delivery or Special Care Nursery). The first week of orientation is spent at the HealthEast General Orientation, HealthEast Nursing Orientation, and Site Orientation. The first day on the unit is spent with the preceptor without a patient care assignment. Orientees and preceptors spend time reviewing department-specific policies, touring the unit, reviewing equipment, and establishing a plan for orientation based on the new nurse's self-assessment. The length of orientation is based on previous experience and how quickly the orientees complete the identified competencies for the specific competence level at which they will be expected to perform after orientation. These competence levels are used for determining expectations for individual nurses and for staffing schedule needs. The competence level categories that have been identified and used for HealthEast Perinatal Nurses are as follows:

- A = Mother-Baby/Gynecological Surgery (expectations for all nurses who might work in HealthEast Perinatal Services, including in-house float and agency nurses)
- B = Mother-Baby/Gynecological Surgery (expectations applied to all nurses who had a Perinatal position, including LPNs and on-call staff)
- CP = Core Pediatric Expectations
- CL = Core Labor and Birth Expectations
- DL = Advanced Labor and Birth Expectations (amniotomy, application of fetal scalp electrode and insertion of intrauterine pressure catheter, providing postanesthesia recovery care, and circulating for cesarean births)
- CS = Core Special Care Nursery Expectations
- DS = Advanced Special Care Nursery Expectations (drawing blood from umbilical lines, chest tube management, caring for stable infants on a ventilator)
- ES = Level III Special Care Nursery Expectations (initial stabilization of an infant on a ventilator)
- L = Lactation Specialist (role that requires skills beyond what is expected of Mother-Baby Nurse but not those of a certified lactation consultant)
- F = Charge Nurse (required highest level of advanced competence for the speciality)

Preceptors assist the new employees with completing their competence checklists. However, it is ultimately the orientees' responsibility to ensure that the checklist is completed, signed, and turned in to their manager at the end of orientation. A copy of the competence checklists is sent to Human Resources after orientation, while the original remains in the work area where it should continue to be used to document additional experiences as they occur (see Display 7-3).

The competence checklists are arranged in four columns:

A. The first column is titled "Position Competence." It lists general and specific knowledge, technical, and critical thinking competence to be addressed during orientation.

B. The second column, titled "Self-Assessment," is to be filled out by the individual, and reflects competence in the new department. If the orientee checks "can function independently," the area might not be reviewed unless a validation tool is required. However, orientees should review any referenced policies to familiarize themselves with the culture of this organization

C. The third column, titled "Action Plan," is to be filled out by the preceptor, orientor, orientee, or anyone else involved in the orientation process. They initial and date the small squares as applicable.

Under the Expectation/Action column there are letters that correspond with the expected level of competence to help clarify what the minimal requirement is for completion of orientation. All involved should take advantage of

DISPLAY 7-3

Mother/Baby Competance Checklist

NAME: _____   DEPT/SITE: _____

EXPECTED COMPETENCE LEVEL (circle)   A   B   CL   CS   CP

POSITION / AREA OF COMPETENCE	SELF-ASSESSMENT			EXPECTATIONS/ACTION PLAN				COMMENTS/RESOURCES
	Can Function Independently	Need Review	Have Not Done	Class or Learning Module	Discussed Information or Reviewed Policy	Assisted or Observed	Return Demonstration	Performed Independently

A=Required for ALL nurses to include float pool nurses working on the Perinatal unit.
B=Required for all Perinatal nursing staff to include on-call and LPN nursing staff.
C=Required for Core Competent staff:
  CL=Labor & Birth
  CS=Special Care Nursery
  CP=Pediatrics

RESOURCE KEY
@ = HEPS Policy Book
M = Learning Module or Resource
SOC = Standard of Care
V = Validation Tool
OM = Operation Manual

I. EQUIPMENT, LOCATION, USE & CLEANING OF:								
A. Birthing Bed to include stirrups (Adel 2100)		X		A 10/8/97 ME			B 10/8/97 ME	CL	OM
B. Blanket warmer		X		A 10/10/97 HH					OM
C. Blood warmer	X				B		CL	CL	OM
D. Breast pump (Egnell)		X		A 10/7/97 ME			B 10/7/97 ME	B 10/8/97 ME	OM, @B-1A
E. CR (Cardio-Respiratory) Monitor) Lead application, use, & alarm limits		X		M-1 10/7/97 NN	B 10/7/97 ME		CS 10/8/97 ME	CS 10/9/97 ME	@C-8

The competence checklists usually are multiple pages. The complete HealthEast Mother-Baby Nurse Competence Checklist is 26 pages, most are 3-6 pages. The signature box in only on the last page with the list of required validation tools.

Competence Checklist reviewed: Date/Year: _____
Employee: _____
Preceptor/Orientor/Educator: _____
Manager: _____

---

*Initial and signature boxes for preceptors or other staff assisting with orientation or training:

Initials/Symbol	Signature
ME	Molly Expert, RNC
HH	Hope Helpful, RN
_____	_____

List of Validation Tools	Date Done
PCA Pump	10/5/97
IV Starts	10/6/97
IV Starts with Lidocaine	10/6/97
Chemsticks on infants	10/3/97
Bulb/Wall suction-infant	10/4/97
Metabolic screen	10/8/97
Circumcision	10/14/97
Breast-feeding Checklist	10/14/97
Urine/Meconium toxicology	10/12/97

and document additional opportunities as they arise. The orientee is expected to complete the preceding competence area as well. (Example: a "D" must also complete all the "C" expectations as well.)

A "V" under return demonstration indicates that the orientee must also complete a validation tool regardless of the self-assessment. A complete list of validation tools required for each competence checklist is located on the last page of the checklist. Ideas for validation tools came from quality assurance/risk management issues, new products, new equipment, new practices, and new patient populations.

D. The fourth column, titled "Comments/Resources," is used for various comments and to list department/job specific resources available such as policies, procedure cards, standards of care, and so on.

The competence checklist is used both for establishing the orientation plan and for documenting orientation needs being met. Other tools are used in addition to the competence checklists and validation tools during orientation. They are

- The cover sheet, which provides a summary of expectations with a time goal, summary of progress on completing checklists, classes, and validation tools required, and narrative notes for orientation progress and changes in the orientation plan.
- The orientation journal, which can be used by the orientee and/or preceptor to make daily narrative notes about experiences, progress, and questions. This tool has helped to record daily information that may be helpful for the weekly formal follow-up with the preceptor.
- Evaluation of Clinical Observation was designed for use when the preceptor was unexpectedly absent and the orientee was paired with a nurse who was not familiar with the orientation plan or when the new orientee is observed by the Clinical Nurse Specialist during and after orientation. The tool provided feedback to the preceptor and manager to be used for formal follow-up. It became a peer review tool that was used for and by all staff to communicate observations to the manager. These observations are about clinical concerns and celebrations/congratulations on a job well done.
- The Orientation Follow-Up Expectations and Need Assessment (OFENA) form is used to update the orientation plan during orientation. It is also used after orientation to detail what competencies still need follow-up after formal orientation is completed. This tool has been vital in ensuring the overall consistency of orientation and meeting needs that are not easily met during formal orientation.
- The Orientation Evaluation form is used by the orientees to provide feedback on the CBO/E program and their personal orientation experience. This information is used to further develop the CBO/E program and preceptor competence.

During orientation the new nurse spends most of the time in the clinical setting with the preceptor, but time is also spent completing identified learning modules, discussing scenarios and expectations with the preceptor, and doing return demonstrations to complete validation tools. On a weekly basis the preceptor spends time with the orientee updating the competence checklists and orientation plan. The Clinical Nurse Specialist minimally meets formally with the orientee at the beginning, middle, and end of the scheduled orientation to ensure that all the orientee's needs are being met. The manager meets formally with the orientee initially and as needed throughout the process, based on the feedback from the preceptor, CNS, or orientee.

MAP FOR DEVELOPING CBO/E PROGRAM

- Establish task force (identify chairperson, typist, and time line).
- Collect resources (present orientation tools, department policies, AWHONN standards, and so on).
- Evaluate unique needs and identify skill levels. Develop competence checklists for "job/position" with expectations and resources.

SUMMARY OF CBO/E PROCESS

Preemployment	Organization & Facility Orientation	Department & Position Orientation	Evaluation/ Reassessment	Identify Learning Needs & Goals

(Initial Comprehensive Competence Assessment)

```
                            Plan to      Plan to
                            Meet         Teach
                            Needs        Others

                              Practice
                              Competence
```

- Core level competence should include all items expected to be completed by the end of orientation in order to function as a team member.
- Identify areas of competence requiring validation and develop tools (high-risk/high-volume, high-risk/low-volume, or problem-prone aspects of the position). A validation tool should include: a competence statement (objective), critical behaviors (steps/criteria), learning options, and evaluation method.
- Establish the follow-up process.
- Determine the pre-employment process.
- Create the Annual Review Expectations and Needs Assessment (ARENA) form to be used with the annual performance appraisal to address ongoing competence assessment. Include areas of competence that may be infrequently used, but must be maintained for the position; are new expectations; and/or may be high-risk/problem prone and need to be assessed routinely.
- Identify and develop resources/learning modules.
- Compile orientation forms into a folder or binder for orientee.
- Create needed policies.
- Establish review/revision process for tools and program.
- Establish system to track staff compliance.

Clinical practice is enhanced when nurses are competent and when they have the resources to provide care that meets the patients emotional and physical needs. This is the ultimate goal of comprehensive Competence-Based Orientation/Education program at HealthEast. Initially it is an overwhelming task, but it is worth the investment of time and energy. A designated program coordinator at each hospital is essential for program success.

Acknowledgments

Acknowledgments to all the HealthEast Perinatal preceptors and nurses whose input and ideas have contributed to the CBO/E program, especially Karen McConville, Maureen Beaverson, Colleen Hart, Jan Johnson, Sandy Gerber, Rita Kruschwitz, Kay Gardner, Joanne Kallstrom, Lisa Kjeseth, Ruth Peterson, Lois Score, Marlette Hoxmeier, Kae Stender, Evva Kelcher, Diana Smith, Jean Landon, Kristine Keefer, Helen Sullivan, Sue Byron, and Mary Robins.

Reference

Del Bueno, D., Barker, F. & Christmyer, C. (1980). Implementing a CBO Program, Nurse Educators, 5(3), 16–20.

Bibliography

Brookfield, S. (1993). On impostership, cultural suicide, and other dangers: How nurses learn critical thinking. The Journal of Continuing Education in Nursing, 197–205.

Gurvis, J. P., & M. T. Grey. (1995). The anatomy of a competency. Journal of Nursing Staff Development, 247–252.

O'Grady, T., & A. O'Brien. (1992, May/June). A guide to competency based orientation—develop your own program. Journal of Nursing Staff Development, 128–133.

Redus, K. M. (1994). A literature review of competency-based orientation for nurses. Journal of Nursing Staff Development, 239–243.

Robinson, S. M., & C. Barberis-Ryan. (1995). Competency assessment: A systematic approach. Nursing Management, 40–44.

PART II

Professional Roles and Responsibilities and Competence Validation for Unlicensed Assistive Personnel

CHAPTER 8

Registered Professional Nurses and Unlicensed Assistive Personnel: Delegation, Supervision, and Staffing Resources

Kathleen Rice Simpson

INTRODUCTION

Despite the lack of positive data about patient outcomes to support changes in professional registered nurse to patient ratios, an increase in the use of unlicensed assistive personnel (UAP) for direct patient care appears to be reality in most healthcare institutions in the United States. A rigorous evaluation of the effects of nursing care and professional/nonprofessional caregiver skill mix on patient outcomes does not exist. Until then use of guidelines for integrating UAPs (American Nurses' Association [ANA], 1996; Association of Women's Health, Obstetric, and Neonatal Nursing [AWHONN], 1997; 1998) into the practice of perinatal nursing can provide a framework for increasing the likelihood that women and newborns will receive the best care possible from the most appropriate caregivers. This chapter reviews current issues about the use of UAPs in the perinatal healthcare setting, including delegation and supervision of UAPs, practice models that have shown to be safe and effective, standards of care for management of staffing resources, and strategies for action.

REVIEW OF AVAILABLE DATA

Limited healthcare financial resources and intense scrutiny of resource allocation by hospital administrators have contributed to consideration of the bottom line in making decisions about the quality and quantity of patient care providers. Typically, nurses represent over two-thirds of a hospital's total workforce and a substantial portion of the budget, thus nursing practice in any institution is a likely target for redesign efforts and cost-containment strategies (Krapohl & Larson, 1996). However, when a number of professional registered nurses are replaced by unlicensed assistive personnel, there is no guarantee that institutional costs will decrease. Staffing and skill mix reductions may set other forces in motion that may actually increase the cost of care, such as increased training and supervision costs for unskilled workers, increased patient complication rates, and decreased caregiver productivity (Robertson, Dowd, & Hassan, 1997).

The failure of "reengineering" in American hospitals to enhance either productivity or efficiency is similar to outcomes of this type of strategy in other American industries. When major American corporations were surveyed about the effects of "downsizing," there was widespread disappointment that the anticipated cost reductions and increase in profits had not been realized and some corporations reported that they had to replace up to 20% of the employees who were dismissed (Shindul-Rothschild, Long-Middleton, & Berry, 1997). The large cost reductions in healthcare promised by many management consultants advocating cost cutting by staffing reductions have not materialized (Robertson et al., 1997).

Unfortunately, data are limited about the impact on patient outcomes of decreasing the nurse to patient ratio and the replacement of registered professional nurses with unlicensed assistive personnel (Aiken, Sochalski, & Anderson, 1996; Hall, 1997; Houston, 1996; Russo & Lancaster, 1995). However, several recent studies indicate that higher nurse to patient ratios improve patient outcomes. The American Nurses' Association (ANA, 1997) study *Implementing Nursing's Report Card: A Study of RN Staffing, Length of Stay and Patient Outcomes* conducted in California, New York, and Massachusetts, found that higher nurse to patient ratios were associated with shorter lengths of stay and a reduction in comorbid conditions such as pressure sores, pneumonia, urinary tract infections, and postoperative infections (ANA, 1997). A review of hospital mortality studies suggested that a higher ratio of RNs to other nursing personnel was associated with lower patient mortality (Prescott, 1993).

Understaffing and underskilling may have indirect costs that offset the benefits of payroll reductions (Robertson et al., 1997). Although the "redesign" efforts in American hospitals that were responsible for a decrease in the percentage of RNs in the caregiver skill mix were implemented to reduce costs, if these efforts result in poor patient outcomes there can actually be an increase in costs and a negative effect on other indices of care such as patient satisfaction and the likelihood of patients to return to the healthcare institution for future care when given a choice (National Coalition on Healthcare [NCH], 1997). Publication of patient satisfaction results in individual hospitals in the lay press can adversely influence the ability to attract patients and negotiate managed care contracts. In a recent poll, only 44% of patients indicated that they had confidence in the healthcare system and 58% agreed that hospital care is not very good and could actually make them sicker due to overworked and poorly trained staff (NCH, 1997).

CURRENT TRENDS IN USE OF UAPS

Definitive data about the changes in number of RN full-time equivalents (FTEs) in the United States over the past 2 years are not yet available; however, there are reports of increased use of UAPs by nurses in the nursing literature in survey format and in the lay press. Almost half of the 7500 nurses in the United States who returned the *American Journal of Nursing* (AJN, 1996) Patient Care Survey reported part-time or temporary nurses have been substituted for full-time RNs in their institution and two out of five of these nurses reported the substitution of UAPs for RNs (Shindul-Rothschild, Berry, & Long-Middleton, 1996). Findings suggest that the most deleterious labor trend affecting professional nursing practice is forcing fewer RNs to do more in less time (Shindul-Rothschild et al.,1997). Results of this study are based on nurses who completed and returned the survey that was published in the March 1996 issue of the *American Journal of Nursing*, so this may not reflect what is happening in all institutions. An informal survey of perinatal nurses was conducted by the Association of Women's Health, Obstetric, and Neonatal Nurses (AWHONN) in 1997 at nursing conferences and through their Internet home page. Based on this survey there is concern about UAPs replacing RNs and how to handle delegation and supervision responsibilities. Most nurses reported use of UAPs in their practice setting with percentage of UAPs as a component of nursing personnel varying by area of the country and individual institutions (AWHONN Lifelines, 1997). It is possible that most survey respondents were those who had been directly affected by the introduction of UAPs in their practice setting, and nonrespondents did not feel this was an issue in their institution; however, the AJN and AWHONN surveys are consistent with other informal data. A recent study of nursing role changes and satisfaction with UAPs found that registered nurses were dissatisfied with UAPs' ability to perform delegated nursing tasks, communicate pertinent information about patient status, and provide more time for professional nursing activities (Barter, McLaughlin, & Thomas, 1997).

UAP DESCRIPTION AND REGULATION

There are at least 50 different titles for UAPs that have been identified in the literature and in clinical practice by the ANA. The multiple titles and responsibilities of UAPs have caused confusion for both professional registered nurses and the public. In general, "UAPs are individuals who have no licensure process and who do not represent a group with a defined body of knowledge, educational process, or method of competence validation (AWHONN, 1997)." They are "trained to function in an assistive role to the registered professional nurse in the provision of patient care activities as delegated by and under the supervision of the registered professional nurse (ANA, 1996)." The legal definition of nursing practice as determined by each state nursing practice act defines the scope of nursing within that state. Professional regulation of nursing practice is based on nursing's contract with society to provide competent care (ANA, 1996). When RNs provide, delegate, assign, and oversee patient care activities, these functions must occur in the context of the profession's responsibility to the public (ANA, 1996). Many state boards of nursing are using their powers to regulate nursing practice involving UAPs by issuing advisory opinions or regulations that provide direction and guidance for delegation of nursing responsibilities to UAPs. A critical first step in developing a patient care model involving UAPs is review of the state nurse practice act and any advisory opinions or regulations about UAPs that may have been promulgated.

PROFESSIONAL ACCOUNTABILITY

The nursing profession is directly accountable to the public for its practice (ANA, 1996). The nursing profession determines the scope of nursing practice and defines and supervises the education, training, and use of UAPs involved in providing direct patient care (ANA, 1996). UAPs can contribute as members of the healthcare team under the direction of the professional registered nurse; however, the RN is ultimately responsible for the coordination and delivery of nursing care to women and newborns (AWHONN, 1998). It is important to remember that the role of the UAP is to assist, not replace, the professional registered nurse (ANA, 1996; AWHONN, 1997; 1998). Certain nursing functions are solely within the scope of nursing practice, thus oversight of the activities of the UAP is integral and necessary to implementation of UAP roles (ANA, 1996; Rhodes, 1997).

FRAMEWORK FOR DELEGATION AND SUPERVISION

The AWHONN (1997) Position Statement *The role of unlicensed assistive personnel in the nursing care for women and newborns* and *Registered professional nurses and unlicensed assistive personnel* (ANA, 1996) provide a framework for determining which tasks may be appropriate for delegation in selected clinical situations and examples of nursing care activities for women and newborns that cannot be delegated based on that framework. Review of these publications prior to development and implementation of a patient care model using UAPs is essential.

The nursing process is traditionally described as including four essential components: assessment, planning, implementation, and evaluation. It is not appropriate to delegate nursing activities that comprise the core of the nursing process and that require specialized knowledge, judgment, competence, and skill (ANA, 1996). Thus, in selecting certain aspects of nursing care that can be delegated to UAPs, it is critical to consider if the tasks meet those exclusion criteria. The delegated task must be a subcomponent of the total nursing process. The registered professional nurse is accountable when delegating nursing tasks and supervising UAPs who carry out those nursing tasks. It is generally agreed that the RN remains legally responsible for the nursing activities delegated to the UAP, although individual state laws may vary (ANA, 1996).

A review of the National Council of State Boards of Nursing ([NCSB],1995) definitions is useful in understanding the role of the registered professional nurse when working with UAPs. **Delegation** is the transferring to a competent individual of the authority to perform a selected nursing task in selected situations (NCSB, 1995). It is important to remember that delegation passes on the responsibility for task performance, but not the accountability for the outcome of the task (ANA, 1996). **Accountability** is being responsible and answerable for actions and inactions of self or others in the context of delegation (NCSB, 1995). **Supervision** is the provision of guidance or direction, evaluation, and follow-up by the registered professional nurse for accomplishment of a nursing task delegated to UAPs (NCSB, 1995). Supervision as used in the clinical context of oversight of overall patient care is very different from supervision as used in the context of the National Labor Relations Act, the federal law that protects employees who engage in concerted activities related to wages and terms and conditions of employment (ANA, 1996). Thus, although RNs supervise UAPs in terms of clinical oversight, according to the ANA, they are not supervisors as defined by the NLRB and should be protected. This issue has not been entirely resolved and continues to be litigated in the federal courts.

Patient assessment is a professional nursing responsibility and thus cannot be delegated to UAPs (JCAHO, 1997). Confusion seems to exist about the difference between collecting data and assessment. **Data** are uninterpreted observations or facts reported to the registered professional nurse (JCAHO, 1997). **Assessment** is the process of transforming data into useful information by analyzing the data (JCAHO, 1997). For example, UAPs can collect data about patients by taking blood pressures, temperatures, and respiratory and pulse rates (AWHONN, 1997). Professional registered nurses analyze that data using critical thinking skills to make an assessment about patient status. Assessment requires nursing judgment, an intellectual process that the RN uses to analyze data and determine the next course of nursing actions (ANA, 1996).

Nursing diagnosis, establishment of nursing care goals, and development of the nursing care plan are central to nursing practice and thus cannot be delegated (ANA, 1996). Selected tasks that fall within the implementation component of the nursing process may be appropriate for delegation if the nursing intervention does not require professional nursing knowledge, judgment, and skill (ANA, 1996). Evaluation of the patient's progress in relation to the plan of care cannot be delegated (ANA, 1996); however, the UAP can contribute data to assist the RN in making that evaluation.

To determine if these tasks are appropriate for delegation in selected clinical situations, the registered professional nurse must consider the following factors:

- patient condition
- capabilities of the UAP
- potential for harm
- complexity of task
- problem solving ability and critical thinking required
- unpredictability of outcome
- amount of clinical oversight the RN will be able to provide
- level of caregiver-patient interaction
- practice setting
- available staffing resources

(AWHONN, 1997)

"Delegated activities must be clearly defined and thoroughly described repetitive tasks that do not require nursing judgements" (AWHONN, 1997). "The knowledge base and clinical skills of the registered professional nurse provide the foundation for nursing assessments and diagnosis, critical thinking and decision making, outcome identification, planning, implementation, and evaluations that are requisite for high-quality outcomes for women and newborns" (AWHONN, 1997). This is not to imply that UAPs are not capable of critical thinking or that they are lacking knowledge and clinical skills (Simpson, 1997). However, the fundamental difference between these two care providers is the type and amount of education, depth of knowledge, and level of critical thinking possessed by the registered professional nurse when compared to the UAP (AWHONN, 1997).

When the professional registered nurse delegates a selected nursing task to a UAP, the nurse is responsible for

1. Determining if the task is suitable for delegation

    The task must:

    be clearly defined and thoroughly described

    be repetitive and represent routine care

    be performed with predictable outcome

    require little or no modification from one patient care situation to another

    not involve ongoing assessment or any significant interpretation, and

    be within the training and competence of the UAP

2. Determining if the UAP is competent to perform the task
(AWHONN, 1998)

PRACTICAL APPLICATION OF THE FRAMEWORK

Using the framework just described, consider the UAP's possible role in application of an electronic fetal monitor (EFM). At first glance, it may seem that application of an external EFM could be appropriate for delegation; however, careful analysis of the nursing process involved precludes this task as appropriate (AWHONN, 1997). Initial steps in application of external EFM require critical nursing assessments including performing Leopold's maneuvers, palpation of the uterine fundus, and determining if the heart rate tracing is fetal or maternal (Menihan, 1997). The data generated by EFM about characteristics of the fetal heart rate and uterine activity can only be assessed by the registered professional nurse who is knowledgeable about the physiologic basis for fetal heart rate monitoring, interpretation of the fetal heart rate pattern, reassuring versus nonreassuring fetal heart rate patterns, and appropriate nursing interventions based on those data (Simpson, 1997). Essentially, there are no aspects of EFM that could be delegated to a UAP because UAPs are lacking the requisite in-depth knowledge and clinical skills to participate in this perinatal nursing activity (AWHONN, 1997). The task is complex, the level of problem solving and critical thinking required is beyond the UAP based on knowledge and education, and there is significant potential for harm to the mother and fetus if EFM data are not correctly interpreted and/or acted upon appropriately (Simpson, 1997).

Data-gathering activities such as vital signs and measurement of oral intake and urinary output may be appropriately delegated to a UAP who has been adequately trained to assume these clinical tasks (AWHONN, 1997). The tasks are repetitive, not complex, and the potential for harm is minimal for the healthy mother and full-term newborn. Critical thinking and problem-solving skills are not required given that these data are reported to the registered professional nurse. However, data gathering involving other than routine patients such as women with preeclampsia, cardiac disease, or respiratory problems is not appropriate because the potential for harm is significant if the data are inaccurate (Simpson, 1997). The registered professional nurse must decide which patients are appropriate candidates for UAP care based on multiple factors. Some aspects of care that may be appropriate for healthy women and newborns are clearly beyond the scope of a UAP when the woman or newborn develops complications (Simpson, 1997).

Registered professional nurses are responsible for directly supervising UAPs as they participate in selected nursing care activities (AWHONN, 1997; 1998). Clear and precise instructions for how and when to report information about completed tasks and data-gathering activities to the RN are essential (Simpson, 1997). For example, the UAP needs to know that abnormal variations in vital signs and changes in the patient's condition require immediate notification of the RN team leader. If medical record documentation is the method of communicating data within normal limits and completed tasks, the UAP needs appropriate instructions. Ongoing discussion, evaluation, and positive reinforcement by the RN is required.

There are special challenges in supervising unlicensed workers because UAPs have no identified career path, receive relatively low wages, and seem to have a higher turnover rate than licensed professionals. Clearly, there are distinct differences between a job and a career. These differences are evident in many aspects of supervising UAPs; however, there are opportunities for RNs to nurture the UAP's interest in patient care by acting as role models and encouraging UAPs who are appropriate candidates to further their education in a healthcare career.

SUCCESSFUL RN-UAP MODELS OF CARE

Critical to the successful implementation of a nursing practice model using UAPs is advance planning and a multidisciplinary team approach.

Representatives from ancillary departments that will be affected such as dietary services, the laboratory, respiratory therapy, and housekeeping are important members of the planning team. Involving the medical staff during the developmental phase is crucial. Encourage representatives from the obstetric, pediatric, and anesthesia departments to actively participate. The quality of these efforts will have a direct impact on the RNs' level of comfort in supervising UAPs and on the physicians' concerns about UAPs providing selected aspects of nursing care for their patients. (See Display 8-1.)

Clear delineation of aspects of care that can be delegated and those that require a registered professional nurse is important. Each institution must develop guidelines for UAPs based on state nurse practice acts or board of nursing rules and regulations, JCAHO standards, publications from professional nursing organizations, and established institutional policies and procedures (Simpson, 1997). Institutional guidelines for UAPs provide the framework for developing unit-specific UAP job descriptions. (See Display 8-2 for a sample job description for a UAP working in the perinatal clinical setting.)

Use of UAPs as members of the healthcare team is not a new concept. The team nursing model was used successfully for many years before primary nursing became popular. However, nurses who graduated after the mid 1980s may not have skills necessary for delegation and supervision of UAPs because of their prior experience with all-RN staffs (ANA, 1996; Johnson, 1996). Much of the focus on implementation of models of care involving skill mix has been on training of UAPs. Adequate training and evaluation of UAPs are crucial components of successful staff integration (see Chapter 9), but before implementation of a model of care involving UAPs, it is essential to provide RNs with guidance on delegation and supervision of these workers (Simpson, 1997). Nurses could benefit from a formal session on decision-making skills about what tasks are appropriate to delegate, how to follow-up, and what steps to take if the UAP is not functioning at the expected clinical skill level. It is important to provide concise written materials as part of the educa-

DISPLAY 8-1

Essential Steps Prior to Implementing a Nursing Care Model Using UAPs

- Use a multidisciplinary team approach.
- Review current guidelines on use of UAPs from professional organizations such as JCAHO, AAP & ACOG, ANA, AWHONN, and NANN, and rules and regulations for individual states' boards of nursing.
- Review institutional guidelines, policies, and regulations.
- Develop job description and evaluation criteria for UAPs based on above review and unit needs.
- Develop patient outcome measures that are sensitive to the use of UAPs such as patient satisfaction and selected aspects of clinical care.
- Provide didactic content on delegation, accountability, responsibility, and supervision for perinatal nurses.
- Provide didactic content, preceptorship, knowledge base evaluation, and clinical skills verification for UAPs.
- Establish a periodic review of how the practice model is working based on established criteria.

Adapted from: Simpson, K. R. (1997). Unlicensed assistive personnel: What nurses need to know. AWHONN Lifelines, 1(3), 26–31.

tion process that can be used as a reference if questions arise later.

Outcome criteria for evaluation of the RN/UAP model should be established prior to implementation. Setting specific time frames for ongoing evaluation are critical for identifying opportunities for improvement and developing strategies to further refine the patient care model. If possible, preliminary analysis of the model should be done within six months after implementation and periodically thereafter. At a minimum, a

DISPLAY 8-2

UAPs: List of Sample Activities for an LDRP Unit

Activities that can be delegated after completion of orientation and successful competence validation include but are not limited to

- Transport of stable mothers and newborns
- Phlebotomy
- Foley catheter insertion and removal (varies from state to state)
- Ambulation assistance
- Assisting women to the bathroom
- Assisting women using a bedpan
- Acting as the scrub person for cesarean birth
- Stocking and cleaning rooms
- Cleaning and sterilizing instruments
- Taking specimens to the laboratory
- Entering orders into the computer
- Printing laboratory results from the computer and providing these data to the nurse
- Answering the unit telephone and patient call system
- Passing out menus
- Serving meals and retrieving trays
- Vital signs for stable patients and documentation in the medical record
- Assisting with pericare and applying ice to the perineum
- Assisting the new mother with breastfeeding
- Bathing mothers and newborns

comprehensive evaluation process should occur on an annual basis (JCAHO, 1997). Suggestions for patient outcomes are nosocomial infection rates, patient injury rates, maintenance of skin integrity, and patient satisfaction. Personnel outcomes appropriate for evaluation are job satisfaction for all staff, career development, performance evaluation, staff retention and turnover, and recruitment success. Institutional outcomes that provide valuable information about overall success of the model are costs of service, length of stay, compliance with accreditation standards, risk management indicators, market share, and recruiting costs (ANA, 1996).

THE IMPACT OF USE OF UAPS ON CURRENT PUBLISHED GUIDELINES FOR MANAGING STAFFING RESOURCES FOR PERINATAL UNITS

Of all aspects of the issue of use of UAPs in the practice setting, registered professional nurse to patient staffing ratios are probably of most concern for the RN. Currently, there are little research-based data to support specific staffing ratios for various clinical situations. Therefore, a reasonable approach to balancing the needs of the patients with the limited financial resources in most healthcare institutions must provide a framework for setting criteria for professional nursing staff to patient ratios.

Patient Acuity

Acuity is defined as the degree of care required by the patient's condition. As acuity increases, requirements for nursing care increase (AWHONN, 1998). Because clinical settings have various patient volume and acuity levels, the provision of safe and effective care must be based on a logical system for staffing that considers resource allocation, acuity assessment, and the education and skill of available care providers. Acuity is an essential component of the decision-making process for defining the level of nursing care and staffing resources. Each institution should have a defined method for evaluating patient acuity (AWHONN, 1998). It is important to note that no one system has been shown to work better or be more reliable in predicting staffing resource needs than another. There is no need for institutions to purchase an expensive computerized acuity system if one is not already in place. Although hospitals have relied on nursing workload or patient classification systems to determine the appropriate level of RN staffing (Shindul-Rothschild et al., 1997), an extensive review of workload instruments found little scientific evidence to support the validity of these types of systems, especially some of the most widely used (Edwardson & Giovannetti, 1994). Thus, the traditional method of evaluating staffing needs based on patient census and clinical condition can be as effective as a computerized acuity system using predictive models. The most important issue is to have some type of system for addressing the dynamic staffing needs of the clinical setting.

Attendance at prepared childbirth classes, level of social support, mental state, and clinical condition of the mother and fetus are factors that contribute to the nursing care needs of the woman during labor and birth. For some women, one-to-one nursing care may be required during the intrapartum period. The primiparous woman who has a cesarean birth after a long labor with oxytocin augmentation has different needs postpartum than a multiparous woman who has a normal labor and spontaneous vaginal birth. There are also different needs for each of these women in the ability to assume care for her newborn during the postpartum period. For all women after birth, the level of parenting skills and choice of feeding method has a direct influence on how much time is required to prepare the new mother and baby for discharge. A woman who suffers perinatal loss may need more intensive nursing time than a mother who has an uncomplicated labor and birth. Each patient and clinical situation is unique and should be evaluated individually for necessary staffing resources. In certain clinical situations, selected aspects of nursing care can be safely delegated to adequately trained, competent UAPs.

Registered Professional Nurse-to-Patient Staffing Ratios

When determining the appropriate registered professional nurse-to-patient ratios for perinatal units, refer to *Guidelines for Perinatal Care* (American Academy of Pediatrics [AAP] and American College of Obstetricians and Gynecologists [ACOG], 1997, p. 19). These RN to patient ratios were developed in the early 1980s by a NAACOG task force of perinatal nurses (E. Knox; A. Ropp, personal communication, April 1997) and were first published in 1983 by AAP & ACOG in *Guidelines for Perinatal Care*. Although there is no evidence that they have been evaluated using scientific methods since they were introduced, these staffing ratios are reasonable in the context of the complexity and nature of nursing care required for women and newborns. They were initially developed based on models of care involving UAPs and were recently reviewed by nursing representatives from AWHONN for the fourth edition of *Guidelines for Perinatal Care*, again considering the role of the UAP as contributing to the nursing care of women and newborns.

There is a misconception among some nurses that the AWHONN (NAACOG)/AAP and ACOG RN to patient ratios are based on a primary nursing model where the RN is the sole provider of nursing care. This misconception has led some administrators to believe that the addition of UAPs to perinatal unit staffing resources allows for a change in the ratios to include more patients per RN. The professional organizations' goal in providing suggestions for RN to patient staffing ratios is the provision of safe and effective perinatal nursing care. For most areas of perinatal nursing care, the contribution to the patient care workload that can be provided by a UAP, while valuable, is not such that it would change the currently accepted safe and effective registered professional nurse to patient ratios (AWHONN, 1998).

Proactive Strategies for Perinatal Nurses

The suggestions provided and resources discussed can be used as a basis for evaluating nursing care models involving UAPs in the perinatal setting. When expressing concerns about safe and effective nursing care and the role of UAPs, the amount and quality of data and background information provided to administrators and key decision makers could make a difference. An opinion from the institution's risk management department based on available data may be an important contribution to the decision-making process. Consider that both administrators and nurses have the best interests of patients in mind, but that administrators have the additional perspective of assessing and allocating limited financial resources. This additional perspective contributes to administrators' focus on costs per patient day when considering RN to patient staffing ratios.

Accuracy in Patient Census Reporting

Perinatal nurses caring for pregnant women always have at least a 1 to 2 RN to patient ratio, yet when considering numbers in staffing patterns, the pregnant woman is generally considered as one patient. Administrators need to be aware that the nurse is actually caring for two patients with the requisite nursing care and medical record documentation that is consistent with caring for these two distinct individuals. When providing information about antepartum and intrapartum census and acuity for budget and staffing purposes to administrators, consider including all patients (both the pregnant woman and her fetus). Avoid use of the terms couplet and mother-baby pair when presenting data about postpartum census and acuity. An RN to couplet care ratio of 1 to 4 can be misleading to administrators. Women who are in the immediate postpartum period and newborns adapting to extrauterine life should be considered in staffing patterns as would any other newly postoperative patient because there are many similarities in acuity. Other units in the hospital do not routinely plan staffing patterns with 1 RN to 8 new postoperative patients. Use of the terms couplet and pair gives a false impression to administrators when evaluating RN to patient ratios for staffing and financial resource allocation. Provide data in terms of actual number of patients for a more realistic view of caring for childbearing women and newborns. As costs per patient day become more scrutinized with the focus on managed care contracts and reimbursement issues, the ability to accurately define acuity based on patient needs is even more critical to ensure adequate staffing and financial resource allocation for perinatal nursing units.

SUMMARY

Perinatal nurses have been and must continue to be advocates for women and newborns (AWHONN, 1998). Participating in the development of RN/UAP models of nursing care that ensure safe and effective RN to patient ratios and include competent and skilled nursing personnel is a critical aspect of the patient advocacy role (Simpson, 1997).

REFERENCES

Aiken, L. H., Sochalski, J.,& Anderson, G. F. (1996). Downsizing the hospital nursing workforce. Health Affairs, 13(4), 88–92.

American Nurses' Association. (1996). Registered professional nurses and unlicensed assistive personnel. Washington, DC: Author.

American Nurses' Association. (1997). Implementing nursing's report card: A study of RN staffing, length of stay, and patient outcomes. Washington, DC: Author.

American Academy of Pediatricians and Gynecologist and American College of Obstetricians and Gynecologists. (1997). Guidelines for Perinatal Care (4th ed.). Elk Grove Village, IL: Author.

Association of Women's Health, Obstetric, and Neonatal Nurses. (1997). The role of unlicensed assistive personnel in the nursing care of women and newborns. Position Statement. Washington, DC: Author.

Association of Women's Health, Obstetric, and Neonatal Nurses. (1998). Standards and guidelines for professional nursing practice in the care of women and newborns (5th ed.). Washington, DC: Author.

Barter, M., McLaughlin, F. E., & Thomas, S. A. (1997). Registered nurse role changes and satisfaction with unlicensed assistive personnel. Journal of Nursing Administration, 27(1), 29–38.

Edwardson, S. R., & Giovannetti, P. B. (1994). Nursing workload measurement systems. Annals and Review of Nursing Research, 12, 95–123.

Hall, L. M. (1997) Staff mix models: Complementary or substitution roles for nurses. Nursing Administration Quarterly, 21(2), 31–39.

Huston, C. L. (1996). Unlicensed assistive personnel: A solution to dwindling health care resources or the precursor to the apocalypse of registered nursing? Nursing Outlook, 44(2), 67–73.

Johnson, S. H. (1996). Teaching nursing delegation: Analyzing nurse practice acts. Journal of Continuing Education in Nursing, 27(2), 52–58.

Krapohl, G. L., & Larson, E. (1996). The impact of unlicensed assistive personnel on nursing care delivery. Nursing Economics, 14(2), 99–109.

Menihan, C. A. (1996). Intrapartum fetal monitoring. In K. R. Simpson and P. A. Creehan (Eds.). AWHONN's Perinatal Nursing. Philadelphia: Lippincott–Raven.

National Coalition on Health Care. (1997). How Americans perceive the health care system. Washington, DC: Author.

Prescott, P. A. (1993). Nursing: An important component of hospital survival under a reformed health care system. Nursing Economics, 11, 192–199.

Rhodes, A. M. (1997). Liability for unlicensed personnel. American Journal of Maternal Child Nursing, 22(6), 327–328.

Robertson, R. H., Dowd, S. B., & Hassan, M. (1997). Skill-specific staffing intensity and the cost of hospital care. Health Care Management Review, 22(4), 61–71.

Russo, J. M. K., & Lancaster, D. R. (1995). Evaluating unlicensed assistive personnel models. Journal of Nursing Administration, 25(9), 51–57.

Shindul-Rothschild, J., Berry, D., & Long-Middleton, E. (1996). Where have all the nurses gone? Final results of our patient care survey. American Journal of Nursing, 96(11), 25–39.

Shindul-Rothschild, J., Long-Middleton, E., & Berry, D. (1997). 10 keys to quality care. American Journal of Nursing, 97(11), 35–43.

Simpson, K. R. (1997). Unlicensed assistive personnel: What nurses need to know. AWHONN Lifelines, 1(3), 26–31.

CHAPTER 9

Unlicensed Assistive Personnel: Orientation and Competence Validation in the Perinatal Clinical Setting

Kathleen Rice Simpson

INTRODUCTION

Over the years, nurses have voiced concerns about the amount of time they spend on nonnursing or indirect patient care activities such as clerical work, ordering supplies, transporting specimens to the laboratory, stocking rooms, cleaning and checking equipment, and other tasks that do not require the special knowledge and clinical skills that can only be obtained through a formal nursing education. Yet there is resistance among some registered nurses (RN) to working with UAPs for fear that UAPs may replace RNs. Job security for RNs and quality of patient care are two of the common issues raised. Using established guidelines and standards for staffing resources (AAP & ACOG, 1997; ANA, 1996; AWHONN, 1997; 1998) ensures that UAPs assist, rather than replace RNs. It is possible to develop a practice model incorporating UAPs into perinatal care that is well within accepted standards and guidelines from professional organizations, state nurse practice acts, and other regulatory agencies. This type of practice model can be beneficial for both perinatal nurses and their patients. Patients get more direct care from registered nurses who are available to do so because they are assisted by trained personnel in accomplishing the many important, but labor intensive, indirect care activities. Nurses have the opportunity to do what they do best: focus on the clinical and psychosocial aspects of caring for childbearing women and newborns.

Consider the following scenarios in an LDR unit: Nurse A cleans and prepares the LDR for the next woman admitted in labor, checks supplies, restocks as needed, admits the woman in labor, draws admission laboratory blood samples, enters the patient's data into the computer, carries the blood specimen to the laboratory, cares for the woman during labor, checks the laboratory results and places the laboratory forms in the medical record, prepares the LDR for birth, acts as the circulator for birth, removes the instruments and delivery table and cleans and sterilizes the equipment when there is time, assesses maternal and newborn vital signs and other clinical characteristics, retrieves and prepares a crushed ice pack for the perineum, completes the required medical record documentation, prepares the woman and newborn for transport to the mother-baby unit, transports the patients including their luggage, cleans the LDR, mops the floor, makes the bed, and restocks and prepares the room for the next patient. Nurse B escorts the woman who is admitted in labor to a fully prepared and stocked LDR, completes the admission assessment, cares for the woman in labor, is notified by the UAP of the laboratory results of blood drawn on admission by the

UAP, acts as circulator for birth after the UAP has prepared the room and equipment, assesses maternal and newborn vital signs during the immediate postpartum period working with the UAP, applies a fresh ice bag to the perineum that has been brought to the LDR by the UAP, assists the woman during the first breastfeeding experience, completes the required medical record documentation while the UAP gives the woman a bath, is assisted by the UAP in the transfer of the woman and newborn to the mother-baby unit, is confident that the LDR is ready and stocked for the next patient and the instruments have been cleaned and sterilized. Having experienced both the Nurse A and Nurse B role over the years, it seems that the latter scenario is preferable. However, to ensure success with this type of practice model, the UAP orientation and competence validation process must be well-designed and comprehensive.

Delegation of selected nursing tasks and supervision of unlicensed assistive personnel (UAPs) have been discussed in detail in Chapter 8, "Registered Professional Nurses and Unlicensed Assistive Personnel: Delegation, Supervision, and Staffing Resources." Standards and guidelines for developing a practice model that incorporates the use of UAPs are also outlined. This chapter provides an overview of suggested orientation and competence validation methods for UAPs in the perinatal clinical setting. In addition, there are examples of UAP position descriptions, competence validation tools, and skills checklists from several healthcare institutions provided in text appendices.

UAP ORIENTATION

During the interview process, it is important to review a list of expected UAP skills and responsibilities. Many UAPs have an unrealistic expectation of the role in a perinatal setting. For example, the UAP position in the full-term nursery usually involves much more than rocking babies and transporting babies to mothers. A pre-employment skills self-assessment tool works well to determine previous experience and clinical skills that the UAP may already possess. Although not always available in all areas of the country, pools of potential candidates for the UAP position, in addition to nursing students, include individuals who have completed a nurses aide program at a community college and are credentialed as a certified nurses' aide (CNA). These UAPs have demonstrated commitment to learning the essentials skills required for the role. Unfortunately, not all community colleges in all areas offer this curriculum. Hiring an experienced UAP with a proven track record and good references from the previous employer can work equally well. This is not meant to imply that hiring a UAP without previous experience is to be avoided; however, the time involved for training and competence validation will be more extensive. Nursing students are ideal because they are usually enthusiastic and motivated to learn and there are opportunities for the employing institution to evaluate the student who chooses to request a position as a registered nurse after graduation. However, the limitations of relying on nursing students as a primary source of UAPs are that their length of employment as UAPs is limited to their years as students and there may be less flexibility in scheduling due to school commitments.

Ideally, before the UAP is oriented to a speciality unit such as perinatal services, the UAP has successfully completed a skills laboratory course and basic classes provided by the institution's department of education. Thus, basic content and clinical skills such as hand washing, vital signs, measuring intake and output, bed making, baths, assisting with ambulation, phlebotomy, foley catheter insertion, medical record documentation, using the computer, handling and labeling laboratory specimens, and interacting with patients and families have already been taught and validated. When the UAP begins orientation to the speciality unit, basic clinical skills can be reinforced and new skills specific to perinatal care such as newborn vital signs, umbilical cord care, preparing the newborn for circumcision, newborn heel sticks for PKUs, assisting with Sitz baths, perineal care, preparing the LDR and OR for birth, acting as a scrub technician for cesarean birth, and cleaning and sterilizing instruments can be introduced. The amount of formal didactic content and clinical skills verification prior to unit orientation influences the type and amount of clinical preceptorship required.

Selecting the most appropriate preceptor is important. Probably a combination of an RN and UAP as preceptors works best. On the unit, the perinatal RN provides basic instruction for clinical skills that have not been covered in the skills laboratory course. The RN must feel confident that the UAP can accurately perform all expected clinical skills, while the UAP preceptor can provide a general orientation to the unit and expectations of how the UAP functions as a team member. As with the preceptor selection process for any job category, the UAP preceptor should be clinically competent and a role model for expected behavior.

The best approach is a 4- to 8-week preceptorship combined with didactic content in a classroom setting. See Appendix 9-1 for a complete description of a patient care associate training course. On days that content is covered that is not applicable to the speciality such as ECG procedures and ostomy care, the UAP who is hired for perinatal services follows a preceptor in the clinical area. Didactic content and the length of the preceptorship are based on the UAP job description, expected skills, and prior experience of the UAP. For example, if the duties of the UAP will be limited to vital signs for stable patients, assisting with baths, ambulation, dietary duties, and patient transport, 4-week preceptorship may suffice. A more comprehensive role of the UAP as described in Display 8-2 is best covered in a 6- to 8-week preceptorship.

Some skills may require repetitive and thorough practice opportunities before competence is achieved. For example, when acting as a scrub person for cesarean birth, the UAP may need to initially review instruments and sterile technique, observe several cases, and then act as the scrub person numerous times with close supervision before he or she is comfortable in this role. Of course it is helpful if all involved display patience and understanding during this process and provide feedback and encouragement after each case. Technical skills related to preparing the room for birth, cleaning and sterilizing instruments, and stocking rooms may also take time. There are multiple minute steps to remember for each of these tasks that, if omitted, can have serious consequences especially during emergent situations. Providing a written list of essential steps involved can be very helpful as a reference for the UAP.

Interactions with patients and families are critical aspects of the UAP role. This area of competence validation should not be diminished or overlooked. The UAPs represent the institution when they interact with patients and lack of clear guidelines in this area can potentially have an adverse effect on patient satisfaction. For example, it is particularly important to discuss appropriate language when caring for women who experience a perinatal loss. Well-meaning phrases that the registered professional nurse knows are not appropriate may seem like comforting words to the UAP who has not been provided education about the grieving process. The importance of accurately identifying newborns by checking identification bracelets with the mother before giving newborns to mothers must be explained in great detail. It must be emphasized that the process is to be repeated each time the newborn is transported to the mother's room. Allowing a woman to breastfeed another woman's infant can have potential adverse outcome if the steps of newborn identification are not completely and routinely followed. Avoidance of routinely sharing the details of their own labor and birth or breastfeeding experiences with patients should also be discussed. Review of guidelines for maintaining patient confidentiality cannot be overemphasized. The inappropriateness of discussions among peers about private patient issues should be thoroughly explained and reinforced.

REGISTERED PROFESSIONAL NURSE ORIENTATION TO THE UAP PRACTICE MODEL

If the role of the UAP is new to the unit, it is important to provide formal guidance about delegation and supervision to the registered nurse staff. Many nurses may not be experienced at working with UAPs, especially if they entered practice when all-RN staffs were the norm. This information can be presented at unit staff meetings or inservices. Common concerns can be addressed and questions clarified. Examples can be provided such as what aspects of care can be delegated, how to follow-up, and what steps should be taken if the UAP is not functioning at the expected skill level.

COMPETENCE VALIDATION

The UAP job description (see Display 9-1 and text appendices) and skills checklists can be used to develop a UAP competence validation tool (see Display 9-2 and text appendices). Competence validation for UAPs involves both knowledge base evaluation and clinical skills verification (Simpson, 1997). Requisite knowledge can be evaluated by traditional paper and pencil tests during the classroom portion of orientation and through informal discussions during the clinical preceptorship. Skills checklists using a step-by-step approach developed for each delegated task can be helpful in evaluating the UAP during the orientation period. It is not enough to document that the UAP can take a blood pressure. It is also important to know if the UAP follows a series of steps that demonstrate a logical, organized, and accurate method of doing so and is aware of what blood pressure parameters require immediate notification of the RN responsible for that patient's care (Simpson, 1997). The nurse can not assume that the UAP has the knowledge and background to know what is appropriate and how to handle individual patient variations.

Successful completion of orientation based on the competence validation criteria is essential before beginning the new role. A follow-up meeting between a member of the management team and the UAP within 3 to 6 months after completion of orientation works well. Patient and family feedback (see text appendices) and peer review processes can be used to discuss progress. Complete and accurate documentation of all aspects of the UAP competence validation process should be maintained. Annual competence validation provides a framework for feedback about performance and allows an opportunity to reinforce excellence. If there are areas that need improvement, close supervision or an additional preceptorship may be necessary.

SUMMARY

Integration of UAPs into the unit practice model is facilitated by a clear understanding of roles and responsibilities of all staff members. Providing formal guidance to RNs about delegation and supervision of UAPs is important, especially for nurses who are only familiar with the primary nursing model. A team approach to interviewing and selecting UAPs including managers, staff nurses, and UAPs works well. Developing and maintaining a comprehensive orientation and competence validation program for UAPs is challenging. The benefits of having assistance to accomplish the nonnursing tasks that are essential to support quality nursing care and unit operations are innumerable. The key is to design a program that is within established standards and guidelines, follow-up as appropriate, and encourage and mentor those in the UAP role. Within this framework, the UAP can make an important contribution in the care of women and newborns.

REFERENCES

American Nurses' Association. (1996). <u>Registered professional nurses and unlicensed assistive personnel</u>. Washington, DC: Author.

American Academy of Pediatricians and Gynecologist and American College of Obstetricians and Gynecologists. (1997). <u>Guidelines for Perinatal Care</u> (4th ed.). Elk Grove Village, IL: Author.

Association of Women's Health, Obstetric, and Neonatal Nurses. (1997). <u>The role of unlicensed assistive personnel in the nursing care of women and newborns</u>. Position Statement. Washington, DC: Author.

Association of Women's Health, Obstetric, and Neonatal Nurses. (1998). <u>Standards and guidelines for professional nursing practice in the care of women and newborns</u> (5th ed.). Washington, DC: Author.

Simpson, K. R. (1997). Unlicensed assistive personnel: What nurses need to know. <u>AWHONN Lifelines, 1</u>(3), 26–31.

DISPLAY 9-1

St. John's Mercy Medical Center
St. Louis, Missouri

JOB DESCRIPTION

Job Title: OB Technician
Department: Nursing Service (Labor and Delivery)
Date: November, 1996   **Job Class #:** 086

Summary: Using sterile techniques, prepares delivery rooms for C-section cases; surgically assists physicians with procedures and functions effectively in obstetrical emergencies. Responsible for the sterilization and maintenance of all sterile equipment. Prepares and turns over delivery rooms after delivery. Assists with patient care, especially the recovery phase of delivered patients. Assists with the collection and transport of specimens. Performs duties and responsibilities in a manner consistent with our mission, values and guiding principles.

Mission: Provide general acute, ambulatory, health promotion, long term and home care services to individuals and families
Continuing commitment to health research and to health education at all levels.
Innovative health and social services to improve quality of life of the communities.

VALUES: DIGNITY, JUSTICE, SERVICE, EXCELLENCE, AND STEWARDSHIP.

GUIDING PRINCIPLES:

Live the Values - We foster a climate of respect, support and service
Be an Organization of Opportunity and Growth - We value difference and support differences in an effort to be culturally diverse in our organization.
Commit to Personal Development - Values and seeks opportunities to learn
Practice Empowerment - Builds and maintains positive relationships. Works cooperatively and listens effectively.
Require Performance and Contribution - Sets challenging objectives, takes initiative
Foster Communication - Promotes and provides courteous and effective communication with internal and external customers.

Principle Accountabilities

30%   1. Surgically assists with scheduled and emergency C-sections (surgical delivery of a baby through an abdominal incision). Maintains surgical delivery rooms, which includes checking all equipment and gathering supplies, rotating sterile supplies and maintaining aseptic technique.

30%   2. Uses autoclave to sterilize instruments kept in department, sterilizes supplies for other units, sterilizes set-up of all tables for vaginal deliveries, breaks down supplies and equipment in LDR rooms after delivery and re-sets room for next patient. Stocks linen supplies in LDRs.

25%   3. Assists in the recovery of delivered patients on a rotating basis. Includes vital signs, fundal checks, assessment of bleeding status,   I & O and the transporting of patients and patients' belongings to room following release from L&D or OBRR.

15%   4. Relieves unit secretary as needed. Cuts monitor belts, baby hats. Stores placentas in freezer, assists with placenta pick-up. Assists maintenance with broken equipment in department. Retrieves lost equipment, miscellaneous, etc.

   5. Performs other work duties as assigned.

DISPLAY 9-1 (cont.)

Knowledge, Skills and Abilities:

High school diploma or equivalent required. More than three months, but less than one year experience required.

The assessment, care and treatment provided by the OB Technologist will be consistent with the specific age related needs of the patient. The OB Technologist is competent to care for patient age groups including the neonatal/infant, adolescent, and adult patient

Working Conditions:

Employee is required to sit occasionally; stand and walk frequently. Employee must lift/carry light (20# max) and medium (50# max) frequently. Employee is required to bend, squat, reach forward, reach overhead and lift floor to waist frequently; lift waist to overhead occasionally. For repetitive action, employee is required to use one or both hands for simple grasping, pushing/pulling and fine manipula-tion. Employee is exposed to the following environmental conditions: temperature changes (heat, cold, wet, damp) frequently; noise, fumes, electrical hazards and hazardous waste occasionally. Employee is frequently exposed to blood borne pathogens.

(occasionally - 1 to 33%; frequently - 34 to 66%; continuously - 67 to 100%).

The most significant of duties are included but this does not exclude occasional work assignments not mentioned or developmental duties.

DISPLAY 9-2

Women and Newborns Services
St. John's Mercy Medical Center, St. Louis, Missouri
Unlicensed Assistive Personnel Core Competence Assessment Tool

General Description of UAP: The UAP works under the direction of the registered professional nurse as part of a multidisciplinary team. The UAP can make a positive contribution as part of the team caring for women and newborns. When nursing activities or tasks are delegated to UAPs, registered nurses are responsible and accountable for overall nursing care. Thus, patient assessment, care planning, and appropriately delegating tasks and interventions remain the responsibility of the registered nurse. The registered nurse is also accountable for ongoing supervision of UAPs and for evaluation of delegated activities including patient outcomes.

Key: Competence Assessment
Needs Further Practice: Preceptor Reassessment Required
Competence: Has Demonstrated Requisite Knowledge and Skill to Perform Under Supervision of RN

Key: Method of Evaluation and Follow-Up
Preceptor Observation: PO
Written Assessment: WA
Return Demonstration: RD
Patient/Family Feedback: PF
Peer Review: PR
None Needed: NN
Skills Checklist: SC
Not Applicable: NA

Name _____ Evaluator Signature/s _____

Expected Outcome/Skill	Needs Further Practice	Competent	Method of Evaluation	Follow-Up	Evaluator Initials/ Date
Maintains patient privacy and confidentiality.					
Demonstrates ability to maintain a poised, calm, and composed manner.					
Communicates in a courteous manner using a pleasant tone of voice.					
Presents a neat and clean appearance in accordance with medical center dress code policy.					
Accepts delegation of appropriate tasks.					
Prioritizes appropriately and demonstrates good judgement in use of time.					
Demonstrates ability to provide accurate and thorough documentation in the medical record.					

DISPLAY 9-2 (cont.)

Expected Outcome/Skill	Needs Further Practice	Competent	Method of Evaluation	Follow-Up	Evaluator Initials/ Date
Administers hygiene measures such as bathing, mouth and skin care. Changes linens.					
Observes changes in patient's condition and reports them immediately to patient's RN.					
Gathers and records data including vital signs, calorie counts, appetite, intake and output, stools, simple dressing changes/decubitus care, weights, specimens, and all assigned patient care activities.					
Performs routine daily activities. Assists with passing trays, snacks, ice water, and feeding patients. Performs passive and active ROM. Turns and positions patients as needed.					
Provides patients and families with explanation of care and psychological support under direction of RN.					
Demonstrates knowledge of newborn identification/security policy and follows procedure appropriately.					
Assists patients with breastfeeding/bottle feeding and refers patient questions or problems to RN as needed.					
Assists patients to the bathroom after birth. Provides patients with information about pericare and refers questions or problems to RN as needed.					
Provides information about maternal-newborn care in preparation for discharge according to mother-baby unit teaching guidelines. Refers questions or problems to RN as needed.					
Demonstrates knowledge of and practices sound infection control techniques including universal precautions and biohazardous waste disposal.					
Evaluates safety needs and provides for a safe environment for patients and coworkers.					
Participates in admission, discharge and transfer of patients and their belongings. Orients patients to their environment.					
Performs clerical duties as necessary (i.e., answers telephones, monitors call lights, displays working knowledge of selected computer functions, ordering equipment and laboratory tests)					

DISPLAY 9-2 (cont.)

Expected Outcome/Skill	Needs Further Practice	Competent	Method of Evaluation	Follow-Up	Evaluator Initials/ Date
Maintains supplies and restocks as needed.					
Demonstrates proficiency in Foley catheter insertion, removal, and measurement of output.					
Demonstrates proficiency in phlebotomy techniques, labeling specimens, computer functions, and transporting specimens to laboratory.					
Sets up sterile vaginal birth instrument table.					
Handles soiled instruments and sterile supplies appropriately. (Uses steam autoclave correctly and prepares soiled instruments for Central Services pick-up).					
Sets up room prior to case following department procedures. Checks spotlights and suction canister, gathers all needed supplies, sutures, and sets up table using sterile technique.					
Functions effectively as a scrub technician. Maintains sterile technique, passes correct instruments, demonstrates accurate sponge and needle counts, collects specimens, and conserves supplies.					
On completion of case, cleans room according to established guidelines. After patient transfer, removes all linen, trash, and equipment; collects placenta and EFM tracings and places in appropriate location.					
Notifies unit secretary of additional procedures and use of supplies.					
Demonstrates knowledge of emergency procedures, maintains control and efficiency in routine and/or difficult situations.					

APPENDIX 9-1.

Patient Care Associate Training Course

A. PURPOSE

The purpose of the Patient Care Associate Training course is to educate and train the inexperienced person to the role of PCA at St. John's Mercy Medical Center. Course content will include fundamental patient care skills, phlebotomy, respiratory, EKG and rehabilitation skills outlined in the task list. No unit specific tasks will be included in this course.

B. GOAL

The goal of PCA Training course is to facilitate the employee's integration into the appropriate Care Center and healthcare team. The course is designed to prepare the candidate in all the required skills outlined on the task list. The program will be 8 weeks in length, with scheduled didactic and clinical sessions. Skills labs will be set-up to check competency of candidates periodically throughout the course. The overall goal is to produce a competent, well-prepared candidate who will be ready to function in his or her clinical area.

C. COURSE STRUCTURE

1. **Patient Care Associate -- Week 1**
   A. **Objectives:** At the completion of week 1, the PCA candidate will be able to:
   > Describe the expectations and duties of the PCA at SJMMC.
   > Discuss medical terminology in broad terms, identify word parts and resources available to the employee.
   > Identify policies and procedures related to the functions of a PCA.
   > Discuss basic human anatomy of the circulatory, musculoskeletal, respiratory, gastrointestinal and genitourinary systems.
   > Demonstrate techniques for bedmaking, vital signs, body mechanics and documentation.
   > Describe patient rights, techniques for personal care of the patient and guest relations.
   > Discuss proper skin care techniques, nutritional needs, accurate intake/output measurement and urine/bowel elimination.
   > Identify the responsibilities of the PCA in admitting, transferring and discharging patients.

APPENDIX 9-1. Cont.

> Demonstrate the proper techniques for ordering/updating information in the computer.

2. **Practicum Experience -- Weeks 2 & 3**
   A. **Purpose**
   To assist the novice PCA with application of basic patient care skills for an 80-hour clinical experience under the direction of a qualified RN designated by the Department of Organizational Development.

   B. **Objectives:** At the completion of the practicum experience, the PCA candidate will be able to:
   > Comfortably and safely care for up to four patients.
   > Define the scope of responsibility for the PCA.
   > Describe his or her own performance strengths and areas for improvement.

   C. **Time Frame for Completion**
   The practicum experience will be Monday - Friday, day shift, the 2 weeks immediately following the didactic session.

3. **Patient Care Associate -- Week 4**
   A. **Objectives:** At the completion of week 4, the PCA candidate will be able to:
   > Discuss the differences between medical and surgical asepsis.
   > Review the anatomy of the GI tract and demonstrate the techniques needed to administer enteral feedings.
   > Demonstrate the techniques of tracheostomy care.
   > Review the anatomy of the bowel and identify different types and care of the ostomy patient.
   > Describe the different types of dressing changes and when they are used.
   > Review the anatomy of the GU tract and demonstrate the technique for insertion of an indwelling catheter.
   > Identify the importance of documenting and practice writing a FOCUS note.

   B. **Practicum Experience**
   1. **Purpose**
   To assist the novice PCA with application of technical patient care skills. These clinical experiences are scheduled to follow the didactic sessions on Tuesday, Wednesday and Thursday. A qualified RN or keytrainer designated by the Department of Organizational Development will oversee these clinicals.

APPENDIX 9-1. Cont.

2. **Objectives**
At the completion of the practicum experience, the PCA will be able to:
   > Comfortably and safely perform the identified procedures.
   > Complete a skills lab experience to assist with competency validation.
   > Describe his or her own performance strengths and areas for improvement.

4. **Phlebotomy Skills -- Week 5**
   A. **Objectives:** At the completion of week 5, the participant will be able to:
   > Identify proper procedures for labeling and collecting blood bank specimens.
   > Demonstrate the One Touch procedure for blood glucose testing.
   > Demonstrate venipuncture techniques for collecting specimens.
   > Discuss possible complications of the venipuncture procedure.

   B. **Practicum Experience**
   1. **Purpose**
   To assist the novice PCA with developing competence in designated phlebotomy procedures. These clinical experiences are scheduled Tuesday, Wednesday and Thursday during a.m. pickup under the supervision of a proficient phlebotomist. A.m. pickup will be held in the areas that currently have a PCA enrolled in the course. Each area will be notified to communicate to staff when pickups will be held by DOD. In the event a previously designated area will not be used as planned, the lab will notify them so a.m. draws can be performed by that area.

   2. **Objectives**
   At the completion of the practicum experience, the PCA candidate will be able to:
   > Comfortably and safely perform the phlebotomy procedures defined.
   > Complete a minimum number of procedures on the skills checklist.
   > Describe his or her own performance strengths and areas for improvement.

APPENDIX 9-1. Cont.

3. **Written Posttest**
A written posttest will be administered at the completion of each lecture session. These tests will be scored and returned to the candidate for review. The tests serve as a review tool for the comprehensive final to be given the final day of the course.

5. **Respiratory Skills -- Week 6**
   A. **Objectives:** At the completion of week 6, the PCA candidate will be able to:
   > Identify a nasal cannula, venti mask, simple mask, partial rebreather mask and a nonrebreather mask.
   > Insert a flowmeter into a wall outlet and adjust the oxygen flow as ordered.
   > Demonstrate how to open and regulate a portable oxygen tank.
   > Calibrate the pulse oximeter.
   > Demonstrate placement of the pulse oximeter on a patient.
   > Accurately read the pulse oximeter and report observations.
   > Demonstrate how to adjust the goal marker to the predicted volume on the incentive spirometer.
   > List the instructions patients are to be given when using the incentive spirometer.
   > Demonstrate the correct procedure for nasotracheal suctioning.
   > Demonstrate the correct procedure for tracheal suctioning.
   > Identify the need for a nasal trumpet.
   > List possible complications associated with the suctioning procedure.

   B. **Practicum Experience**
   1. **Purpose**
   To assist the novice PCA with application of respiratory skills. These clinical experiences are scheduled on Wednesday and Thursday under the direction of a respiratory therapist.

   2. **Objectives**
   At the completion of the practicum experience, the PCA candidate will be able to:
   > Comfortably and safely perform the respiratory procedures defined.
   > Complete a minimum number of procedures on the skills checklist.

APPENDIX 9-1. Cont.

> Describe his or her own performance strengths and areas for improvement.

3. **Written Posttest**

   A written posttest will be administered at the completion of each lecture session. These tests will be scored and returned to the candidate for review. The tests serve as a review tool for the comprehensive final to be given the final day of the course.

6. **EKG/Rehabilitation Skills -- Week 7**
   A. **Objectives:** At the completion of week 7, the PCA candidate will be able to:
   > Demonstrate how to use and restock the EKG machine.
   > Demonstrate the procedure for 12-Lead EKG on an adult patient.
   > Identify when to repeat the procedure.
   > Describe what to report to the healthcare team.
   > Demonstrate proper body mechanics when transferring patients.
   > Demonstrate proper technique in positioning patients in bed.
   > Demonstrate passive and active range of motion.
   > Demonstrate proper technique when ambulating patients.

   B. **Practicum Experience**
   1. **Purpose**

      To assist the novice PCA with application of the EKG procedure and rehabilitation skills. The candidate will spend time with a designated keytrainer performing the EKG procedure either on the unit or in the cardiopulmonary department on Thursday. The rehabilitation practicum will occur during the day on Wednesday in the department under the supervision of a physical or occupational therapist.

   2. **Objectives**

      At the completion of the practicum experience, the PCA candidate will be able to:
      > Comfortably and safely perform the EKG procedure.
      > Comfortably and safely perform identified rehabilitation skills.
      > Complete a minimum number of procedures on the skills checklist.
      > Describe his or her own performance strengths and areas for improvement.

APPENDIX 9-1. Cont.

    3. Written Posttest
A written posttest will be administered at the completion of each lecture session. These tests will be scored and returned to the candidate for review. The tests serve as a review tool for the comprehensive final to be given the final day of the course.

    C. Team Training and MedStar Practice
On Friday, the format for class will be instruction on team training and communication skills in the morning, with a supervised practice for MedStar in the afternoon. PCA candidates will be asked to complete practice scenarios similar to those in their clinical area.

7. Final Clinical Wrap-Up -- Week 8
    A. Objectives: At the completion of week 8, the PCA candidate will be able to:
- Demonstrate competence in all technical skills.
- Complete written posttesting successfully.
- Organize patient work flow and complete tasks with minimal supervision from the clinical instructor.

    B. Practicum Experience
    1. Purpose
To assist the PCA candidate with integration of skills for a 32-hour clinical experience under the direction of a qualified RN designated by the Department of Organizational Development.

    2. Objectives
- Integrate patient care skills into flow of care.
- Chart observations and tasks accurately.
- Complete minimum number of procedures for assigned skills if not previously documented.
- Function with minimal supervision from the clinical instructor as part of the healthcare team.

    C. Course Testing and Wrap-Up
On Friday, the day will be spent performing the following:
- Completion of comprehensive written test
- Completion of a course evaluation
- Individual feedback on performance from the clinical instructor
- Return of test scores and skills checklist to clinical instructor for forwarding to nurse manager

APPENDIX 9-1.   Cont.

> Identification of areas for development and written action plan completed
> Graduation!!

D.   DOCUMENTATION

Documentation and feedback mechanisms for the PCA candidate will include the following.

1. **Written Posttests** - Written tests developed by the clinical experts for given modules will be administered throughout the first 7 weeks. There will be a comprehensive final written exam the last day of the course. This test will be graded by the DOD instructor coordinating the course, or a designee, and returned to the PCA for their review. A score of **80%** will be considered as passing. In the event the candidate does not score an 80%, the instructor will review the content with the candidate, who will then retest. If the candidate is unsuccessful after two attempts, the manager will be notified for further direction.

2. **Competency Skills Checklist** - A comprehensive skills checklist will be given to the PCA candidate the first week of the course. It is the responsibility of the clinical instructor to evaluate the tasks performed and provide feedback to the participant on his or her level of performance throughout the entire course. At the completion of the week 7, the checklist will be collected by the clinical instructor. Any deficient areas must be addressed and completed during the final week of the program. When the checklist is completed, it will be forwarded to the nurse manager with additional documentation by the Department of Organizational Development. *Unit specific skills checklists should be attached as an addendum to the standard checklist.*

3. **Clinical Performance Evaluation-** The clinical instructor will complete a clinical performance evaluation on each PCA candidate during his or her practicum experience. The evaluation will be reviewed and signed by the candidate and the instructor at the completion of the clinical experience.

4. **Management Feedback** - The DOD coordinator or designee will follow-up with the nurse manager when there are performance or safety concerns with individual candidates. The instructor will **not** routinely follow-up with the nurse manager if the candidate is functioning at the expected level of competence identified by the clinical instructor.

APPENDIX 9-1. Cont.

At the conclusion of the course, the nurse manager can expect to receive documentation of candidate's transcript of course attendance, comprehensive test score, skills checklist and clinical performance evaluation from the DOD coordinator. This paperwork should be kept in the employee's file.

E. **COURSE GUIDELINES/RESPONSIBILITIES**
   1. **Nurse Managers**
      > Managers will enroll PCA candidates through the Department of Organizational Development.
      > Managers will **not** utilize the PCA candidate on the floor during the 8-week orientation period.
      > Managers will ensure the skills taught during the PCA course will be utilized in the clinical setting.
      > Managers will ensure the mentor for the new PCA is competent in his or her clinical skills and utilize appropriate communication techniques for giving feedback.
      > Managers will provide feedback to the DOD course coordinator as needed to ensure the course is meeting the needs of the manager, staff and PCA candidate.

   2. **PCA Candidate**
      > The candidate will arrive to all didactic and clinical sessions on time and prepared.
      > The candidate will attend all sessions and will be responsible for notifying the appropriate instructor if unable to participate.
      > The candidate will be responsible for asking questions and participating in all didactic and clinical activities.
      > The candidate will be receptive to feedback regarding performance.
      > The candidate will acknowledge when assistance is needed and seek assistance as necessary.
      > The candidate will operate under all Medical Center policies when in the clinical areas.
      > The candidate will seek out opportunities to perform skills in the clinical areas.
      > The candidate will successfully complete all written testing by the end of the course.
      > The candidate will successfully complete all mandatory requirements by the end of the course.

   3. **Clinical Instructors**
      > The clinical instructors will communicate performance expectations to the candidate and provide feedback on a routine basis.

APPENDIX 9-1. Cont.

> The clinical instructors will educate the candidates according to Medical Center policies, accepted clinical standards of care and current research, when it impacts clinical practice.
> The clinical instructors will document performance of each candidate on a standardized form.
> The clinical instructors will provide feedback to the DOD coordinator on a routine basis, or if performance issues are identified.
> The clinical instructors will guide the development of the candidate during the clinical experiences and document progress on the skills checklist.

4. **Department of Organizational Development**
   > The Department of Organizational Development will provide coordination for each 8-week course.
   > The Department of Organizational Development will track attendance of PCA candidates through the Registrar system.
   > The Department of Organizational Development will continually evaluate the course and modify as needed.
   > The Department of Organizational Development will store the course curriculums and have available for review.
   > The Department of Organizational Development will ensure the clinical competence and expertise of any clinical instructor assisting with the didactic or clinical aspects of this course.
   > The Department of Organizational Development will keep the skills checklist current and revise as needed.
   > The Department of Organizational Development will communicate dates/times and locations of upcoming courses.
   > The Department of Organizational Development will reserve the right to cancel any course where there are insufficient numbers enrolled.

5. **General Guidelines**
   > A PCA candidate with little or no patient care experience should be enrolled in the entire 8-week course.
   > In the event a nursing student is hired, it will be at the manager's discretion as to which modules they will attend.
   > If a candidate has CNA or other patient care experience when hired, it will be at the manager's discretion as to which modules they will attend.
   > A PCA deficient in phlebotomy, respiratory, EKG or rehabilitation skills can be enrolled for those specific modules by notifying the DOD.
   > The Skills Lab days will be used to validate competency of skills according to the standard of care indicated for that skill.

APPENDIX 9-1. Cont.

> The Skills Lab days can be used to validate the competency of a PCA candidate who is not attending the entire 8 weeks. For example, the nursing student or CNA who needs verification of fundamental patient care skills.
> The skills checklist developed by the DOD will be the standard checklist for any areas utilizing PCA's. **Any unit specific PCA tasks will need to be attached and filed with the standard checklist upon completion of the skill.**
> In the event performance problems persist, the nurse manager is ultimately responsible for any disciplinary action that may occur.
> The PCA candidate will need designated time with a mentor in his or her area of practice to become oriented to the patient types, routines and staff. However, his or her unit-based orientation should be significantly decreased from previously.
> The PCA candidate will need minimal supervision during this orientation period, unless otherwise communicated to the manager.

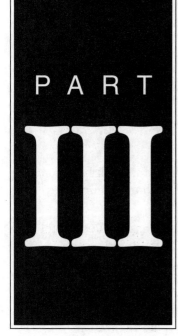

PART III

Appendices

CHAPTER 1

MULTIPLE CHOICE

1. The United States consistently ranks unfavorably with other developed countries in perinatal care outcomes because
   A. health care dollars are not evenly distributed across populations
   B. pregnant women in the U.S. have greater stress than in other countries
   C. there are greater harmful environmental hazards for women

2. One major concern of health care providers and consumers regarding policy changes from proposed federal legislation is that
   A. care will be less accessible
   B. educational requirements will change for health care workers
   C. it will lead to decreased quality and quantity of care

3. Patient's expectations of the quality of care they receive most often focuses on the
   A. caring and empathetic attitude of the nurses
   B. technical aspects of their care
   C. type and timeliness of their care

4. Reduced length of stay for postpartum families has necessitated many changes for nurse managers including
   A. decreasing the number of registered nurses
   B. redefining quality outcomes based on current length of stay
   C. reorganizing unit structure

5. With current managed-care reimbursement practices
   A. billing for services provided does not effect reimbursement
   B. the charge for specific services should reflect the actual cost of service
   C. reimbursement is based on the number of patients and their length of stay

6. If a woman has had consistent prenatal care for which you have complete prenatal records, it is likely that she will need
   A. no additional blood testing
   B. only a complete blood count and blood typing
   C. only a urinalysis

7. Review of current literature will help health care providers eliminate unnecessary products such as
   A. breast creams for breastfeeding mothers
   B. analgesics for episiotomy discomfort
   C. petroleum jelly for circumcisions

8. A clinical indicator is a/an
   A. episodic monitor used to evaluate individual nurses' quality of care
   B. quantitative measure of an aspect of care that can be used to monitor quality
   C. subjective means of collecting data for accreditation review

9. Care paths designed from professional standards of care and practice guidelines are useful in
   A. counseling nurses during annual evaluation
   B. obtaining accreditation from JCAHO
   C. tracking, measuring, and evaluating patient outcomes

10. Variance tracking can provide an important data base for continuous quality improvement by
    A. assessing errors by individuals at a given point of time
    B. defining the standard of care for the institution
    C. identifying where changes in practice can improve patient outcomes

FILL IN THE BLANK

11. The traditional fee-for-service did not provide incentive to practice cost-effectively because _____.

12. Overall patient satisfaction with hospitalization is often determined by the patient's perception of the quality of _____ they received.

13. The scope of care traditionally offered in the hospital to childbearing families has

become increasingly more difficult to provide due to _____.

14. It is important that health care providers evaluate practices and services to determine if they are based on _____.

15. Hospitals can begin using reusable rather than disposable items such as gowns, shoe covers, wash cloths, etc. as long as care is taken to protect individuals from _____.

16. Work redesign projects and decreased length of stay have forced health care providers to design practice models more efficient than the _____.

17. Perinatal centers should consider eliminating frills that do not have a direct impact on _____.

18. One of the earliest proponents of outcomes evaluation, _____, used morbidity and mortality statistics to identify substandard care.

CHAPTER 2

MULTIPLE CHOICE

1. Which organization ensures nurses practicing in all areas of the United States have met the same educational criteria before entering into clinical practice?
   A. American Nurses Association (ANA)
   B. Joint Commission on Accreditation of Healthcare Organizations (JCAHO)
   C. National Council of State Boards Licensing Exam (NCLEX)

2. The legal basis for which of the following is the government's power to protect the public's health, safety and welfare?
   A. certification
   B. licensure
   C. malpractice

3. Which of the following indicates to the public and healthcare community that an individual has demonstrated qualification and special knowledge in a defined clinical area of nursing?
   A. certification
   B. credentialing
   C. licensure

4. In a case of professional negligence, the most difficult entity for the claimant to prove is
   A. breach of duty
   B. causation
   C. damages

5. Professional nursing liability is most commonly increased by the absence of
   A. documentation
   B. unit policies and procedures
   C. validation of core competencies

6. Incident management
   A. includes "near misses" with potential for adverse outcome
   B. increases hospital and nursing liability
   C. involves prospective evaluation of patient concerns

7. JCAHO validation of core competencies in nursing practice requires
   A. a general hospital-wide skills checklist evaluation
   B. assessment at completion of unit orientation and every 2 years thereafter
   C. both skills verification and knowledge-based evaluations

8. Nurse/physician conflict about a patient's management should
   A. be presented to the patient's family
   B. not occur in a professional setting
   C. utilize effective communication techniques

9. After repeated requests for assistance, a physician fails to respond to deteriorating maternal condition. The nurse should
   A. again request the physician to evaluate the patient
   B. call in another obstetrician for consult
   C. institute the unit's chain of command

APPENDIX A • AWHONN'S PERINATAL NURSING ITEM BANK WITH ANSWER KEY

FILL IN THE BLANK

10. Perinatal nursing is unique among nursing specialties because nurses caring for pregnant women always have a minimum nurse patient ratio of _____ .

11. In the United States nursing licensing is governed by _____ enacted by the state legislatures.

12. The _____ process validates an individual registered nurses qualifications and special knowledge in a defined clinical area of nursing.

13. The perinatal nurse is responsible for decisions and actions within the domain of _____ practice.

14. To be found guilty of professional negligence, facts that first must be established are
    1. _____
    2. _____
    3. _____
    4. _____

15. When a nurse deviates from the standard of care and an injury occurs to the patient that was caused by the nurse's negligence, it is referred to as _____.

16. A retrospective process that involves examination of all of the events surrounding an adverse outcome is _____.

17. Subscribing to professional journals, use of computer-assisted instructional programs (CAI's), completing self-study programs and attending perinatal nursing conferences are all examples of _____ _____.

18. Whenever a nurse is uncertain about how to proceed in a situation of conflict she should initiate the _____.

19. A nurse who purchases her own liability insurance in addition to employer-provided coverage may find herself at _____ risk to become involved as an individual in a malpractice action.

CHAPTER 4

MULTIPLE CHOICE

1. By 32 weeks of gestation in a normal pregnancy, blood volume increases by approximately
   A. 1000 ml.
   B. 1300 ml.
   C. 1600 ml.

2. The maternal position for optimum cardiac output is
   A. right lateral
   B. sitting
   C. supine

3. During labor, cardiac output
   A. decreases dramatically
   B. increases progressively
   C. remains the same

4. An intravenous fluid bolus is given prior to epidural anesthesia to
   A. increase blood pressure
   B. increase cardiac output
   C. insure adequate hydration

5. Normally during pregnancy, the blood pressure
   A. decreases
   B. increased progressively
   C. remains at prepregnancy values

6. The volume of the maternal autotransfusion immediately after birth is
   A. 600 ml.
   B. 800 ml.
   C. 1000 ml.

7. The normal range for PaO_2 levels in late pregnancy is
   A. 94-98 mm Hg.
   B. 99-103 mm Hg.
   C. 104-108 mm Hg.

8. The slight increase in pH that occurs during pregnancy is due to
   A. decrease in hemoglobin and hematocrit
   B. increase in renal excretion of bicarbonate
   C. large increase in respiratory rate

9. During pregnancy serum urea and creatine levels
   A. decrease
   B. increase
   C. remain constant

10. Heartburn is common during pregnancy due to
    A. decreased gastric motility
    B. increased secretion of hydrochloric acid
    C. relaxation of the esophageal sphincter

11. The following physical finding may occur during pregnancy in response to normal cardiovascular changes.
    A. dependent edema
    B. elevated blood pressure
    C. decreased heart rate

12. Average blood loss at vaginal birth ranges from
    A. 200-300 ml.
    B. 500-600 ml.
    C. 800-900 ml.

13. Average blood loss at cesarean birth ranges from
    A. 1300-1500 ml.
    B. 800-1200 ml.
    C. 400-700 ml.

14. During pregnancy cardiac output increases
    A. 10-20%
    B. 30-50%
    C. 60-80%

15. Cardiac output is greatest during which period of the birth process?
    A. active phase
    B. second stage
    C. immediately after birth

16. Which cardiovascular parameter decreases during pregnancy?
    A. systemic vascular resistance
    B. stroke volume
    C. heart rate

17. An average white cell count during labor and early postpartum is
    A. 5,000–10,000/mm^3
    B. 13,000–20,000/mm^3
    C. 25,000/mm^3 or greater

18. Which of the following coagulation factors do not increase during pregnancy?
    A. fibrin
    B. platelets
    C. plasma fibrinogen

19. Which of the following decreases during pregnancy?
    A. glomerular filtration rate
    B. renal blood flow
    C. colloid oncotic pressure

20. By term, blood flow to the uterus is approximately
    A. 200 ml./min.
    B. 500 ml./min.
    C. 800 ml./min.

21. The line in the skin that divides the abdomen longitudinally from the sternum to the symphysis is known as
    A. linea nigra
    B. striae gravidarum
    C. spider nevi

22. Which of the following changes occur in the respiratory system during pregnancy?
    A. tidal volume decreases 30-40%
    B. oxygen consumption increases 15-20%
    C. respiratory rate decreases

23. Which of the following can be a normal finding during pregnancy?
    A. glycosuria
    B. proteinuria
    C. hematuria

24. Which respiratory system parameter decreases during pregnancy?
    A. tidal volume
    B. minute ventilation
    C. functional residual capacity

25. Identify the clotting factor that decreases during pregnancy.
    A. fibrin
    B. plasma fibrinogen
    C. coagulation factors XI, XIII

FILL IN THE BLANK

26. The increase in cardiac output and decrease in heart rate following delivery is due to _____.

27. The greater increase in plasma volume than in red cell volume results in a state called _____.

28. The hypercoagulability state of pregnancy is due to the _____.

29. During pregnancy, oxygen consumption _____.

30. The primary determinant of volume hemostasis is _____.

31. The renal clearance of many substances is increased during pregnancy due to the _____.

32. Normal stretching of the skin and hormonal changes during gestation may produce "stretch marks" that are called _____.

33. The hormone, released from the anterior pituitary, that is responsible for initiating lactation is _____.

34. The hormone crucial in maintaining pregnancy is _____.

35. Management of the pregnant woman with diabetes requires blood glucose values rather than urine glucose values because _____.

36. The _____ system undergoes the most profound changes during pregnancy.

37. After childbirth, the contracted uterus shunts blood from the uterine vessels into the systemic circulation causing an _____ of approximately 1000 ml.

38. Increases in plasma volume and red cell mass result in an increase in _____ during pregnancy.

39. Cardiac output progressively decreases and returns to nonpregnant levels by _____.

40. The _____ accommodates one-third of the additional blood volume at term.

41. _____ produces relaxation of smooth muscle and vasodilation.

42. Blood pressure reaches its lowest point in the _____ trimester.

43. During pregnancy, the woman becomes resistant to the pressor effects of _____.

44. Pregnancy is considered a _____ state due to the increases of several essential coagulation factors.

45. The pregnant woman is at increased risk for venous _____ due to coagulation changes and venous stasis.

46. _____ are lipid substances that affect smooth muscle contractility, play an important role in the mechanism of labor, and are potent vasodilators.

47. Irregularly shaped brown blotches on the face are known as _____, or the "mask of pregnancy."

48. The bluish discoloration of the cervix is known as _____.

CHAPTER 5

MULTIPLE CHOICE

1. The developmental task of the first trimester is
   A. identification of the maternal role
   B. movement from conflict and ambivalence to acceptance
   C. resolution of the approach-avoidance conflict related to childbirth and loss of control

2. A necessary element for the development of a therapeutic relationship with a perinatal client is
   A. kind and sympathetic judgments to guide the woman toward an appropriate maternal role
   B. sharing of relevant personal information that demonstrates the empathy of the perinatal nurse
   C. the establishment of healthy, clear boundaries between the woman and the nurse

3. The changes and transitions affecting the mind, body and soul during pregnancy are best defined using a
   A. holistic model
   B. physiological model
   C. psychosocial model

4. A major issue during the third trimester is/are
   A. physical changes of pregnancy
   B. infant's well-being
   C. ambivalence about the maternal role

5. Symptoms of postpartum depression include
   A. agitation and anger
   B. anxiety and irritability
   C. hallucinations and delusions

6. When the length of postpartum hospitalization is short, discharge planning should include
   A. a brief psychiatric assessment to rule out postpartum psychosis
   B. directing the new mother to look up the telephone numbers of health care providers
   C. identifying with the new mother and her partner key support people

7. Reva Rubin suggests that during the postpartum period it is helpful for the new mother to
   A. accept constructive criticism from the nurse so that she can learn to correctly care for her infant
   B. be encouraged to focus on the infant's needs exclusively so that she can provide care following discharge
   C. put meaning into the childbirth experience by verbalizing her reality

8. The estimate of new mothers experiencing "baby blues" is
   A. 20-30%
   B. 40-50%
   C. 70-80%

9. Discharge teaching for the new mother and family includes information that labile moods should stabilize and organization and confidence increase by
   A. 3 weeks
   B. 8 weeks
   C. 12 weeks

FILL IN THE BLANK

10. Ten elements of a comprehensive psychosocial assessment include
    1. _____
    2. _____
    3. _____
    4. _____
    5. _____
    6. _____
    7. _____
    8. _____
    9. _____
    10. _____

11. Participants included in the psychosocial assessment are _____ , _____ , and _____.

12. The data obtained during a psychosocial assessment is used to develop _____ and _____ .

13. There is a strong correlation between mood and anxiety disorders prior to pregnancy and _____ .

14. A critical aspect of holistic-care planning for the perinatal client involves coordination of _____ .

15. During the second trimester, women are increasingly vulnerable to _____ .

16. When conducting a psychosocial assessment it is important to determine the _____, _____, and _____ of mood or emotional disturbances.

17. Most women do not seek help with depressive disorders following delivery because _____.

18. Maternal role attainment is a process that takes _____ to develop.

19. The mother is better able to meet the needs of her infant when _____.

CHAPTER 6

MULTIPLE CHOICE

1. Over the past 40 years, the incidence of preterm birth has
   A. declined significantly
   B. remained the same
   C. increased slightly

2. Recommended weight gain for an underweight pregnant woman is
   A. 15-25 lbs.
   B. 24-35 lbs.
   C. 28-40 lbs.

3. If both parents are positive for sickle cell trait, the risk of sickle cell disease in each infant is
   A. 25%
   B. 50%
   C. 100%

4. In a normotensive pregnant woman, blood pressure is lowest in the
   A. first trimester
   B. second trimester
   C. third trimester

5. Measurement of maternal fundal height in centimeters (±2) should correlate with gestational age
   A. after 20 weeks gestation
   B. between 22 and 34 weeks gestation
   C. between 35 and 40 weeks gestation

6. During pregnancy, the blood pressure recorded with an automatic blood pressure device
   A. alters mean arterial blood pressure
   B. underestimates diastolic blood pressure
   C. underestimates systolic blood pressure

7. The biochemical evaluation of every woman should include
   A. glucose challenge test
   B. group B streptococcus culture
   C. tuberculin screen (PPD)

8. A nonreactive non-stress test
   A. is reassuring
   B. indicates the need for further testing
   C. is ominous

9. Health promotion and education to improve pregnancy outcome in the next generation should begin
   A. when children are in school
   B. when teens become sexually active
   C. in the first trimester of pregnancy

10. The appropriate time for a glucose screening test is between
    A. 20 and 24 weeks gestation
    B. 24 and 28 weeks gestation
    C. 28 and 32 weeks gestation

11. Risk assessment for all women during the initial prenatal visit should include
    A. Tay Sachs screening
    B. family, individual, and reproductive health history
    C. ultrasound for fetal anomalies

12. The recommended weight gain during pregnancy is
    A. 28-40 lbs.
    B. 25-35 lbs.
    C. 15-25 lbs.

13. A significant effect of cigarette smoking during pregnancy is
    A. increased incidence of pregnancy-induced hypertension
    B. increased incidence of maternal lung cancer
    C. increased incidence of low birth weight and prematurity

14. Maternal serum alpha-fetoprotein screens for
    A. heart defects
    B. multiple gestation
    C. neural tube defects

15. If two parents are affected by sickle cell disease
    A. 25% of children will have sickle cell disease
    B. 50% of children will have sickle cell disease
    C. 100% of children will have sickle cell disease

16. A primary method of fetal surveillance for all pregnancies is
    A. ultrasonography
    B. non-stress tests
    C. kick counts

17. The most significant food shortages for low income women occur
    A. before their WIC eligibility is determined
    B. at the end of the month when federal/local resources diminish
    C. because they do not have adequate education regarding economical food preparation

18. A key component of preterm birth prevention education is
    A. permission to call the health care provider
    B. identification of the hospital admission procedure
    C. instruction of the significant other

FILL IN THE BLANK

19. The monitoring of fetal activity by "kick counts" is initiated at _____ weeks gestation.

20. It is recommended that every woman have an initial serology and GC culture, and that the tests be repeated at ___ weeks.

21. The recommended weight gain for an obese woman during pregnancy is _____.

22. Approximately ___% of human malformations are caused by genetic factors alone.

23. Agents that cause congenital malformations are called _____.

24. A biophysical profile summative score of _____ or greater is considered a sign of fetal wellbeing.

25. In the fetus, male and female genitalia are recognizable by _____ weeks.

26. Tay-Sachs disease is a recessive disorder common in families of _____ ancestry.

27. The anticoagulant _____ is a known teratogen.

28. A _____ contraction stress test is reassuring.

29. Amniocentesis for genetic evaluation is usually done between ___ and ___ weeks gestation.

30. The three basic components of prenatal care are
    1. _____
    2. _____
    3. _____

31. Moderate physical activity during an uncomplicated pregnancy maintains _____ and _____ fitness.

32. Diagnosis of gestational diabetes mellitus is made when there are _____.

33. Maternal serum alpha-fetoprotein is offered between ___ and ___ weeks gestation.

34. A healthy fetus usually has ___ perceivable movements in one hour.

35. The five parameters assessed in the Biophysical Profile are:
    1. _____
    2. _____
    3. _____
    4. _____
    5. _____

CHAPTER 7

MULTIPLE CHOICE

1. Proteinuria in severe preeclampsia is defined as the excretion of how many grams/liter in a 24-hour period?
   A. 1.0 g/L
   B. 3.0 g/L
   C. 5.0 g/L

2. An early indication of impending magnesium sulfate toxicity in the patient with preeclampsia is the absence of
   A. deep tendon reflexes
   B. fetal movement
   C. urine output

3. The therapeutic range of serum magnesium during magnesium sulfate therapy to prevent eclamptic seizures is
   A. 1–4 mg/dl
   B. 5–8 mg/dl
   C. 8–11 mg/dl

4. The immediate care of the patient during an eclamptic seizure is to
   A. administer an anticonvulsant agent
   B. ensure a patent airway
   C. establish IV access

5. Invasion of the trophoblastic cells into the uterine myometrium is termed placenta
   A. accreta
   B. increta
   C. percreta

6. The majority of cases of failure of prostaglandin f2 alpha to control hemorrhage occurs in women with
   A. chorioamnionitis
   B. multiple gestation
   C. previous cesarean section

7. The incidence and severity of neonatal complications decrease to almost zero after how many weeks of completed gestation?
   A. 30
   B. 32
   C. 34

8. What fetal heart rate pattern is associated with fetal movement beginning in the second trimester?
   A. accelerations
   B. decelerations
   C. tachycardia

9. The only agent currently approved by the FDA for use as a tocolytic in the United States is
   A. magnesium sulfate
   B. terbutaline
   C. ritodrine

10. Preterm premature rupture of the membranes with documented premature labor is most commonly followed by birth within
    A. 24-36 hours
    B. 48-72 hours
    C. 72 hours-1 week

11. Preeclampsia is the presence of hypertension and
    A. edema
    B. headaches
    C. proteinuria

12. Severe preeclampsia is defined by a
    A. diastolic blood pressure of at least 110 mm Hg
    B. excretion of 4500 gms protein in a 24-hour urine collection
    C. serum BUN of 10 with a serum creatinine of 1.0

13. A woman at 28 weeks of gestation reports painless, bright red vaginal bleeding. The most likely diagnosis is
    A. abruptio placentae
    B. placenta previa
    C. uterine rupture

14. A clinical finding seen with a dehiscence of a prior low segment cesarean scar during labor is
    A. cessation of uterine contractions
    B. fetal heart rate changes
    C. lowering of intrauterine pressures

APPENDIX A • AWHONN'S PERINATAL NURSING ITEM BANK WITH ANSWER KEY

15. The initial drug of choice for a postpartum hemorrhage is
    A. methergine injection
    B. oxytocin infusion
    C. prostaglandin 15-MF$_{2a}$ injection

16. The risk factor most predictive of a preterm birth is
    A. prior preterm birth
    B. prior preterm labor
    C. uterine irritability

17. Betamimetic tocolytic agents work by
    A. blocking oxytocin release
    B. interfering with calcium uptake
    C. relaxing smooth muscle

18. A fundamental principle for a successful maternal-fetal transport is
    A. accomplishing the transport as quickly as possible
    B. assessing maternal and fetal stability
    C. having a physician present for the transport

FILL IN THE BLANK

19. _____ disorders of pregnancy are the most common medical complication of pregnancy.

20. A diastolic blood pressure of _____ mm Hg on two occasions of at least 6 hours apart is necessary for the diagnosis of severe preeclampsia.

21. The blood pressure should be recorded with the woman in a _____ position.

22. _____ is the drug of choice to prevent seizure activity in the patient with preeclampsia.

23. Vasa previa is the result of a _____ insertion of the cord.

24. For the fetus to maintain adequate oxygenation, the maternal oxygen saturation must be at least _____ %.

25. Systolic blood pressures of less than _____ mm Hg are associated with acute renal failure.

26. Betamimetic agents are contraindicated in the patient with known _____ disease.

27. _____ impairs fetal renal function which may result in oligohydramnios.

28. Antenatal _____ administration has been associated with approximately a 50% reduction in neonatal respiratory distress syndrome.

29. Maternal morbidity from hypertension in pregnancy includes
    1. _____
    2. _____
    3. _____
    4. _____

30. The goals of antihypertensive therapy in the woman with preeclampsia are _____ _____ and to _____ _____ .

31. Laboratory markers for HELLP Syndrome are _____ , _____ _____ , and _____ _____ .

32. A leading cause of maternal morbidity following an eclamptic seizure is _____ .

33. _____ is a late sign of hypovolemia in the woman experiencing bleeding during pregnancy.

34. Obstetrical factors predisposing a woman to disseminated intravascular coagulation are
    1. _____
    2. _____
    3. _____
    4. _____
    5. _____
    6. _____
    7. _____

35. Nonuterine symptoms of preterm labor include
    1. _____
    2. _____
    3. _____
    4. _____
    5. _____

36. Maternal physical side effects of prolonged bedrest include
    1. _____
    2. _____
    3. _____
    4. _____
    5. _____

37. Current treatment modalities to decrease the incidence of respiratory distress syndrome in the preterm neonate are
    1. _____
    2. _____
    3. _____

CHAPTER 8

MULTIPLE CHOICE

1. Second stage labor begins with
   A. complete dilation of the cervix
   B. fetal head at +1 station
   C. urge to push

2. The urge to push alerts the nurse to
   A. complete cervical dilation
   B. imminent birth
   C. +1 or greater station

3. An absolute contraindication to induction is
   A. grand multiparity
   B. multiple gestation
   C. non-reassuring fetal status

4. The most common adverse effect of oxytocin administration is
   A. fetal distress
   B. rapid labor
   C. uterine hyperstimulation

5. Amnioinfusion was first used for
   A. diluting thickly stained amniotic fluid
   B. treatment of oligohydramnios
   C. treating variable and prolonged decelerations of the fetal heart rate

6. Vaginal examination should be avoided when one of the following is present:
   A. chorioamnionitis
   B. maternal hepatitis
   C. unexplained bleeding

7. A rare but serious complication of amniotomy in women with polyhydramnios is
   A. cord prolapse
   B. placental abruption
   C. uterine rupture

8. Use of low forceps is characterized by
   A. station of at least +2 but not on pelvic floor
   B. rotation less than 45 degrees
   C. scalp visible at introitus

9. Primigravidas are more likely to have one of the following labor deviations:
   A. prolonged latent phase
   B. secondary inertia
   C. uterine hypotonus

10. The normal length of the pregravid cervix is
    A. 2.5–3 cm.
    B. 3.5–4 cm.
    C. 4–4.5 cm.

11. Prostaglandin gel for cervical ripening may be administered every
    A. 3 hours
    B. 4 hours
    C. 6 hours

12. Prostaglandin gel should be administered with caution in women with a history of
    A. asthma
    B. chorioamnionitis
    C. rapid labors

APPENDIX A • AWHONN'S PERINATAL NURSING ITEM BANK WITH ANSWER KEY

13. Maternal water intoxication from oxytocin infusion can be prevented by utilizing
    A. low dose oxytocin
    B. maintaining intravenous intake at 125 cc/hr
    C. physiologic electrolyte solutions

14. The most effective technique for relieving shoulder dystocia is
    A. firm, perpendicular fundal pressure
    B. gentle, horizontal fundal pressure
    C. suprapubic pressure applied over the symphysis, behind the pubic bone

15. Research has demonstrated that the presence of a labor support person is important because
    A. laboring women will feel less alone
    B. fewer perinatal complications occur
    C. mothers report a more positive birth experience

16. Following an amniotomy, signs and symptoms of maternal infection include
    A. uterine tenderness, fetal tachycardia, and fever
    B. uterine hypotonia, fetal bradycardia, and cloudy amniotic fluid
    C. decreasing WBC, non-periodic FHT changes, and maternal anxiety

17. An absolute contradiction for labor induction is
    A. active genital herpes
    B. grand multiparity
    C. chorioamnionitis

18. According to ACOG standards, fetal heart rate is evaluated in the low-risk woman during the first stage of labor every
    A. 10 minutes
    B. 15 minutes
    C. 30 minutes

19. During an amnioinfusion, if 250 cc of fluid infuse with no return, the nurse should
    A. continue the infusion for another 250 cc and observe for fluid return
    B. discontinue the infusion until the fluid is returned
    C. increase the rate of the infusion and observe for fluid return

20. Contraindication to vaginal birth after cesarean section is
    A. horizontal uterine scar
    B. maternal anxiety related to labor
    C. twin gestation

21. According to ACOG standards, maternal bladder status should be assessed during labor at least every
    A. hour
    B. 2 hours
    C. 3 hours

22. Surgical birth places additional strain on the maternal-newborn relationship. The following would facilitate bonding:
    A. allow the father contact with the newborn in the nursery
    B. calling the infant by name and promising to bring the mother and baby together as soon as possible
    C. early and sustained contact with the newborn

FILL IN THE BLANK

23. The occiput of the fetal head should be _____ to be engaged or zero station.

24. Physiologic second stage management differs from traditional second stage management by _____ _____.

25. The McRoberts maneuver is a technique used _____.

26. Two techniques for relieving shoulder dystocia are
    1. _____
    2. _____

27. Potential neonatal complications of shoulder dystocia are
    1. _____
    2. _____

28. Three methods for cervical ripening are
    1. _____
    2. _____
    3. _____

29. Four signs and symptoms of chorioamnionitis are
    1. _____
    2. _____
    3. _____
    4. _____

30. Uterine hyperstimulation is defined as a uterine resting tone _____ mmHg.

31. The Bishop Score evaluates these five parameters
    1. _____
    2. _____
    3. _____
    4. _____
    5. _____

32. Determination of the position of the fetal head becomes necessary when _____.

33. Vaginal examination of the cervix to assess labor progress includes assessment of
    1. _____
    2. _____
    3. _____

34. Signs of placental abruption include
    1. _____
    2. _____
    3. _____

35. Three fetal factors thought responsible for the onset of labor are
    1. _____
    2. _____
    3. _____

36. Stripping of the amniotic membranes to ripen the cervix and stimulate labor has been most successful in women with the following characteristics
    1. _____
    2. _____
    3. _____
    4. _____

37. During an amnioinfusion, the infusion should be discontinued if the uterine resting tone exceeds _____ mmHg.

38. Oligohydramnios is often reflected by variable decelerations of FHR due to _____.

39. Signs and symptoms of water intoxication due to prolonged oxytocin infusion include
    1. _____
    2. _____
    3. _____
    4. _____
    5. _____
    6. _____
    7. _____

40. During labor maternal temperature should be monitored at least every ___ hours.

41. A _____ degree perineal laceration involves skin, mucus membrane, fascia and muscles of perineum.

42. Operating rooms located on perinatal units must maintain the same standards of care as the _____.

43. _____ pushing has less impact on uteroplacental blood flow and allows for perineal relaxation.

44. In the absence of an intrauterine pressure catheter, it is necessary to _____ the uterus to assess strength of uterine contractions.

45. _____ is the primary drug used to treat malignant hyperthermia.

CHAPTER 9

MULTIPLE CHOICE

1. According to the NAACOG Practice Resource, when auscultation is used for fetal assessment during labor for a low-risk woman, the fetal heart rate should be auscultated in the first stage of labor every
   A. 5 minutes
   B. 15 minutes
   C. 30 minutes

APPENDIX A • AWHONN'S PERINATAL NURSING ITEM BANK WITH ANSWER KEY

2. For a low-risk woman in the second stage of labor, the fetal heart rate should be auscultated every
   A. 5 minutes
   B. 10 minutes
   C. 15 minutes

3. Types of changes in fetal heart rate baseline rate include
   A. a persistent rise or fall in rate
   B. accelerations
   C. periodic decelerations

4. Fetal bradycardia in the second stage of labor following a previously normal tracing may be caused by
   A. fetal hypoxemia
   B. increased fetal vagal stimulation
   C. uteroplacental insufficiency

5. A common cause of fetal tachycardia with average short-term variability is
   A. fetal hypoxemia
   B. maternal fever
   C. vagal stimulation

6. Loss of short-term variability may be due to
   A. fetal stimulation
   B. medication administration
   C. uterine activity

7. The goal in treatment for late decelerations is to
   A. correct cord compression
   B. improve maternal oxygenation
   C. maximize uteroplacental blood flow

8. The most frequently observed fetal heart rate deceleration is the
   A. early deceleration
   B. late deceleration
   C. variable deceleration

9. Amnioinfusion may be useful in correcting
   A. early decelerations
   B. late decelerations
   C. variable decelerations

10. Non-reassuring fetal heart rate patterns that may indicate progressive hypoxemia may be characterized by
    A. a rising baseline rate and absence of short-term variability
    B. late decelerations, average short-term variability and a stable baseline rate
    C. prolonged decelerations with recovery to baseline with average short-term variability

11. An example of fetal metabolic acidemia would be
    A. pH 7.20 with base deficit of 6
    B. pH 7.15 with base deficit of 3
    C. pH 7.19 with base deficit of 12

12. A fetal condition that can result in fetal bradycardia is
    A. anemia
    B. prematurity
    C. vagal stimulation

13. While caring for a laboring woman who is HIV seropositive, the external fetal heart rate tracing is difficult to interpret and possibly non-reassuring. The best nursing action would be to
    A. apply fetal scalp electrode to assess short term variability
    B. auscultate for presence of fetal heart rate accelerations
    C. call for midwife or physician to evaluate

14. Which type of fetal heart rate decelerations results from changes in fetal cerebral blood flow secondary to a vagal reflex?
    A. early
    B. late
    C. variable

15. Which type of fetal heart rate deceleration results from decreased uteroplacental blood flow?
    A. early
    B. late
    C. variable

16. Which type of fetal heart rate deceleration results from umbilical cord compression?
    A. early
    B. late
    C. variable

17. Brief accelerations of the fetal heart rate that may either precede and/or follow variable decelerations are called
    A. overshoots
    B. shoulders
    C. uniform accelerations

18. Just prior to fetal bradycardia and death, the electronic fetal monitoring tracing shows absent short-term variability and
    A. absence of late deceleration
    B. baseline tachycardia
    C. overshoots

19. Which of the following fetal heart rate patterns will likely develop with severe fetal anemia?
    A. lambda
    B. saltatory
    C. sinusoidal

20. A work-up for maternal systemic lupus erythematosus is ordered following the assessment of which fetal dysrhythmia?
    A. complete atrioventricular heart block
    B. premature ventricular contractions
    C. supraventricular tachycardia

FILL IN THE BLANK

21. Late decelerations are characterized by deceleration of the fetal heart rate that begins at the _____ of the contraction, does not return to the baseline rate until _____ the contraction ends, and occurs repetitively.

22. Variable decelerations are characterized by decelerations that have _____ timing in relation to the contractions, but always have an _____ change in rate.

23. Early decelerations are characterized by a drop in fetal heart rate that begins at the _____ of a contraction, recovers to the _____ by the end of the contraction. Early decelerations are _____ and do not require intervention.

24. Nursing intervention for late decelerations generally require _____ oxytocin if it is infusing.

25. Reassuring fetal heart rate tracings have an absence of decelerations, may show accelerations, and/or _____ short-term variability as recorded by a fetal scalp electrode.

26. Whenever a very unusual fetal heart rate pattern occurs that cannot be easily characterized, the possibility of a fetus with _____ should be considered.

27. Most fetal dysrhythmias are not life-threatening, except for _____, which may lead to fetal congestive heart failure.

28. Decreased short-term variability may be caused by multiple factors including _____, _____, and hypoxemia.

29. In the presence of variable decelerations, progressive hypoxemia may be characterized by an increasing baseline rate, loss of short-term variability and the presence of _____.

30. Late decelerations associated with acute placental changes are caused by uterine _____, placental _____ and/or maternal _____.

31. If the fetal heart rate tracing does not return to a reassuring tracing following interventions for late decelerations, administration of _____ to stop uterine activity may be indicated.

32. Uterine resting tone and the intensity of contractions are measured in mmHg only when an _____ is being used.

33. A sinusoidal pattern may develop in the Rh sensitized fetus or the fetus who is _____.

34. In the presence of maternal and/or fetal risk factors, auscultation of the fetal heart rate should occur every _____ minutes in the active phase of the first stage of labor and every _____ minutes in the second stage of labor.

35. Average long-term variability is defined as _____ bpm.

36. Attempts to correct variable decelerations can best be accomplished by _____ .

37. When assessing late or variable decelerations, two parameters that reassure the nurse of adequate fetal oxygenation are _____ and _____.

38. When an electronic fetal monitoring tracing is interpreted to be non-reassuring or indicative of fetal stress, a well-oxygenated newborn is delivered at least _____ % of the time.

39. In the presence of fetal heart rate accelerations greater than 15 bpm above baseline and lasting more than 15 seconds, the fetal condition is comparable to the fetal blood gas pH of at least _____ and is considered reassuring.

40. Baseline fetal heart rate tachycardia or bradycardia is assessed over a minimum of a ____ minute time frame.

41. In predicting fetal status, the most important characteristic of the fetal heart rate is _____.

42. Nursing interventions to maximize uteroplacental blood flow in the presence of late decelerations include

    1. _____
    2. _____
    3. _____
    4. _____

CHAPTER 10

MULTIPLE CHOICE

1. Pain during the first stage of labor is caused by
   A. cervical and lower uterine segment stretching and traction on ovaries, fallopian tubes, and uterine ligaments
   B. pressure on the bony pelvis, urethra, bladder, and rectum
   C. uterine muscle hypoxia, lactic acid accumulation, and distention of the pelvic floor muscles

2. The success of tactile stimulation to decrease pain during labor is explained by
   A. large sensory nerve fibers carrying impulses more quickly than small sensory nerve fibers
   B. myelinated nerve fibers carry impulses from the uterus, cervix, and pelvic joints
   C. unmyelinated sensory nerve fibers carry cutaneous stimulation to the spinal cord

3. The release of maternal catecholamines during labor results in
   A. increased cardiac output and decreased blood pressure
   B. decreased cardiac output and decreased blood pressure
   C. increased cardiac output and increased blood pressure

4. The role of "coach" during labor is associated with activities such as
   A. assisting the woman with breathing and relaxation techniques
   B. observing the birth process
   C. responding to requests for physical and emotional assistance

5. Effleurage is defined as
   A. firm massage over the uterus
   B. light massage over the uterus
   C. light massage over any area of the body

6. Tranquilizers such as Phenergan, Vistaril, and Largon are frequently administered during labor to
   A. decrease the pain of contractions
   B. potentiate the effects of narcotics
   C. relieve anxiety and increase sedation

7. The epidural catheter for labor pain management is generally placed between the
   A. 1st and 2nd lumbar vertebrae
   B. 3rd and 4th lumbar vertebrae
   C. 4th and 5th lumbar vertebrae

8. Symptoms of an intravascular injection of a local anesthetic agent include
   A. lightheadedness, tinnitus, and bradycardia
   B. tachycardia, numbness of the tongue, and decreased blood pressure
   C. tachycardia, tinnitus, and palpitations

9. Continued use of the same breathing technique during labor may provide insufficient stimulation or distraction to interfere with pain perception. This phenomena is referred to as
   A. habituation
   B. repetition
   C. monotony

10. A woman in prolonged early labor is given which of the following medications to produce a period of sleep
    A. butorphanol (Stadol)
    B. pentobarbital (Nembutal)
    C. promethazine hydrochloride (Phenergan)

11. Neonatal respiratory depression could result from the use of IV Stadol if birth occurs
    A. anytime within 12 hours of administration
    B. 2 or 3 hours after administration
    C. within 1 hour of administration

12. The advantage of using Nubain to relieve pain associated with labor is
    A. less effect on frequency and duration of contractions
    B. less nausea and vomiting than with opioids
    C. shorter onset of action and longer duration of action than opioids

13. Current research suggests that increase in length of labor associated with epidural infusion may be related to
    A. hypotension and failure to maintain right uterine displacement
    B. intravenous fluid bolus given prior to catheter placement
    C. use of narcotics in the infusion

14. During that period of time when epidural anesthesia is being initiated, the nurse-patient ratio should be
    A. one to one
    B. one to two
    C. there are no standards for nurse-patient ratio

15. One of the first interventions the perinatal nurse might suggest for a woman experiencing pain on one side during a continuous epidural infusion is to
    A. lay toward the side with pain
    B. maintain the woman in a lateral position, off the painful side
    C. request that anesthesia reevaluate the woman

16. Ephedrine is used to correct which side effect of epidural anesthesia/analgesia?
    A. hypotension
    B. nausea and vomiting
    C. pruritus

17. What medication can be given to reverse the symptom of a distended bladder during a continuous epidural infusion?
    A. bupivacaine
    B. epinephrine
    C. naloxone

APPENDIX A • AWHONN'S PERINATAL NURSING ITEM BANK WITH ANSWER KEY

FILL IN THE BLANK

Using the Gate Control Theory, explain how each non-pharmacologic pain management strategy interrupts the transmission of painful stimuli

18. _____ hydrotherapy
19. _____ focal point
20. _____ breathing techniques
21. _____ labor support
22. _____ relaxation

   A. use of auditory or visual stimulation to block the transmission of the painful stimuli
   B. use of cutaneous stimuli to relieve painful stimuli
   C. use of memory or cognitive processes to control degree to which a sensation is interpreted as painful

Complications associated with epidural anesthesia are related to the type of medication and amount of medication used

23. _____ hypotension
24. _____ late decelerations
25. _____ neonatal hyperthermia
26. _____ persistent occiput posterior
27. _____ urinary retention
28. _____ pruritus

   A. local anesthesia
   B. narcotic

29. Another word for imagery is _____.

30. Effleurage involves _____ massage that glides over the skin.

31. Following administration of an opioid during early labor, frequency and duration of contractions and fetal heart rate variability may _____.

32. IV push narcotics should be given _____ _____ uterine contractions to decrease transfer of medication to the fetus.

33. Birth should optimally occur within 1 hour or after _____ hours following administration of pain medication to decrease the potential for neonatal respiratory depression.

34. Medications such as Nubain and Stadol are considered _____.

35. A patient receiving epidural anesthesia will begin to feel relief within _____ minutes following medication injection.

36. Respiratory depression following epidural anesthesia with a combination of narcotic and local anesthetic is most likely related to the _____.

37. A fluid bolus of 500-1000 ml of an isotonic solution should be administered ____ minutes prior to the initiation of regional anesthesia to decrease the potential for maternal hypotension.

38. Auditory and visual stimulation serve as a _____ during labor, decreasing the perception of painful stimuli.

39. Prenatal education and labor support are effective pain management strategies because they _____.

CHAPTER 11

MULTIPLE CHOICE

1. Hemodynamic/hematologic changes occurring during the postpartum period include
   A. elevated blood pressure for 48 hours after birth
   B. elevated cardiac output for at least 48 hours after birth
   C. decreased white blood cell count during first 72 hours after birth

2. During the postpartum period, respiratory and acid-base changes include
   A. hypercapnia
   B. increased PCO_2
   C. decreased base excess

3. Teaching about postpartum sexual activity includes the information that
   A. K-Y jelly is preferred if additional vaginal lubrication is needed
   B. sexual arousal inhibits the release of milk from the breasts
   C. sexual intercourse may be resumed 2 to 4 weeks after vaginal or cesarean birth

4. Which of the following physiologic responses during the immediate postpartum period is normal?
   A. complaints of dizziness when sitting up prior to ambulation
   B. saturation of the peripad with blood every 15 minutes
   C. urinary output of 25 cc/hour

5. Nursing interventions for postpartum hemorrhage include
   A. continuous fundal massage to decrease bleeding and facilitate uterine muscle contraction
   B. bladder catheterization to maintain uterine contraction and accurate measurement of output
   C. Trendelenburg position to facilitate cardiac function and oxygenation of vital organs

6. During the postpartum assessment, the nurse notes hypotension, dyspnea, fever, and abdominal pain. These symptoms suggest the development of
   A. endometritis
   B. pulmonary embolism
   C. pyelonephritis

7. Normal metabolic changes occurring during the postpartum period include
   A. decreased plasma renin and angiotensin II levels
   B. increased blood glucose levels
   C. increased prolactin levels due to placental delivery

8. The greatest factor influencing a woman's successful transition to motherhood is
   A. resumption of a positive and satisfying sexual relationship with her partner
   B. regular attendance at parent support group meetings
   C. emotional support and physical involvement in child care by a significant other

9. Postpartum endometritis is
   A. associated with invasive procedures, such as internal monitoring or amnioinfusion, prolonged labor, and prolonged rupture of membranes
   B. effectively treated with a single dose of ampicillin or cephalosporin
   C. less frequent following cesarean birth due to sterile technique used during surgery

10. Disruptions in the integrity of the anal sphincter, third-degree tears, and sphincter weakness are
    A. associated with increased incidence of being incontinent of flatus
    B. prevented through the judicious use of instrumentation during birth
    C. a problem freely discussed by women with their health care providers

11. The nurse can positively affect a new mother's self-concept and mothering abilities by
    A. encouraging supportive family and friends to become participants in learning opportunities and infant care during hospitalization
    B. encouraging the mother to adopt mothering behaviors and attitudes similar to those of other new mothers
    C. encouraging the mother to accept procedures and routines of the maternity care center

12. Postpartum fundal massage should include
    A. force needed to effect uterine contraction using two hands for procedure
    B. forceful one-handed pressure on fundus until clots expressed
    C. pressure on uterus using two hands until bleeding stops

APPENDIX A • AWHONN'S PERINATAL NURSING ITEM BANK WITH ANSWER KEY

13. Stress incontinence during postpartum may be associated with the management of the
    A. first stage of labor
    B. second stage of labor
    C. third stage of labor

14. No more than 800 cc of urine should be removed during postpartum catheterization because of the potential for
    A. hypertension
    B. hypotension
    C. infection

15. The most effective method to prevent endometritis is
    A. antibiotics
    B. handwashing
    C. nutrition

16. A decline in sexual interest/activity during the postpartum period is most likely caused by
    A. bleeding from the vagina
    B. fear of pregnancy
    C. postpartum psychosis

17. Which drug can cause postpartum hemorrhage
    A. Dicloxicillin
    B. Methadone
    C. Nifedipine

18. Cardiac output after birth peaks at
    A. 1-4 minutes
    B. 5-9 minutes
    C. 10-15 minutes

19. Which anesthetic provides the most hemodynamic stability after cesarean birth?
    A. epidural with epinephrine
    B. epidural without epinephrine
    C. general

20. Nutritional counseling for women who breastfeed should include consuming how many more calories than before pregnancy?
    A. 300
    B. 400
    C. 500

FILL IN THE BLANK

21. To increase venous return during postpartum hemorrhage, the woman is positioned with _____.

22. A white blood cell count of 28,000/mm with polymorphonuclear leukocytes on post partum day 2 would be considered _____.

23. Hematocrit values indicating adequate fluid volume following postpartum hemorrhage is _____.

24. _____ is the most sensitive and specific bedside diagnostic tool for deep vein thrombosis.

25. If a postpartum woman displayed dyspnea and chest pain, the nurse would suspect _____.

26. Restlessness, shaking, tachycardia and fearfulness are suggestive of _____.

27. Counseling regarding contraception must include information about transmission of _____.

28. Symptoms of postpartum blues include _____.

29. During the initial postpartum period, nursing interventions should include assessment of _____, _____, and _____ every 15 minutes for at least 1 hour or more often if indicated.

30. Typically, postpartum blues occur at _____ days postpartum and continue for no more than _____ days.

31. Causes of late postpartum hemorrhage are _____, _____, and _____.

32. The acronym BUBBLERS, used to organize postpartum assessment, stands for _____, _____, _____, _____,

_____, _____, _____, _____.

33. For each _____ ml of blood loss, the hematocrit will decrease 2 to 4%, and the hemoglobin will decrease 1 to 1.5 g/dl.

34. Assessment findings suggesting the development of mastitis include _____, _____, _____, and _____.

35. Topics that should be discussed during postpartum teaching with a woman include _____, _____, _____, and _____.

36. A major factor affecting emotional adjustment during the postpartum period in low-risk women is _____.

37. The first hour after birth is the time of greatest risk for postpartum hemorrhage because _____ _____.

38. Prodromal symptoms of a postpartum eclamptic seizure include _____, _____, _____, and _____.

39. It is important that the nurse has the drug _____, readily available when patients are receiving heparin therapy for thrombophlebitis.

CHAPTER 12

MULTIPLE CHOICE

1. Miscarriage occurs in what percentage of pregnancies?
   A. 15
   B. 20
   C. 25

2. Tim and Ann have experienced the death of their 2-day-old son Tyler from meconium aspiration. During this acute phase of grief, the nurse would expect all of the following grief responses?
   A. acceptance
   B. guilt
   C. somatic distress

3. The nurse provides parents with special momentos and pictures of their deceased newborn to make the experience more real. This should be helpful based on which acute symptom of grief work?
   A. anger
   B. inability to maintain organized patterns of activity
   C. preoccupation with the deceased

4. When asked "why did this happen," the nurse's best response is to
   A. ignore the question
   B. listen and provide comfort
   C. offer explanations

5. When parents decide that they do not want photographs to take home of their infant, the nurse should
   A. file them in case they change their minds
   B. pack the pictures in their belongings
   C. throw them away

FILL IN THE BLANK

6. Losses can be divided into four types
   1. _____
   2. _____
   3. _____
   4. _____

7. _____ grief occurs when parents experience grief prior to the death of their child.

8. Parents may experience _____ grief when their child has a deformity or is chronically ill because they are continually reminded that the child is not "perfect."

9. Bereaved parents can take pleasure in the memories of their child, who has died, through _____ grief which brings gentle sadness in remembering.

10. Participating in a _____ provides parents with the emotional support of others who have experienced a similar loss.

11. The nurse should preserve special mementos for the parents such as _____, _____ and _____.

12. Nursing care of the bereaved family during acute grief work, when the family is irritable or angry, would be to _____.

13. When a mother expresses thoughts about having caused the death of her baby, the nurse should _____ .

14. An _____ support group is one where bereaved parents can enter and leave at will.

15. Nurses often repress their feelings after caring for a family who has experienced a loss. Repressed feelings may cause the nurse to feel _____, _____, and _____ .

16. When nurses experience overload in caring for bereaved families, they may be helped by talking with skilled members of the _____ to process their feelings.

17. Novice nurses who want to work with bereaved families can gain experience by

    1. _____
    2. _____
    3. _____

CHAPTER 13

MULTIPLE CHOICE

1. Metabolism of brown fat occurs
   A. immediately after birth
   B. in response to cold stress
   C. when oxygen saturation is below 90

2. A 10-minute apgar is assigned when the
   A. 1-minute apgar is less than 7
   B. 5-minute apgar is less than 7
   C. newborn has required resuscitation immediately after birth

3. Performing chest physiotherapy as the newborn transitions to extrauterine life
   A. is common practice in the presence of thick meconium
   B. is indicated anytime breath sounds are moist
   C. may decrease newborn oxygen levels

4. During the first week of life, newborns are at risk for bleeding from a variety of anatomical sites because
   A. several clotting factors are being underproduced by the spleen
   B. the liver is immature and not yet producing several clotting factors
   C. Vitamin K is not available from the GI tract

5. According to the American Academy of Pediatrics, the optimal time to administer Vitamin K is
   A. after 2 hours of life
   B. after the infant is bathed
   C. within 1 hour of birth

6. Excess erythromycin ophthalmic ointment in a newborn's eyes is
   A. left in place until absorbed or eventually removed during the bath
   B. removed using sterile water for irrigation
   C. wiped away after 1 minute with a sterile cotton ball

7. Research has shown that use of which of the following products is associated with shorter separation time for the umbilical cord stump
   A. alcohol alone
   B. a combination of alcohol and triple antibiotic dye
   C. triple antibiotic dye alone

8. The key to preventing infant abductions from taking place is
   A. a state of the art electronic infant security system
   B. carefully obtained newborn footprints
   C. implementation of a systematic infant safety program

9. Vitamin K is produced by the newborn
   A. as a normal compensatory mechanism whenever bleeding occurs
   B. as the GI tract becomes colonized with bacteria following initiation of feeding
   C. in response to the parenteral injection of vitamin K

10. As part of the algorithm for performing neonatal resuscitation, medications are initiated when the newborn's
    A. heart rate is below 80 after 30 seconds
    B. heart rate is 60-80 and not increasing
    C. physician identifies they are necessary

11. Initiation of respiration is triggered in the brain by
    A. decreased carbon dioxide concentration
    B. decreased oxygen concentration
    C. decreased surfactant production

12. In utero, pulmonary vascular resistance in the fetus is
    A. equal to neonatal
    B. higher than neonatal
    C. lower than neonatal

13. In the fetus, most blood is diverted away from the lungs through the
    A. ductus arteriosus
    B. ductus venosus
    C. foramen ovale

14. Clamping the umbilical cord at birth causes
    A. decrease in blood pressure and decrease in systemic vascular resistance
    B. increase in blood pressure and decrease in systemic vascular resistance
    C. increase in blood pressure and increase in systemic vascular resistance

15. The major contributing factor to closure of the ductus arteriosus is sensitivity to
    A. decreasing arterial carbon dioxide concentration
    B. decreasing arterial oxygen concentration
    C. rising arterial oxygen concentration

16. In a healthy newborn, the ductus arteriosus will have closed or be closing by
    A. 0–6 hours of life
    B. 12–24 hours of life
    C. 48–72 hours of life

17. The premature infant is more susceptible to evaporative heat loss due to
    A. decreased body surface area
    B. decreased muscle tone
    C. increased permeability of skin

18. Hemorrhagic disease of the newborn is prevented by administration of
    A. vitamin A
    B. vitamin D
    C. vitamin K

19. Velamentous insertion of the umbilical cord may result in
    A. birth trauma
    B. blood loss
    C. congenital anomaly

20. A complication of polyhydramnios may be
    A. meconium aspiration
    B. prolapsed cord
    C. respiratory distress

FILL IN THE BLANK

The following nursing interventions support the newborn's transition to extrauterine life by interrupting what mechanism of heat loss?

21. _____ dry newborn thoroughly, remove wet linen
22. _____ when necessary use humidified, warmed oxygen
23. _____ place cover between newborn and metal scale
24. _____ preheat radiant warmer
25. _____ use of warmed blankets for swaddling
    A. evaporation
    B. convection
    C. conduction
    D. radiation

26. Maternal intrauterine transmission of _____ antibodies protects the newborn from bacterial and viral infections for which the mother has already produced antibodies.

27. The best way to protect newborns from infection is to encourage _____.

28. A 2000-gram infant should receive _____ mg of vitamin K.

29. Erythromycin ophthalmic ointment protects newborns from the organisms _____ and _____.

30. Immediately following birth, in the absence of spontaneous respirations, a nurse begins giving the newborn positive pressure ventilation. The second nurse should _____.

31. Respiratory adaptations during the transition to extrauterine life are dependant on _____, _____, and _____ stimuli to the brain.

32. In utero, oxygenated blood flows from the placenta to the fetus through the _____.

33. During fetal life, the placenta is an organ of _____.

34. The umbilical cord has ___ vein(s) and artery(ies).

35. The four main mechanisms of heat loss in the neonate are _____, _____, _____, and _____.

36. Nonshivering thermogenesis generates heat in the newborn through metabolism of _____.

37. Hypothermia in the neonate increases _____ consumption.

38. Surfactant _____ surface tension in the alveoli.

39. In neonatal resuscitation, chest compressions should be initiated if the heart rate is below _____.

40. A potential neonatal complication of maternal ingestion of alcohol is _____.

CHAPTER 14

MULTIPLE CHOICE

1. A hypospadias has
   A. a meatus on the dorsal surface of the glans
   B. a meatus on the tip of the glans
   C. a meatus on the ventral surface of the glans

2. Short fingers, incurving of the fifth finger, and a wide space between the big toe and second toe is often seen in
   A. Beckwith syndrome
   B. Down syndrome
   C. Turner syndrome

3. The moro reflex should
   A. disappear by 1 month of age
   B. disappear by 3 months of age
   C. disappear by 6 months of age

4. Telangiectatic nevi
   A. are usually elevated, rough, and dark red
   B. most often are seen on the neck, forehead, and eyelids
   C. will not blanch with pressure

5. Tears are usually absent in the newborn until
   A. 2–4 weeks of age
   B. 2–3 months of age
   C. 4–6 months of age

6. Femoral pulses may be decreased or absent in
   A. congestive heart failure
   B. patent ductus arteriosus
   C. shock

7. In the neonate, the trigeminal nerve is assessed by
   A. blinking in response to light
   B. presence of rooting and sucking reflexes
   C. symmetry of facial movement with crying

8. An infant with choanal atresia will
   A. be cyanotic at rest
   B. be cyanotic with crying
   C. have a flat nasal bridge

9. A thin upper lip, smooth philtrum, and a short palpebral fissure are often seen with
   A. Down syndrome
   B. Fetal Alcohol Syndrome
   C. Pierre Robin syndrome

10. A persistent bradycardia of less than 100 beats per minute is most often seen in a newborn with
    A. congenital heart block
    B. congestive heart failure
    C. vagal stimulation

11. Using the Silverman Index to assess a newborn's respiratory effort, a score of zero indicates
    A. moderate respiratory distress
    B. no respiratory distress
    C. severe respiratory distress

12. In the neonate, blood pressure in the lower extremities is
    A. usually higher than in the upper extremities
    B. usually lower than in the upper extremities
    C. usually no different than in the upper extremities

13. The umbilical cord should contain
    A. one artery and one vein
    B. two arteries and one vein
    C. two veins and one artery

14. Talipes equinovarus
    A. is caused from positioning in utero and is easily correctable
    B. is outward turning of the foot
    C. usually requires casting for correction

15. In the term infant the popliteal angle will be
    A. less than 90 degrees
    B. 140–120 degrees
    C. 180–160 degrees

16. The bluish discoloration of a newborn's hands and feet seen in the first 24–48 hours and up to 10 days of life is
    A. acrocyanosis
    B. central cyanosis
    C. circumoral cyanosis

17. Jaundice within the first 24 hours of life may be related to
    A. asphyxia
    B. cardiac disease
    C. sepsis

18. Edema over the presenting part of a newborn's head that feels spongy and resolves within a few days of life is most likely
    A. caput succedaneum
    B. cephalhematoma
    C. related to placement of a scalp electrode during labor

19. Which of the following observations made during the gestational age assessment indicates the greatest degree of physical maturity
    A. labia majora cover clitoris and labia minora
    B. labia majora large and minora small
    C. prominent clitoris and enlarging labia minora

20. In the newborn, jaundice first appears on the
    A. head and face
    B. trunk and extremities
    C. sclera

21. To measure fontanels accurately, a ruler or measuring tape is placed
    A. after 24 hours of age when molding has resolved
    B. diagonally from bone to bone
    C. from suture line to suture line

22. The crossed-eyes appearance of many newborns is called
    A. hypertelorism
    B. nystagmus
    C. strabismus

23. Candida albicans (thrush) is transmitted to the fetus/newborn
    A. rarely after the first month of life
    B. via the placenta
    C. when caregivers fail to wash their hands

24. Bowel sounds are present in the newborn
    A. after passage of first meconium stool
    B. immediately after birth
    C. within 1 hour of birth

25. A prominent xiphoid process identified during a newborn physical assessment is
    A. a normal finding
    B. associated with intrauterine growth retardation
    C. indicative of respiratory distress

FILL IN THE BLANK

26. At birth, newborns are covered with an odorless, white, cheesy, protective coating called _____.

27. Changes in _____ may be the first sign of sepsis, cardiopulmonary, or hematologic diseases.

28. Presence and clarity of the _____ indicates an intact lens, and is assessed using an ophthalmoscope.

29. Congenital hip dislocation is evaluated by _____ and _____ maneuvers.

30. Whitish yellow cysts called _____ containing epithelial cells may be present on the hard palate at birth, but disappear within a few weeks.

31. Constant, rapid involuntary movement of the eye, which usually disappears by four months of age is _____.

32. _____ is an asymmetrical neck deformity due to injury of the sternocleidomastoid muscle.

33. Black or white spots on the periphery of the iris are called _____.

34. "Sniffles" or persistent, profuse mucopurulent or bloody discharge from the nose may indicate _____.

35. Acrocyanosis is the result of _____ _____ and tends to worsen if the newborn becomes chilled.

Identify the following variations seen in the integument of newborns.

36. _____ "lace-like" pattern in response to chilling, stress, or over stimulation

37. _____ dependent side of the body becomes pink, upper half of the body is pale

38. _____ red-to-purple macular lesion, which is permanent and does not blanch to pressure

39. _____ blotchy rash of small yellow vesicles surrounded by an erythematous area
    A. erythema toxicum
    B. Harlequin's sign
    C. mottling
    D. port wine stain

CHAPTER 15

MULTIPLE CHOICE

1. A woman with a history of breast augmentation should be informed that her chances of breastfeeding successfully are
    A. dependent upon the type of surgical procedure
    B. greatly decreased because of the surgery
    C. not altered by the surgery

2. The onset of milk production in a postpartum woman is triggered by
    A. periodic stimulation of oxytocin
    B. a rapid rise in prolactin
    C. a sudden decrease in estrogen

3. Compared with mature breast milk, the fat content of colostrum is
    A. about the same
    B. higher
    C. lower

4. A pregnant woman asks what she should do to prepare her nipples for breast feeding. She is informed that nipple exercises
    A. do little to prevent nipple soreness
    B. improve nipple erectility
    C. increase the nursing mother's confidence

5. Frequent breastfeeding during the first 24 hours postpartum increases
    A. maternal fatigue
    B. newborn weight gain
    C. nipple tenderness

6. Breast engorgement in the breast-feeding mother is minimized by
    A. pumping after the newborn nurses
    B. avoiding unnecessary nipple stimulation
    C. eliminating strict time limits for feedings

7. During a home visit to a 4-day old breast-feeding newborn, the nurse observes jaundice. Which of the following interventions should be suggested to the mother?
    A. increasing the frequency of breast feeding
    B. supplementing breast feeds with water
    C. temporarily pumping and discarding her breast milk

8. A newborn is reported to have breast-fed very well during the first hour after birth. The baby is now 12 hours old and has not had a second successful feeding. The nurse should
    A. advise the mother to give water every 2 to 3 hours
    B. review with the mother the newborn's sleep cycles and hunger cues
    C. teach the mother to pump her breasts for stimulation

9. A woman calls the hospital asking what she should do for her 10-day-old breast-feeding newborn who wants to nurse "all the time." The nurse should recommend that the mother
    A. continue breastfeeding based on the newborn's cues
    B. offer formula if the newborn is still hungry after breastfeeding
    C. use other comforting techniques to space feedings at least 2 hours apart

10. A bottle-feeding mother asks if she should give her baby water. The nurse should instruct her to
    A. add a little extra water to the formula on hot days
    B. feed the newborn only properly mixed formula
    C. give the newborn water between feedings if fussy

11. The hormone responsible for milk production is
    A. human placental lactogen
    B. oxytocin
    C. prolactin

12. Colostrum is rich in
    A. fat
    B. IgG
    C. protein

13. As human milk matures, the concentration of immunoglobins and proteins
    A. decreases
    B. increases
    C. remains the same

14. The main constituent of mature milk is
    A. fat
    B. protein
    C. water

15. A mother holds her breast with her thumb on top and fingers below. This hold is called
    A. "C"
    B. cigarette
    C. cup

16. The most effective method to relieve nipple pain is
    A. cabbage leaves
    B. warm water compresses
    C. tea bags

17. Formula feeding is recommended for newborns with
    A. galactosemia
    B. jaundice
    C. thalassemia

18. After opening a can or bottle of formula, the contents should be used within
    A. 24 hours
    B. 48 hours
    C. 72 hours

19. The most economical formula preparation is
    A. concentrate
    B. powder
    C. ready-to-feed

20. Methods to suppress lactation include
    A. applying warmth to the breast
    B. limiting fluid intake for 48 hours
    C. wearing a firm-fitting bra

FILL IN THE BLANK

21. Long-term milk production is regulated by _____.

22. Colostrum's yellow color is due to its high _____.

23. Breast-feeding mothers should be advised to base the frequency they feed their newborns on _____.

24. By 5 days of age, a breast-feeding newborn can be expected to have _____ stools each day.

25. Chronic nipple tenderness and breast pain are signs of _____.

26. A hard, tender area in the breast of a breast-feeding woman should be treated with _____.

27. The recommended amount of formula per feeding for a bottle-fed newborn under 24 hours of age is _____ ml.

28. Formula stored in the refrigerator is safe to use for a period of _____.

29. When the breast-feeding baby is correctly latched onto the mother's breast, the tongue covers _____.

30. Factors that influence a woman's decision to breast feed include _____, _____, _____.

31. Which childhood illnesses are reduced when breastfeeding? _____, _____, _____, and _____.

32. The _____ regulates the amount of breast milk produced so it matches the infant's intake.

33. The lowest fat content of mature milk is found in the _____ and _____.

34. The process of bringing the newborn's mouth to the breast is called _____.

35. Methods to assess infant intake during breastfeeding include noting the presence of _____, _____, and _____.

36. The consequence of mixing too much water with formula is _____.

37. Early neonatal sucking problems have been documented with the intrapartum use of _____ and _____.

38. Breastfeeding is an effective contraceptive method for the first 6 months postpartum if the woman is _____ and _____.

CHAPTER 16

MULTIPLE CHOICE

1. Newborns who develop transient tachypnea are often born
   A. by cesarean section
   B. preterm
   C. with primary surfactant deficiency

2. In a newborn, tachypnea is defined as a respiratory rate greater than
   A. 40 breaths/minute
   B. 60 breaths/minute
   C. 80 breaths/minute

3. Hypoglycemia associated with hyperinsulinemia, such as in the infant of a diabetic mother, occurs between
   A. 1-3 hours after birth
   B. 5-7 hours after birth
   C. 8-10 hours after birth

4. One etiology of hypoglycemia is decreased production of glucose, which should be suspected in the newborn who is
   A. hypothermic
   B. IDM
   C. small for gestational age

5. Clinical jaundice is apparent at serum bilirubin levels of
   A. 1-3 mg/dl
   B. 5-7 mg/dl
   C. 9-11 mg/dl

6. In a full-term newborn, physiologic hyperbilirubinemia is characterized by a progressive increase in serum bilirubin that peaks at
   A. 24 hours
   B. 72 hours
   C. 5 days

7. Gastrointestinal symptoms associated with neonatal abstinence syndrome include
   A. constipation
   B. diarrhea
   C. voracious appetite

8. Which illegal drug, when used alone, is responsible for the most severe withdrawal symptoms in the newborn?
   A. cocaine
   B. heroine
   C. methadone

9. When ruling out sepsis in the newborn, broad spectrum antimicrobial agents are initiated after cultures have been obtained. The most commonly used agents are
   A. ampicillin/cephalosporin
   B. ampicillin/gentamicin
   C. penicillin/gentamicin

10. Treatment for sepsis should continue for
    A. 5-7 days
    B. 7-10 days
    C. 14 days

11. Hypothermia can cause
    A. decreased metabolic demand
    B. hypoglycemia
    C. metabolic alkalosis

12. A sign of hypoglycemia in the newborn is
    A. increased appetite
    B. plethoric skin tone
    C. temperature instability

13. Which of the following newborns should be screened for hypoglycemia?
    A. infant born at 38 weeks
    B. small-for-gestational-age infant
    C. twins, each weighing 3000 grams

14. In the newborn, physiologic hyperbilirubinemia is characterized by a progressive increase in serum bilirubin to a peak of
    A. 5 mg/dl at 72 hours of age
    B. 10mg/dl at 48 hours of age
    C. 8 mg/dl at 72 hours of age

15. Infants undergoing phototherapy should have axillary temperatures monitored at least
    A. every 30 minutes
    B. every 2 hours
    C. hourly

16. For infants born to cocaine-addicted mothers, frequently exhibit
    A. constipation
    B. feeding difficulties
    C. lethargy

17. Which of the following interventions is useful to support an infant experiencing abstinence syndrome?
    A. increased tactile stimulation
    B. musical mobile placed over the crib
    C. rocking

18. The diagnosis of neonatal sepsis is made in the presence of positive
    A. blood and urine culture
    B. blood culture and clinical symptoms
    C. urine culture and clinical symptoms

FILL IN THE BLANK

19. Surfactant _____ surface tension in the alveoli and functions as a stabilizer to prevent deflation during expiration.

20. When meconium only partially obstructs the airway, a _____ effect results where air enters the lower airways on inspiration but cannot escape on expiration.

21. Glucose homeostasis requires the initiation of various metabolic processes including _____ forming glucose from non-carbohydrate sources and _____, conversion of glycogen stores to glucose.

22. As bilirubin levels rise, there is concern that bilirubin encephalopathy, also known as _____, will develop.

23. In nearly all newborns, phototherapy decreases or blunts the rise in serum _____ bilirubin regardless of gestational age, race or presence or absence of hemolysis.

24. A variety of medications are used to treat neonatal abstinence syndrome. The three most commonly used are _____, _____, and _____.

25. _____ is the one common side effect of all of the medications used to treat neonatal abstinence syndrome.

26. The three most common bacterial agents associated with neonatal sepsis are _____, _____, and _____.

27. The primary neonatal factors influencing the development of sepsis are _____ and _____.

28. Once sepsis has been diagnosed, antibiotic therapy must continue for _____ days.

29. Intrapartum administration of prophylactic antibiotics has proven to be beneficial in preventing _____.

30. Heroine withdrawal in a newborn may last _____.

31. Use of _____ is avoided during phototherapy to eliminate the risk of burns.

32. Skin care is important during phototherapy because the infant often has _____.

33. An infant born to a mother who received tocolytic therapy would be prone to _____.

34. Tachypnea is defined as a respiration rate of _____ breaths per minute.

35. To prevent meconium aspiration syndrome, the mouth and pharynx may be suctioned _____ the head is delivered.

36. Narcotics used to manage labor pain may result in _____ respiratory effort in the newborn.

37. The mortality rate associated with neonatal sepsis increases as birth weight _____.

CHAPTER 17

MULTIPLE CHOICE

1. According to Reva Rubin's classic research, during the first 24 hours postpartum, the new mother is interested in
   A. spending uninterrupted time with her baby
   B. learning to care for herself and her newborn
   C. discussing her labor and birth experience

2. Research has shown that women discharged from the hospital within 24 hours after giving birth feel
   A. angry and dissatisfied with the health care system
   B. more of a sense of control, confidence and competence
   C. very vulnerable, especially if they were primiparous

3. Encouraging parents to complete a learning needs assessment
   A. decreases the amount of time the nurse will spend teaching
   B. helps parents recognize information needed prior to hospital discharge
   C. helps the nurse delegate her work more effectively

4. Follow-up phone calls to families after hospital discharge
   A. are a necessary component of a comprehensive discharge planning program for institutions caring for high-risk populations
   B. is a research-based, cost-effective alternative to 48- or 72-hour hospital stays
   C. should be documented and maintained as a permanent part of the medical record

5. A copy of the clinical pathway is given to childbearing woman and families
   A. as soon as they enter the system
   B. at discharge so it can be used by families to evaluate the care received
   C. to promote collaboration between women and their physicians

6. One of the reasons postpartum length of stay has decreased is
   A. increased need for inpatient hospital beds secondary to an increase in birth rates
   B. shift in consumer attitudes about childbirth to a wellness orientation
   C. significant increase in nosocomial infections on postpartum units

7. The increase in the quality and quantity of prenatal data about the childbearing family provided by a database results in
   A. enhanced individualized care and teaching
   B. more effective use of available nursing staff
   C. more effective use of economic resources

8. The development of effective teaching methods and materials include consideration of
   A. the reading and comprehension levels of the expectant family
   B. staff preferences for class materials and schedules
   C. the use of only group presentations to maximize use of resources

9. The goal of validating the effectiveness of maternal-newborn education is to
   A. document nursing time spent in providing maternal-newborn education to new mothers
   B. evaluate the teaching skills of nurses and provide a basis for their continuing education
   C. verbalize understanding or demonstrate skills related to critical concepts of the program

10. The primary purpose of the clinical pathway is to ensure
    A. that assessments, interventions, and appropriate outcomes are accomplished within a limited time span
    B. that optimal use of nursing time in an era of decreased staffing ratios
    C. uniformity and consistency in maternal-newborn education

11. An essential first step in the evaluation of a prenatal and inpatient education program is the
    A. determination of clinical pathway variance data
    B. identification of the program goals and expected outcomes
    C. retrospective review of medical record data

FILL IN THE BLANK

12. In institutions where the length of postpartum hospitalization is down to 24 hours, prenatal classes need to expand their curriculum to include _____.

13. Use of a _____ involves women and families in childbearing decisions, increases satisfaction, and promotes collaboration between families and health care providers.

14. Encouraging a family to prepare a birth plan will make them aware of _____ and _____.

15. Opportunities to identify the learning needs of families include
    1. _____
    2. _____
    3. _____
    4. _____
    5. _____

16. In any practice model, the _____ plays a key role in postpartum education.

17. Methods of postpartum follow-up after hospital discharge include
    1. _____
    2. _____
    3. _____
    4. _____
    5. _____

18. An advantage of case management is that _____, has comprehensive knowledge of each family and is responsible for ensuring all of their needs are met.

19. Outcome criteria used to evaluate postpartum discharge planning programs includes
    1. _____
    2. _____
    3. _____

20. The focus of prenatal classes has expanded because _____.

21. The prenatal visit is an ideal time for the perinatal nurse to _____ and _____.

22. Prenatal assessment and education programs complement _____.

23. Information that can be included within a prenatal patient data base include _____, _____, _____, and _____.

24. Alternatives to lengthy series of prenatal classes include _____, _____, and _____.

25. The results of involving childbearing families in decisions about the birth experience are _____ and _____.

26. Prior to discharge, maternal-newborn knowledge and skills should be _____.

27. Opportunities for case managers to access expectant women prior to delivery include _____, _____ and _____.

28. A postpartum discharge planning program is cost effective if _____.

29. Qualitative methods of evaluating patient education programs include _____, _____, and _____.

CHAPTER 18

MULTIPLE CHOICE

1. The primary reason for readmission following early discharge is
    A. hyperbilirubinemia
    B. maternal wound infection
    C. sepsis in the newborn

2. Criteria for discharge within 24 hours after the birth include
    A. availability of family or support persons following discharge
    B. presence of community supported hotlines for maternal questions
    C. uncomplicated cesarean delivery and postpartum course

3. It is difficult to use past research to support early discharge today because most current early discharge programs support new mothers with a
    A. greater number of home visits
    B. minimal variability in income levels
    C. shorter length of stay following childbirth

4. Suggested perinatal homecare services following a vaginal birth include
    A. two follow-up phone calls
    B. two to three home nursing visits
    C. 24-hour phone availability of a perinatal nurse for 1 week

5. Suggested perinatal homecare services following a cesarean birth include
    A. three follow-up phone calls
    B. three home nursing visits
    C. 24-hour phone availability of a perinatal nurse for 1 week

6. During the first days at home following childbirth, the physical and emotional changes experienced by the mother are intensified by
    A. changing hormone levels
    B. fatigue
    C. physical discomforts

7. A successful strategy for promoting maternal confidence following childbirth is
    A. a collaborative approach between mother and nurse
    B. firm guidance and teaching from the perinatal nurse
    C. maternal observation of nursing care of the newborn

8. Suggested criteria for employment as a perinatal homecare nurse include
    A. certification in obstetric nursing care
    B. 1-year perinatal nursing experience
    C. 7 contact hours of continuing education in perinatal nursing each year

9. Maternal physical and psychosocial assessments and interventions during the first postpartum home visit include
    A. Homan's sign
    B. interpretation of the birth experience
    C. discussion of weight loss strategies

10. An evaluation of a perinatal homecare program includes
    A. consistent cost reduction
    B. maternal satisfaction
    C. personnel satisfaction

FILL IN THE BLANK

11. Factors influencing the current trend toward shortened length of stay for new mothers include

    1. _____
    2. _____
    3. _____
    4. _____

12. Factors that limit the generalizability of past research about the success of early discharge programs include

    1. _____
    2. _____
    3. _____
    4. _____

13. The goals of perinatal discharge programs and homecare services include

    1. _____
    2. _____
    3. _____
    4. _____

14. Nursing interventions during the first home visit include

    1. _____
    2. _____
    3. _____

15. Nursing interventions during the second and subsequent home visits include _____ and _____.

16. Strategies to ensure adequate rest following discharge include _____ _____ and _____.

17. During the first days following childbirth, a woman has a need to _____ _____.

18. To formulate an individualized plan of care following childbirth, the perinatal nurse performs a thorough _____, _____, and _____.

19. Perinatal nursing interventions during the home visit are directed at

    1. _____
    2. _____
    3. _____
    4. _____
    5. _____
    6. _____

20. Additional services that can be provided by the perinatal nurse in the home following childbirth include _____, _____, _____, and _____.

APPENDIX A • AWHONN'S PERINATAL NURSING ITEM BANK WITH ANSWER KEY

Chapter 1
Key
1. A (page 4)
2. C (page 4)
3. A (page 5)
4. B (page 5)
5. A (page 7)
6. A (page 8)
7. A (page 9)
8. B (page 12)
9. C (page 13)
10. C (page 13)
11. it paid 100% of billed charges (page 4)
12. nursing care (page 5)
13. reduced length of stay (page 5)
14. ritual or reason (page 7)
15. body substance exposure (page 9)
16. traditional practice model (page 10)
17. quality (page 10)
18. Florence Nightingale (page 10)

Chapter 2
Key
1. C (page 16)
2. B (page 16)
3. A (page 17)
4. B (page 19)
5. A (page 20)
6. A (page 21)
7. C (page 21)
8. C (page 23)
9. C (page 23)
10. 1:2 (page 16)
11. nurse practice acts (page 16)
12. certification (page 16)
13. nursing (page 18)
14. 1. duty (page 19)
    2. breach of duty
    3. damages
    4. proximate cause
15. causation (page 19)
16. incident management (page 21)
17. continuing education (page 22)
18. chain of command (page 23)
19. increased (page 24)

Chapter 4
Key
1. C (page 46)
2. A (page 47)
3. B (page 47)
4. B (page 47)
5. A (page 48)
6. C (page 46)
7. C (page 50)
8. B (page 50)
9. A (page 51)
10. C (page 53)
11. A (page 46)
12. B (page 47)
13. B (page 47)
14. B (page 47)
15. C (page 48)
16. A (page 46 and 48)
17. C (page 48)
18. B (page 49)
19. C (page 51)
20. B (page 56)
21. A (page 56)
22. B (page 50)
23. A (page 52)
24. C (page 50)
25. C (page 49)
26. autotransfusion of approximately 1000 ml at birth (page 47)
27. physiologic anemia of pregnancy (page 47)
28. increased levels of coagulation factors (page 49)
29. increases (page 50)
30. renal sodium (page 51)
31. increased glomerular filtration rate (page 51)
32. striae gravidarum (page 55)
33. prolactin (page 55)
34. progesterone (page 55)
35. glucosuria is normal during pregnancy (page 52)
36. cardiovascular (page 46)
37. autotransfusion (page 47)
38. blood volume (page 47)
39. six weeks postpartum (page 48)
40. uterus (page 48)
41. Progesterone (page 48)
42. second (page 48)
43. Angiotensin II (page 48)
44. hypercoagulable (page 49)
45. thrombosis (page 49)
46. prostaglandins (page 55)
47. melasma (page 56)
48. Chadwick's sign (page 56)

Chapter 5
Key
1. B (page 64)
2. C (page 62)
3. A (page 62)
4. B (page 66)
5. B (page 69)
6. C (page 70)
7. C (page 68)
8. C (page 69)
9. A (page 69)
10. family and social history, psychiatric history, mental status, self-concept/self-esteem, support systems, stressors, coping strategies, spirituality, neurovegetative signs, knowledge of the pregnancy experience (page 63)
11. pregnant woman, family, nurse (page 62)
12. nursing diagnoses, care plans, and strategies for nursing care delivery (page 62)
13. exacerbation or reoccurrence in the postpartum period (page 63)
14. the multi-disciplinary team providing care for the woman and her family (page 63)
15. emotional nuances in relationships with family and professionals (page 65)

16. frequency, duration, and intensity (page 70)
17. they believe it is a normal reaction secondary to the stress of becoming a mother (page 69)
18. approximately 10 months (page 68)
19. her own physical and psychological needs have been met (page 68)

Chapter 6

Key

1. B (page 75)
2. C (page 82)
3. A (page 88)
4. B (page 86)
5. B (page 87)
6. B (page 86)
7. C (page 84)
8. B (page 95)
9. A (page 99)
10. B (page 87)
11. B (page 79)
12. B (page 82)
13. C (page 82)
14. C (page 88)
15. C (page 88)
16. C (page 94)
17. B (page 96)
18. A (page 97)
19. 28 (page 95)
20. 36 (page 86)
21. 15 lbs. (page 82)
22. 10 (page 91)
23. teratogens (page 91)
24. 8 (page 96)
25. 12 (page 94)
26. Jewish (page 89)
27. Coumadin (page 92)
28. negative (page 95)
29. 15 and 20 (page 89)
30. risk assessment health promotion intervention (page 78)
31. cardiorespiratory muscular (page 83)
32. two or more abnormally elevated values on the glucose tolerance test (page 87)
33. 15 and 20 (page 88)
34. 10 (page 95)
35. fetal muscle tone, fetal movement, fetal breathing movement, amniotic fluid volume, fetal heart rate (pages 95 and 96)

Chapter 7

Key

1. C (page 114)
2. A (page 117)
3. B (page 117)
4. B (page 119)
5. B (page 124)
6. A (page 127)
7. C (page 131)
8. B (page 135)
9. C (page 137)
10. B (page 139)
11. C (page 112)
12. A (page 114)
13. B (page 121)
14. B (page 125)
15. B (page 127)
16. A (page 133)
17. C (page 137)
18. B (page 141)
19. hypertensive (page 110)
20. 110 (page 114)
21. semi-Fowler's (page 116)
22. magnesium sulfate (page 117)
23. velamentous (page 124)
24. 95% (page 128)
25. 60 (page 130)
26. cardiac (page 137)
27. indomethacin (page 138)
28. corticosteroid (page 139)
29. 1. abruptio placentae
    2. disseminated intravascular coagulation
    3. hepatic failure
    4. acute renal failure (page 111)
30. to prevent maternal cerebral vascular accident; to maintain uteroplacental perfusion (page 118)
31. hemolysis; elevated liver enzymes; low platelets (page 119)
32. aspiration (page 119)
33. hypotension (page 127)
34. 1. abruptio placentae
    2. hemorrhage
    3. preeclampsia
    4. amniotic fluid embolism
    5. sepsis
    6. cardiopulmonary arrest
    7. massive transfusion therapy
    8. saline termination of pregnancy
    9. dead fetus syndrome (page 130)
35. 1. low abdominal pressure
    2. low backache
    3. vaginal bleeding or discharge
    4. a feeling of "something" in the vagina
    5. thigh pain (page 133)
36. 1. muscle atrophy
    2. muscle weakness
    3. bone loss
    4. decreased gastric motility
    5. increased gastric reflux
    6. changes in cardiac output (page 136)
37. 1. antenatal corticosteroid administration
    2. thyrotropin-releasing hormone combined with glucocorticoid
    3. artificial surfactant therapy (page 139)

Chapter 8

Key

1. A (page 160)
2. C (page 160)
3. C (page 170)
4. C (page 171)
5. C (page 173)
6. C (page 157)

7. B (page 170)
8. A (page 173)
9. A (page 153)
10. B (page 157)
11. C (page 168)
12. A (page 168)
13. C (page 171)
14. C (page 165)
15. B (page 167)
16. A (page 169)
17. C (page 170)
18. C (page 159)
19. A (page 176)
20. A (page 177)
21. C (page 159)
22. C (page 177)
23. at the level of the ischial spines (page 157)
24. awaiting spontaneous bearing-down efforts (page 164)
25. to facilitate birth with shoulder dystocia (page 165)
26. McRobert's maneuver, suprapubic pressure (page 165)
27. clavicle fracture brachial plexus injury (page 165)
28. laminaria tents prostaglandin gel low-dose oxytocin (page 168,169)
29. foul-smelling amniotic fluid, uterine tenderness, fever, elevated WBC, fetal tachycardia (page 169)
30. >20 mm Hg (page 171)
31. cervical dilation, cervical effacement, fetal station, cervical consistency, cervical position (page 169)
32. descent is slow in second stage (page 157)
33. dilation, effacement, station of the fetal head (page 157)
34. vaginal bleeding, uterine tenderness, hypertonus (page 170)
35. placental aging, fetal cortisol, prostaglandin (page 152)
36. multiparous, well-applied vertex, some cervical effacement, 1-2 centimeters, dilation (page 168)
37. 20 (page 176)
38. cord compression (page 173)
39. headache, nausea and vomiting, mental confusion, decreased urinary output, hypotension, tachycardia, cardiac arrhythmias (page 171)
40. 4 (page 159)
41. second (page 166)
42. operating room/recovery room (page 176)
43. open-glottis (page 160)
44. palpate the uterus (page 171)
45. Dantrolene (page 179)

Chapter 9
Key
1. C (page 188)
2. C (page 188)
3. A (page 189)
4. B (page 194)
5. B (page 189)
6. B (page 197)
7. C (page 203)
8. C (page 203)
9. C (page 208)
10. A (page 215)
11. C (page 214)
12. C (page 194)
13. B (page 197)
14. A (page 199)
15. B (page 199)
16. C (page 203)
17. B (page 208)
18. A (page 215)
19. C (page 216)
20. A (page 194)
21. peak, after (page 199)
22. variable, abrupt (page 203)
23. beginning, baseline rate, benign (page 199)
24. discontinuing (page 211)
25. average (page 213)
26. congenital anomalies (page 216)
27. supraventricular tachycardia (page 218)
28. two of the following: medications, prematurity, fetal sleep, fetal dysrhythmia, anesthetic agents, CNS or cardiac anomaly (page 199)
29. overshoots (page 215)
30. hyperstimulation, abruption, hypertension (page 199)
31. tocolytics (page 203)
32. intrauterine pressure catheter (page 211)
33. anemic (page 216)
34. 15; 5 (page 188)
35. 6–25 (page 200)
36. changing maternal position (page 206)
37. variability and rate (page 199)
38. 50 (page 213)
39. 7.20 (page 213)
40. 10 (page 189)
41. variability (page 195)
42. 1. increasing IV fluids
    2. maintaining lateral maternal position
    3. administering O_2 by mask
    4. discontinuing oxytocin (page 203)

Chapter 10
Key
1. A (page 228)
2. A (page 228)
3. C (page 229)
4. A (page 230)
5. C (page 234)
6. C (page 235)
7. C (page 238)
8. C (page 238)
9. A (page 231)
10. B (page 235)
11. B (page 236)
12. B (page 236)
13. B (page 238)
14. A (page 239)

APPENDIX A • AWHONN'S PERINATAL NURSING ITEM BANK WITH ANSWER KEY

15. A (page 243)
16. A (page 242)
17. C (page 243)
18. B (page 229)
19. A (page 229)
20. A (page 229)
21. C (page 229)
22. C (page 229)
23. A (page 239)
24. A (page 239)
25. A (page 239)
26. A (page 239)
27. B (page 239)
28. B (page 239)
29. daydreaming (page 232)
30. light (page 234)
31. decrease (page 235)
32. during (page 236)
33. 4 (page 236)
34. agonist/antagonists (page 236)
35. 10 minutes (page 238)
36. narcotic (page 239)
37. 15-30 (page 242)
38. distraction (page 228)
39. increase maternal confidence and sense of control (page 229)

Chapter 11

Key

1. B (pages 253)
2. B (page 254)
3. C (page 265)
4. A (page 253)
5. B (page 258)
6. B (page 261)
7. A (page 252)
8. C (page 268)
9. A (page 259)
10. A (page 255)
11. A (page 250)
12. A (page 258)
13. B (page 252)
14. B (page 252)
15. B (page 259)
16. B (page 263)
17. C (page 257)
18. C (page 253)
19. B (page 254)
20. C (page 256)
21. legs elevated to 20-30° (page 258)
22. elevated or leukocytosis (page 259)
23. 30 (page 258)
24. measurement of affected leg circumference 2 cm larger than unaffected leg circumference (page 261)
25. pulmonary embolism (page 261)
26. shock (page 262)
27. sexually transmitted diseases (page 266)
28. anger, anxiety, fatigue (page 267)
29. vital signs, lochia, uterine tone/position (page 256)
30. 3 to 5, several (page 267)
31. infection, subinvolution, retained placenta (page 257)
32. breasts, uterus, bladder, bowel, lochia, episiotomy/incision, emotional responses, Homan's sign (page 256)
33. 450-500 ml (page 257)
34. fever, localized tenderness, chills, palpable hard mass (page 260)
35. pelvic-floor exercises, postpartum exercise, sexuality, contraception (pages 263-264)
36. fatigue (page 267)
37. there are large venous areas that are exposed after the separation of the placenta (page 257)
38. severe persistent occipital headache, scotomata, blurred vision, photophobia, epigastric or right upper quadrant pain (page 253)
39. protamine sulfate (page 261)

Chapter 12

Key

1. B (page 273)
2. A (page 276)
3. C (page 276)
4. B (page 276)
5. A (page 283)
6. 1. significant other
   2. some aspect of self
   3. stages of growth and development
   4. external objects (page 272)
7. anticipatory (page 277)
8. chronic (page 277)
9. bittersweet (page 278)
10. bereavement support group (page 279)
11. pictures; footprints; lock of hair (page 283)
12. listen (page 276)
13. reassure her that her feelings are normal (page 276)
14. ongoing (page 282)
15. out of control; tearful; self-focused (page 282)
16. multidisciplinary team (page 282)
17. reading books on grief; attending conferences; and working with an appropriate role model (page 282)

Chapter 13

Key

1. B (page 296)
2. B (page 301)
3. C (page 301)
4. C (page 304)
5. C (page 304)
6. C (page 304)
7. A (page 304)
8. C (page 304)
9. B (page 304)
10. A (page 300)
11. B (page 290)
12. C (page 295)
13. A (page 294)
14. C (page 295)
15. C (page 295)
16. B (page 295)
17. C (page 296)
18. C (page 304)
19. B (page 292)
20. B (page 292)
21. A (page 297)
22. B (page 297)

23. C (page 297)
24. C (page 297)
25. C (page 297)
26. IgG (page 297)
27. handwashing (page 297)
28. 1 mg (page 304)
29. Chlamydia and gonococcus (page 304)
30. evaluate the heart rate (page 300)
31. chemical, thermal, sensory (page 290)
32. umbilical vein (page 294)
33. low vascular resistance (page 295)
34. one, two (page 304)
35. evaporation, convection, conduction, and radiation (page 297)
36. brown fat (page 296)
37. oxygen (page 298)
38. lowers (page 293)
39. 80 (page 300)
40. fetal alcohol syndrome (page 291)

Chapter 14

Key

1. C (page 328)
2. B (page 331)
3. C (page 335)
4. B (page 310)
5. C (page 313)
6. C (page 324)
7. B (page 333)
8. A (page 317)
9. B (page 318)
10. A (page 324)
11. B (page 321)
12. A (page 321)
13. B (page 323)
14. C (page 329)
15. A (page 309)
16. A (page 308)
17. C (page 311)
18. A (page 311)
19. A (page 309)
20. A (page 309)
21. B (page 311)
22. C (page 313)
23. C (page 319)
24. C (page 324)
25. A (page 320)
26. vernix (page 308)
27. skin color (page 308)
28. red reflex (page 313)
29. Ortolani's, Barlow's (page 329)
30. Epstein's pearls (page 318)
31. nystagmus (page 313)
32. torticollis (page 320)
33. Brushfield spots (page 315)
34. congenital syphilis (page 317)
35. poor peripheral circulation (page 309)
36. C (page 310)
37. B (page 310)
38. D (page 310)
39. A (page 310)

Chapter 15

Key

1. A (page 343)
2. C (page 338)
3. C (page 339)
4. A (page 339)
5. B (page 342)
6. C (page 346)
7. A (page 345)
8. B (page 342)
9. A (page 346)
10. B (page 347)
11. C (page 338)
12. C (page 339)
13. A (page 339)
14. C (page 339)
15. A (page 340)
16. B (page 345)
17. A (page 347)
18. B (page 348)
19. B (page 347)
20. C (pages 348–350)
21. removal of milk from the breast (page 339)
22. beta carotene content (page 339)
23. hunger cues (page 342)
24. at least three (page 343)
25. thrush or candida infection (page 345)
26. heat and massage (page 347)
27. 15 (page 348)
28. 48 hours (page 348)
29. its lower gum (page 341)
30. education, age, support (page 338)
31. respiratory infections, otitis media, bacteremia, meningitis (page 338)
32. autocrine control mechanism (page 339)
33. morning, beginning of a feeding (page 339)
34. latch-on (page 341)
35. audible swallows, elimination patterns, satiation cues (page 343)
36. oral water intoxication (page 347)
37. Stadol, epidural anesthesia (page 342)
38. amenorrheic, exclusively breastfeeding (page 350)

Chapter 16

Key

1. A (page 358)
2. B (page 359)
3. A (page 361)
4. C (page 360)
5. B (page 363)
6. B (page 363)
7. B (page 366)
8. C (page 367)
9. B (page 373)
10. B (page 373)
11. B (page 360)
12. C (page 361)
13. B (page 362)
14. C (page 363)
15. B (page 364)
16. B (page 367)
17. C (page 367)
18. B (page 368)
19. decreases (page 357)
20. ball-valve (page 357)
21. gluconeogenesis, glycogenolysis (page 361)
22. kernicterus (page 363)
23. unconjugated or indirect (page 364)
24. dilute tincture of opium (DTO), paregoric, pheno-

barbital (page 368)
25. sedation (page 368)
26. Group B B hemolytic strep, *E-coli*, H. flu (page 368)
27. gestational age, birth weight (page 370)
28. 7–10 (page 373)
29. GBS (page 370)
30. 8–16 weeks (page 367)
31. creams and lotions (page 365)
32. loose stools (page 364)
33. hypoglycemia (page 360)
34. 60 (page 359)
35. once (page 357)
36. poor (page 356)
37. decreases (page 370)

Chapter 17

Key

1. C (page 379)
2. B (page 380)
3. B (page 384)
4. C (page 398)
5. A (page 392)
6. B (page 380)
7. A (page 380)
8. A (page 384)
9. C (page 389)
10. A (page 392)
11. B (page 398)
12. postpartum and newborn care (page 379)
13. birth plan (page 384)
14. birthing options; hospital policies (page 384)
15. 1. prenatal classes
   2. prenatal visits
   3. telephone contact
   4. on admission to the hospital
   5. hospital tours (page 384)
16. staff nurse (page 386)
17. 1. telephone calls
   2. home visits
   3. support groups
   4. office visits
   5. community programs (page 389)
18. one person (page 390)
19. 1. family knowledge about maternal-newborn care
   2. ability to identify support persons and community resources
   3. familiarity with signs and symptoms of complications (page 398)
20. shorter hospital stays result in less time for teaching maternal-newborn content (page 379)
21. assess family learning needs; provide one-on-one information (page 379)
22. inpatient postpartum teaching (page 379)
23. demographic information; due dates; family assessment and learning needs; and significant clinical history (page 380)
24. weekend programs, flexible hours, and antepartum home visits (page 380)
25. increased satisfaction and a collaborative relationship between health care providers and patients (page 384)
26. validated through discussion or return demonstration (page 386)
27. referrals from health care providers; third party payers; tours of the maternity facilities (page 390)
28. unnecessary phone calls or return visits to the institution or primary health care provider are decreased (page 398)
29. patient interview, focus groups, and letters or phone calls from program participants (page 398)

Chapter 18

Key

1. A (page 402)
2. A (page 403)
3. C (page 402)
4. A (page 404)
5. A (page 404)
6. B (page 404)
7. A (page 405)
8. C (page 408)
9. A (page 405)
10. B (page 407)
11. 1. emphasis on cost reduction
   2. consumer demand for a more natural experience
   3. increased care participation
   4. favorable outcomes for mothers discharged within 24 hours (page 401)
12. 1. differences in criteria for discharge
   2. inconsistencies in definition of "early"
   3. type of providers
   4. number of visits (page 402)
13. 1. bridging the interests of families, providers, payers, and community
   2. coordination of efforts
   3. minimizing duplication
   4. filling in the gaps in health care (page 403)
14. 1. thorough physical examination of mother and newborn
   2. reinforce postpartum teaching
   3. answering questions from mother and family (page 404)
15. physical assessment of mother and newborn; follow-up of previous questions and concerns

175

(page 404)
16. seeking assistance from family members and friends; sleeping when the baby sleeps (page 405)
17. describe and discuss the labor and birth process (page 405)
18. physical; psychosocial; environmental assessment (page 405)
19. 1. reinforcing earlier teaching
    2. providing assistance with self-care
    3. promoting health education
    4. providing emotional support
    5. validating the childbirth experience
    6. emphasizing community resources (page 406)
20. 1. staple removal following cesarean birth
    2. obtaining laboratory samples
    3. initiating and monitoring newborn phototherapy (page 407)

APPENDIX B • CORE COMPETENCE CHECKLIST FOR PERINATAL UNITS

PERINATAL UNIT CORE COMPETENCIES

NAME _____ EVALUATOR/S _____

DATE COMPLETED _____

KEY: PERINATAL UNIT CORE COMPETENCIES

Advanced Beginner:
Has a basic understanding of the physiology and pathophysiology of pregnancy, accurate assessment skills, and appropriate nursing interventions. Clinical assignment with an experienced perinatal nurse.

Competent:
Has a basic understanding of the physiology and pathophysiology of pregnancy, accurate assessment skills, and appropriate nursing interventions. Able to provide care independently. Knows when to seek consultation of an experienced perinatal nurse.

Proficient:
Has a thorough knowledge base of the physiology and pathophysiology of pregnancy, accurate assessment skills, and appropriate nursing interventions. Able to provide care in complex clinical situations. Acts as preceptor to new orientees and unit charge nurse as assigned.

Expert:
Has a thorough knowledge base of the physiology and pathophysiology of pregnancy, accurate assessment skills, and appropriate nursing interventions. Able to provide care in complex clinical situations. Acts as preceptor to new orientees and unit charge nurse as assigned. Acts as clinical resource in fetal heart rate pattern interpretation, standards of care, and policies and procedures.

KEY: METHOD OF EVALUATION AND FOLLOW-UP

Preceptor Observation	PO	Peer Review	PR	Patient Feedback	PFB
Return Demonstration	RD	Written Self-Assessment	WSE	Computer Assisted Instruction	CAI
Skills Checklist	SC	Medical Record Audit	MRA	None Needed	NN
Video Tape Viewing	VTV	Learning Module Completion	LMC		

St. John's Mercy Medical Center, St. Louis, Missouri

APPENDIX B • CORE COMPETENCE CHECKLIST FOR PERINATAL UNITS

PERINATAL UNIT CORE COMPETENCIES

Competency	Advanced Beginner	Competent	Proficient	Expert	Method of Evaluation	Follow-up	Initials	Date
ANTEPARTUM								
Able to complete a comprehensive assessment of women during the antepartum period experiencing complications of pregnancy including preterm labor, premature rupture of membranes, pregnancy-induced hypertension, preeclampsia, diabetes, bleeding, and infection.								
Plans and delivers care to women with pregnancy complications appropriate to the specific clinical situation.								
Has a thorough understanding of the warning signs of preterm labor and is able to discuss this information with women at risk in a manner that facilitates their understanding.								
Has knowledge of both institutional and community resources available to women with complications of pregnancy and makes referrals as appropriate.								
Able to provide information prior to discharge such as signs and symptoms of specific clinical situation, and when to call the obstetrician/primary healthcare provider, or come to the hospital to women with pregnancy complications.								
Plans and delivers care to women during the antepartum period considering individual diversities related to age, culture, ethnicity and religion.								
INTRAPARTUM								
Able to complete a comprehensive perinatal nursing assessment on pregnant women admitted to labor-delivery-recovery unit.								
Able to identify pregnant women at high risk for pregnancy and/or medical complications.								
Provides supportive care to the woman and her family in situations involving fetal loss or fetal abnormalities.								
Assesses the woman's educational needs during the intrapartum period and provides appropriate information to the woman and her family.								
Plans and delivers care to women who experience labor and birth without complications.								
Plans and delivers care to women with perinatal and/or medical complications including pregnancy-induced hypertension, preterm labor, bleeding in pregnancy, and multiple gestations.								

APPENDIX B • CORE COMPETENCE CHECKLIST FOR PERINATAL UNITS

PERINATAL UNIT CORE COMPETENCIES

Competency	Advanced Beginner	Competent	Proficient	Expert	Method of Evaluation	Follow-up	Initials	Date
INTRAPARTUM continued								
Has a thorough understanding of the physiologic basis for electronic fetal heart rate monitoring.								
Able to interpret electronic fetal heart rate monitor tracings, identify reassuring and nonreassuring FHR patterns, and initiate appropriate nursing interventions.								
Has a thorough understanding of the normal labor and birth process.								
Plans and delivers care to women who labor without analgesia/anesthesia.								
Has a thorough understanding of the nursing care for laboring women with epidural analgesia/anesthesia.								
Has a thorough understanding of the pharmacokinetics of oxytocin.								
Acts as labor coach and circulating nurse for both vaginal and cesarean births.								
Able to complete a systematic assessment of the newborn, including evaluating the need for resuscitation and assigning Apgar scores.								
Plans and delivers care to women during the antepartum period considering individual diversities related to age, culture, ethnicity and religion.								
POSTPARTUM								
Able to perform a comprehensive assessment of the woman in the immediate postpartum period.								
Has a thorough understanding of normal physiologic processes occurring during the postpartum period.								
Plans and delivers care to women without complications during the postpartum period.								
Able to identify women at risk for complications during the postpartum period, including hemorrhage, infection, pregnancy-induced hypertension and preeclampsia.								
Plans and delivers care to women with complications during the postpartum period.								

APPENDIX B • CORE COMPETENCE CHECKLIST FOR PERINATAL UNITS

PERINATAL UNIT CORE COMPETENCIES

Competency	Advanced Beginner	Competent	Proficient	Expert	Method of Evaluation	Follow-up	Initials	Date
POSTPARTUM continued								
Has a thorough knowledge of breastfeeding and supports the woman who wants to initiate breastfeeding in the immediate postpartum period.								
Has a thorough understanding of the physiology of human lactation.								
Facilitates the breastfeeding process including supporting the women during initial breasting as soon as possible after birth, positioning, latch on, satiation cues, breast care, measures to manage engorgement, and use of manual or electric breast pumps.								
Facilitates the formula feeding process including providing information about amount of feeding, satiation cues, demand feeding, positioning, burping, formula preparation and measures to prevent or decrease breast engorgement.								
Promotes maternal-newborn attachment including encouraging examining, touching, talking to newborn, keeping couplet together as much as possible, providing information about newborn behavior states, sleeping and waking patterns, and comforting strategies.								
Provides information about maternal self-care and newborn care prior to discharge including safety issues, feeding techniques, and signs and symptoms indicating need to call the pediatrician, obstetrician, or other primary healthcare provider.								
Plans and delivers care to women during the antepartum period considering individual diversities related to age, culture, ethnicity and religion.								
NEWBORN								
Able to perform a comprehensive assessment of the newborn.								
Has a thorough understanding of normal newborn transitional care including thermoregulation, glucose monitoring, respiratory status.								
Plans and delivers care to the healthy full term newborn.								
Able to identify newborns at risk for complications during the first hours of life including temperature, glucose, and respiratory instabilities.								
Plans and delivers care to the newborn with complications.								

APPENDIX C • SUGGESTED PERINATAL NURSING RESOURCES FOR ORIENTATION AND CONTINUING EDUCATON: COMPUTER-ASSISTED INSTRUCTIONAL PROGRAMS VIDEOTAPE SERIES, SELF-ASSESSMENT LEARNING MODULES, AND CURRENT PERINATAL TEXTBOOKS

SUGGESTED PERINATAL NURSING RESOURCES

Computer assisted instructional (CAIs) programs

AWHONN CAIs:
Bleeding in Pregnancy
Diabetes in Pregnancy
Pregnancy-Induced Hypertension
Cardiac Disease in Pregnancy
Sexually Transmitted Diseases
Psychosocial Aspects of High-Risk Pregnancy
All have self assessments (20-item quiz) at the end of the program

Videotape series

AWHONN Videotape Series: Cross Training for Obstetrical Nurses
Antepartum Care
Intrapartum Care
Postpartum Care
Bleeding in Pregnancy and Preterm Labor
Pregnancy-Induced Hypertension
Diabetes in Pregnancy
Newborn Assessment
Home Follow-up of Early Postpartum Discharge Families
Self assessment booklet is available

AWHONN Videotape Series: Essentials of Electronic Fetal Monitoring Ed.2 (1994)
Principles of Instrumentation
Pattern Interpretation
Nursing Intervention and Documentation
Manual included: Competency Validation

AWHONN Videotape Series: Critical Concepts in Fetal Heart Rate Monitoring Ed. 2 (1996)
Maternal Adaptation
Fetal Adaptation
Case Studies in Maternal Crises
Case Studies in Fetal Crises
Current Issues and Challenges in Documentation
Resource Manual Included

AWHONN Videotape Series: OB-GYN Limited Ultrasound (1996)
Concepts in Limited Ultrasound
Limited Ultrasound in Obstetrical Settings
Limited Ultrasound in Gynecologic and Infertility Settings
Resource Manual Included

APPENDIX C • SUGGESTED PERINATAL NURSING RESOURCES FOR ORIENTATION AND CONTINUING EDUCATON: COMPUTER-ASSISTED INSTRUCTIONAL PROGRAMS VIDEOTAPE SERIES, SELF-ASSESSMENT LEARNING MODULES, AND CURRENT PERINATAL TEXTBOOKS

AWHONN Videotape Series: Women's Healthcare
Breast Disease and Breast Cancer
Gynecologic Cancer
Pelvic Inflammatory Disease and Ectopic Pregnancy
Menopause and Hormone Therapy
Uterine Surgery

Self-paced learning modules
Martin, J., (1996). Intrapartum Management Modules. Williams and Wilkins
Phillips, C. (1996). Family-Centered Maternity/Newborn Care. Mosby
Both have self assessments after each chapter

Self-assessment modules
The National Certification Corporation for the Obstetric, Gynecologic, and Neonatal Nursing Specialities (NCC) has a self-assessment program for nurses that covers various topics in the perinatal nursing specialty. The modules have written material and questions about content that can be used as part of a continuing education or competency validation program.

Self-assessment modules
AWHONN Compendium of Postpartum Care (1996) Free to AWHONN members

Self-assessment modules
The March of Dimes Nursing modules series are available on a wide variety of perinatal and neonatal nursing topics.

Selected current textbooks for perinatal unit library:

Allen, K. M. & Phillips, J. M. (1997). Women's health across the lifespan: A comprehensive perspective. Philadelphia, PA: Lippincott.

Blackburn, S.T. & Loper, L. (1992). Maternal, fetal and neonatal physiology: A clinical perspective. Philadelphia, PA: W. B. Saunders.

Clark, S. L., Cotton, D. B., Hankins, G. D. V., & Phelan, J. P. (1994). Handbook of critical care obstetrics. Boston: Blackwell Scientific Publications.

Datta, S. (Ed) (1997). Anesthetic and obstetric management of high-risk pregnancy. St. Louis: Mosby.

Foley, M. R. & Strong, T. H. (Eds.) (1997). Obstetric intensive care: A practical manual. Philadelphia. PA: W. B. Saunders.

Freeman, R. & Garite, T. (1991). Fetal heart rate monitoring. Baltimore: Williams & Wilkins.

Gabbe, S., Niebyl, J. & Simpson, J. (Eds.) (1997). Obstetrics: Normal and problem pregnancies. New York: Churchhill Livingston.

APPENDIX C • SUGGESTED PERINATAL NURSING RESOURCES FOR ORIENTATION AND CONTINUING EDUCATON: COMPUTER-ASSISTED INSTRUCTIONAL PROGRAMS VIDEOTAPE SERIES, SELF-ASSESSMENT LEARNING MODULES, AND CURRENT PERINATAL TEXTBOOKS

Knuppel, R. & Drukker, J. E. (Eds.) (1993). High risk pregnancy: A team approach. Philadelphia, PA: W. B. Saunders.

Lawrence, R. (1994). Breastfeeding: A guide for the medical profession. St. Louis: Mosby.

Lowdermilk, D., Perry, S. & Bobak, (Eds.). (1997). Maternity and gynecologic nursing. St. Louis: CV Mosby Co.

Mandeville, L. K. & Troiano, N. H. (Eds.) (1998). High risk intrapartum nursing. Philadelphia, PA: J. B. Lippincott.

May, L. & Mahlmeister, L. (Eds.). (1997). Maternal and neonatal nursing: Family centered care. Philadelphia: J. B. Lippincott.

Parer, J. T. (1997). Handbook of fetal heart rate monitoring. Philadelphia, PA: W. B. Saunders.

Ramsay, M. M., James, D. K., Steer, P. J., Weiner, C. P., & Gonik, B. (1997). Normal values in pregnancy. Philadelphia, PA: W. B. Saunders.

Simpson, K. R., & Creehan, P. A. (Eds.). (1996). AWHONN's Perinatal nursing. Philadelphia: J. B. Lippincott.

Tappero, E. & Honeyfield, M. (Eds.). (1996). Physical assessment of the newborn: A comprehensive approach to the art of physical assessment. Petaluma, CA: NICU INK.

Tucker, S. (1996). Fetal monitoring and assessment. St. Louis: Mosby.

Rituals Associated with Pregnancy, Childbirth, Postpartum and Infant Care

From Lipson, J., Dibble, S., & Minarik, P. (Eds.). (1996). <u>Culture & nursing care: A pocket guide</u>. San Francisco: The Regents, University of California.

Filipinos (Cantos & Rivera, 1996)

Pregnancy care

Prenatal care is an expectation for those who can afford it. Family gives much attention to the pregnant woman. She is not allowed to work outside the home. She is encouraged to eat well and is given choice foods when possible. She is encouraged to get plenty of sleep at night. In the last few months, she is discouraged from staying in a dependent position, such as prolonged sitting or sleeping during the day for fear of water retention. Sexual intercourse is taboo during the last two months of pregnancy. As the time of birth draws near, the traditional Filipino woman is encouraged to eat fresh eggs based on the belief that eating slippery foods will allow the baby to "slip" through the birth canal.

Labor practices

If an M.D. is not present during labor, a self-trained "midwife" assists with delivery. Noise and stimulation are minimized for fear that too much commotion will increase labor pains. Father usually not with the wife during labor, unless Lamaze is being practiced. Some fathers remain at work or with their male friends for support. Some pregnant woman may try to walk around the room to promote dilatation. Offer adequate pain relief; some may refuse.

Role of laboring woman during birth process

The soon-to-be-mother assumes an active role during labor, sometimes commanding either the family or the midwife to cover or fan her. Most women will keep moaning or grunting to an accepted social level. Others may scream and become hysterical.

Role of the father and other family members during birth process

The father assumes a passive role during the birth process, except for those who attend Lamaze classes. A female member of the family who is a mother is preferred to be the coach during labor.

Vaginal vs. cesarean section

Vaginal delivery is preferred.

Breastfeeding

Breast feeding is an expectation of all Filipino mothers, sometimes until the child is a toddler. For working mothers, breastfeeding is concurrently practiced with formula feeding until the child is at least a year old. Some seafood, i.e., clams and fish, is avoided for unknown reasons.

Birth recuperation

The new mother is expected to be with the baby 24 hours a day. Most of the new tasks are shared by the mother and a sister and the father. The mother is freed from heavy housework, provided with nourishing soup to drink, and pampered with attention. While recuperating, the mother is encouraged to use a pelvic binder for at least six weeks. New mothers are discouraged from showering immediately; however, hygiene is of utmost importance. Mothers may give themselves a thorough sponge bath, sometimes many times in a day. Peri care is done by washing with soap and water, or by adding some drops of vinegar to the warm water.

Problems with the baby

If there is a problem with the baby, it is best to consult with the father and other family support, such as the mother of the new mother, prior to informing her. The M.D. must be the person telling the new mother.

Male and female circumcision

Male circumcision not traditionally done at birth. However, for working parents, it is now common practice to allow their new baby boy to be circumcised prior to discharge. Female circumcision never performed.

Haitians

(Colin & Paperwalla, 1996)

Pregnancy care

Pregnancy care is not seen as a health problem but a happy time for entire family. Pregnancy does not relieve the woman from her work; she is expected to fulfill her obligations throughout pregnancy. Pregnant women experience an increase in salivation, and Haitian women rid themselves of the excess at places that may seem inappropriate. Sometimes they carry a "spit" cup with them and are not embarrassed by this behavior. They do not believe that they should swallow their saliva. Others need to be tolerant of this behavior since excess salivation is a natural effect of pregnancy. Pregnant women are restricted from eating spices because they may irritate the child. However, they are permitted to eat vegetables and red fruits, believing that this will build up the child's blood. They are encouraged to eat a lot because they are eating for two. Some may seek prenatal care at private physician's office or at a clinic. Generally, however, many Haitian women do not seek prenatal care.

Labor practices

May walk, pace, sit, squat, and rub her belly; will not ask for analgesics.

Role of the laboring woman during birth process
Plays an active role during this process: talks loud, may scream, curse and sometimes even becomes hysterical. Some are stoic, only moaning or grunting.

Role of the father and other family members during birth process.
Father is a non-participant, remaining outside of the process. Believes this a private event best handled by women. Woman not coached; however, female family members will give assistance as needed if midwife involved.

Vaginal vs. cesarean section
Vaginal delivery more common, natural childbirth the norm. Women in higher social strata quicker to have cesarean. C-section feared, however, because it's abdominal surgery.

Breastfeeding
Encouraged for up to 9 months postpartum. Milk of lactating woman believed to be stored in her breast, and can become detrimental to both mother and child if it becomes too thick or too thin. If too thin, it is believed that milk has "turned" and may cause diarrhea in the child, headache and possible postpartum depression in the mother. If milk is too thick, may cause impetigo (*bouton*). Mixed feedings (breast and bottle) very much accepted. If child develops diarrhea, breastfeeding immediately discontinued.

Birth recuperation
Very important period for Haitian woman. Takes an active role in own care, dresses warmly, takes baths (*vapors*), and drinks tea, in order to be rejuvenated. Belief that first three days postpartum should be on bed rest, avoid drafts, and not venture out during the night. One major practice is that of the three baths: special leaves are gathered and boiled to make a special water for hot bathing during the first three days postpartum, and the woman is encouraged to drink tea boiled from these same leaves. For the next three days, the mother bathes in a special water in which leaves have been soaked and warmed by the sun. About 1 month postpartum, the mother takes the third bath, a cold bath. The third bath enhances healing, tightens muscles and bones which have been loosened during delivery.

After childbirth, woman believed to be particularly susceptible to entry of gas (*gaz*) into the body. To prevent this, she must tighten her waist with a piece of linen or a belt. Procedure also important to tighten woman's bones loosened by birth of her child.

Food restrictions important in this phase and include not eating white food (i.e., milk, white lima beans, lobster, tomatoes, etc.), considered cold food. Eating cold food believed to increase vaginal discharge and/or hemorrhage. Acceptable foods include cornmeal mush or porridge, red bean sauce, rice and beans, and plantain.

Problems with baby

Maternal grandmother first person summoned if problems with child. Home remedies tried first.

Male and female circumcision

Females not circumcised. Male circumcision not encouraged. Believed that male circumcision decreases sexual satisfaction.

Mexican Americans

(dePaula, Lagana, Gonzalez-Ramirez, 1996)

Pregnancy care

Barriers to prenatal care include fear of health care system, financial constraints, and lack of transportation. Many women believe pregnancy not an illness and prenatal care unnecessary. Others seek prenatal care for reassurance of fetal well-being. Early and regular prenatal care usually associated with higher socioeconomic and educational levels and acculturation to Western health care belief system. Paradoxically, Mexican American women with late or no prenatal care experience have surprisingly healthy birth outcomes. Many women from lower socioeconomic levels attend clinics staffed by nurse practitioners, physicians or nurse midwives, with physicians and midwives supervising deliveries. Women with adequate financial resources generally choose obstetricians.

Familialism (strong attachment to nuclear and extended family) provides supportive and respectful environment for pregnant women. Women who are attentive mothers are highly respected. Expectant mothers discouraged from heavy work and harmful activities such as smoking, drinking, or drug use. Encouraged to frequently rest, walk, eat well, and get plenty of sleep. Finances permitting, less acculturated women readily relinquish other roles to insure health birth outcome. More acculturated women with outside jobs report more role conflict. Common for grandmothers to move into nuclear family homes during last weeks of pregnancy and for weeks following delivery (sometimes coming from great distances). Grandmothers or other female family members assume domestic roles and assist pregnant woman and new mother in health maintenance and restoration. Prenatal care has very broad meaning to Mexican American women, including informal home care from family members. Pregnant women protected from folk illnesses such as *Mal de ojo* (evil eye), *susto* (fright), and *antojois* (cravings). Often, folk medicine carried from Mexico by mothers and grandmothers and used within confines of extended family. This information usually not shared with practitioners. More acculturated women sometimes reluctantly report belief in these practices as unexplainable but effective.

Labor practices

Walking recommended to ensure quick birth. One folk belief is that inactivity will result in loss of amniotic fluid, causing fetus to stick (*se pega*) to uterus. Fear of unnecessary or dangerous medical interventions, separation from family members, and loss of physical privacy leads many women to labor at home for much of labor with supportive female family members, arriving at hospital in advanced labor. More acculturated women, especially those lacking labor support from experienced women, generally come to hospital earlier and rely on health care providers for labor support.

Role of the laboring woman during birth process

Historically, Mexican American woman portrayed as *la Sufrida*, a passive participant, expected to suffer in silence and deliver child to her husband. This is outmoded and stereotypical. Laboring women seen as strong and forebearing participants in natural a process. Family members usually reinforce this belief, helping woman through periods of fearfulness. Many Mexican American women supplement family support with childbirth classes, making them more informed and active participants.

Role of the father and other family members during birth process

Traditionally, men not present at delivery. Usually wait in another place. Sisters, mothers, mother-in-laws, or grandmothers assist and coach during labor. More acculturated couples attend childbirth preparation classes which encourage active participation of father. Except for father of baby, men not present during active labor and delivery, but may be part of large extended group of friends and family present during early labor. Important to support woman's preferences in labor assistants. Asking about this in private demonstrates sensitivity to concept of "*simpatia.*"

Vaginal vs. cesarean section

Normal spontaneous vaginal delivery preferred. Mexican American women fear unnecessary cesarean delivery, see surgery as life threatening.

Breastfeeding

Most women breastfeed. Formula promotion in Latin America has led some women to believe breastfeeding less nutritious.

Birth recuperation

Traditional 40-day period of recuperation, called *la cuarentena*. Women cared for by other women, but expected to care for newborn. Domestic chores taken on by female relatives or friends. New mothers discouraged from taking showers for several days, also discouraged from getting out of bed for first few hours after birth and then only to use bathroom. Light foods provided, including *caldo de pollo*, herbal teas, and *tortillas*. Beans avoided.

Life in U.S. rarely offers luxury of *la cuarentena*. Economic needs and separation from extended family lead many women to resume domestic or work activities within first two weeks. Some women feel *la cuarentena*, unduly restrictive and old-fashioned, but make efforts to comply to some degree as show of respect to women who assist.

Problems with baby
Traditionally, consultation with head of household expected, as felt that new mothers should be sheltered from worry. Maternal dietary restrictions protect newborn infant from illness or discomfort (e.g., chilies and beans). Family may need information on risks of dehydration (e.g., *Caida de Mollera* and diarrhea) and helpful Western medical interventions. Infants sometimes treated with herbal teas, such as *manzanilla* (chamomile) for colic.

Male and female circumcision
Circumcision in males or females not practiced in traditional Mexican American culture. However, male circumcision sometimes practiced by more acculturated families.

Puerto Ricans

(Juarbe, 1996)

Pregnancy care
Pregnancy is a time of indulgence for women in many families. All favors and wishes granted for well-being of woman and baby. Men behave with tolerance, understanding, and patience at women's preferences. Diet followed carefully. Exercise viewed as inappropriate, and lifting objects prohibited. Rest and plenty of sleep recommended. Nurses should encourage regular exercise and good nutrition rather than too much eating. Many women choose to refrain from *tener relaciones* (sexual intercourse) during and after the second trimester. Men often see this time as opportunity for extramarital sexual activities. With caution and sensitivity, nurses may ask men about this issue and educate men about STD and AIDS risks resulting from multiple sexual partners.

Labor practices
Hygiene and modesty highly respected during labor. Women prefer to have their body covered and not be examined frequently. Prefer bed position for labor. Prefer hospital environment with spouse or family member, mother or sister, present during labor.

Role of the laboring woman during birth process

Active and demanding role assumed. Loud or noisy expressions of pain socially acceptable and encouraged to cope with pain and discomfort. Pain medications desirable. Explain to mother about pain management choices, risks, and benefits.

Role of the father and other family members during birth process

Fathers assume passive, supportive role during labor. Young fathers prefer to attend birth classes to assist during labor. Others prefer not to be present during labor but wish to be informed frequently.

Vaginal vs. cesarean section

Vaginal delivery preferred. For some, cesarean section carries "weak woman" stigma. Discuss options and choices early in pregnancy and educate patient about birth process possibilities. Discourage view of "weak women" with patient and partner.

Breastfeeding

Need to assess for individual beliefs of patient due to generational changes and differences in cultural beliefs between rural and urban women. Women from rural areas may prefer breastfeeding for first year. Women who work outside home may use formula, breastfeeding, or both. Beans, starch products, and eggs avoided during breastfeeding; believed to give colic to infant. Provide education about nutrition, benefits from breastfeeding.

Birth recuperation

Assess support systems available for new mother and assist in using them. First meal after delivery should be homemade fresh chicken soup. Women encouraged to avoid wind, cold temperature, lifting heavy objects, and doing housework during the cuarentena (first 40 days after labor). Some do not wash their hair during this time. Good hygiene highly encouraged with plenty of soaps, body lotions, and light fragrances. Some women who work outside the home may experience great distress when not following some of these cultural values/norms. Assess for individual perceptions and dissatisfaction with working role and birth recuperation.

Problems with baby

Mother wants to be first to know of problem with baby. If information provided by nurses, new mom might ask to talk to pediatrician at once.

Male and female circumcision

Male circumcision traditionally done at birth. Provide information and choices to family before birth. Some rural or traditional families prefer not to circumcise child for fear of causing pain, bleeding, or harm to infant. Female circumcision never performed.

Russians

(Evanikoff, 1996)

Pregnancy care

With some patients, prenatal care not expected unless pregnant mother feels something is wrong. Pregnant women protected from bad news, believed potentially harmful to fetus. Pregnant mother can work outside home until last trimester. During whole course of pregnancy, mother discouraged from lifting any heavy objects, such as chairs or boxes. Also discouraged from performing heavy exercise, such as jumping or jogging. Believed that these activities may harm fetus: umbilical cord may become wrapped around baby and the baby may choke or baby may move to breech position or become past due.

Labor practices

When pregnant mother senses time of delivery is near, she is encouraged to drink castor oil (although practice slowly fading) or is given an enema for easier birth. If M.D. not available, then midwife can assist with delivery. Mother highly encouraged to walk when contractions begin, to promote dilatation. During traditional births, mother discouraged from taking any pain medication during labor for fear of harm to baby or herself (e.g., epidurals), but some may want it. Stimulation and lighting in birthing room should be minimal. Believed that newborn's eyes are not yet strong or mature enough, and too much light will cause baby to develop poor eyesight.

Role of the laboring woman during birth process

Russian women generally assume passive role during birthing process; follow commands of doctor or midwife. Depending on individual, Russian mothers generally are not very loud when giving birth.

Role of the father and other family members during birth process

Traditionally, father plays passive role; is not allowed in birthing room. Only closest female family member allowed, such as maternal mother, sister, or mother-in-law (whoever is available at time), but may vary, depending on level of acculturation.

Vaginal vs. cesarean section

Vaginal delivery highly preferred over cesarean. In Russia, if baby in breech position, all possible measures taken by physician to ensure vaginal delivery.

Breastfeeding

Breastfeeding an expectation of all Russian mothers until milk "runs out" (even to toddler years). Russian mothers know importance of breastfeeding, such as health benefits and immunological properties that can be passed to baby. Russian mothers' partners support and encourage breastfeeding. In Russia, even societal support for breastfeeding is given. Employers provide child care at work site, and average maternity leave is about 25 months. Important for breastfeeding mother to be at peace. Believed that baby may become "hyper" later in life if there is too much noise or stimulation or if mother is nervous when breastfeeding. If breastfeeding mother suddenly shocked or scared for any reason, first breast milk should be expelled before feeding baby again. This milk considered unhealthy, and may cause baby to develop diarrhea. Russian mothers breastfeed in dim light to save baby's eyesight. When breastfeeding, breasts should be kept warm at all times, such as dressing warmly; believed to prevent mother from developing breast cancer later in life.

Birth recuperation

Traditional practices are 15 days of bedrest. Cooking and other various household chores done by mother's mother or other appropriate person for up to 40 days. During these 40 days, new mother should remain at home and not go outside. Believed that new mother's internal organs should heal and return to their pre-pregnant position during birth recuperation to prevent future physical problems. Traditionally, new mother wears pelvic binder to regain her figure. Peri care with warm water important.

Problems with baby

If problem with baby, first notify mother of baby; she may not want anyone else to know.

Important to keep baby warm at all times to keep baby's bones developing normally and to prevent illnesses. Baby's head should always be covered when exposed to cold, wind, or very hot sun.

Male and female circumcision

In general, Russian Christian parents do not believe in male circumcision. Some Jewish parents prefer male circumcision. Discuss with parents. Female circumcision never preformed.

References

Cantos, A. & Rivera, E. (1996). Filipinos. In J. Lipson, S. Dibble, & P. Minarik (Eds.), <u>Culture & nursing care: A pocket guide (pp. 115-125). San Francisco: The Regents, University of California.</u>

Colin, J.M., & Paperwalla, G. (1996). Haitians. In J. Lipson, S. Dibble, & P. Minarik (Eds.), <u>Culture & nursing care: A pocket guide</u> (pp. 139-154). San Francisco: The REgents, University of California.

APPENDIX D • CULTURALLY COMPETENT CAREGIVING TOOLS

de Paula, T., Lagana, K., & Gonzalez-Ramirez, L. (1996). Mexican Americans. In J. Lipson, S. Dibble, & P. Minarik (Eds.), <u>Culture & nursing care: A pocket guide</u> (pp. 203-221). San Francisco: The Regents, University of California.

Evanikoff, L. J. (1996). Russians. In J. Lipson, S. Dibble, & P. Minarik (Eds.), <u>Culture & nursing care: A pocket guide</u> (pp. 239-249). San Francisco: The Regents, University of California.

Juarbe, T. (1996). Puerto Ricans. In J. Lipson, S. Dibble, & P. Minarik (Eds.), <u>Culture & nursing care: A pocket guide</u> (pp. 222-238). San Francisco: The Regents, University of California.

CULTURALLY SENSITIVE CAREGIVING

Instructions: Circle all correct responses for each question:

1. Which of the following are appropriate definitions of the term "race"?

    A. Genetic linkage among individuals of the same nationality.
    B. An inbreeding group of individuals with a specific geographic locus.
    C. A legal-cultural issue based on cultural-behavioral patterns.
    D. Presence of physical similarities in a group of persons who also share similar values.

2. Ethnocentric means that:

    A. An individual is xenophobic.
    B. One believes one's own cultural ways are superior to others.
    C. Assimilation into another culture is not possible.
    D. One is unable to relate to persons of a different ethnic background.

3. The caregiver's own cultural values and beliefs can provide a basis for accepting different lifeways if the caregiver has:

    A. An opportunity to learn about different cultural backgrounds.
    B. A questioning attitude.
    C. Developed self-awareness of his/her own beliefs, values and practices.
    D. Considered the world from the perspective of those in different ethnic groups.

4. Education may fail to help an individual to understand health conditions because:

    A. Ideas learned in early childhood often take precedence over facts.
    B. It is often difficult for patients to trust those who think differently.
    C. A strong faith in a belief opposed to a scientific theory will probably predominate.
    D. The patient has the right to make decisions only when educated on his/her concerns.

5. The nurse should be aware of which of the following potential barriers to seeking health care? The pregnant woman's:

    A. Lack of knowledge of the body and how it functions.
    B. Fear of surgery, especially a cesarean birth.
    C. Belief that pregnancy is normal and valuing of the natural course of events.
    D. Need to remain in complete control, avoiding episodes of loss of consciousness.

APPENDIX D • CULTURALLY COMPETENT CAREGIVING TOOLS

6. An initial cultural assessment includes which of the following major components?

   A. Patient's feelings about death.
   B. Religion.
   C. Treatment expectations.
   D. Norms of etiquette.

7. Which of the following are ways to prepare for giving culturally sensitive care to child-bearing families?

   A. Take courses in transcultural nursing.
   B. Learn a foreign language.
   C. Work with a mentor experienced in ethnic care.
   D. Avoid situations resulting in culture shock.

8. The term "ethnic" means:

   A. The totality of all the person is and does, including cultural values and beliefs.
   B. An individual's nationality and assimilated cultural practices.
   C. The extended family's genetic characteristics as evidenced by race and cultural lifeways.
   D. A group of people of the same race sharing common and distinctive cultural characteristics.

9. Acculturation can best be defined as:

   A. The process in which an ethnic group takes on some of the cultural ways of the dominant ethnic group in the society.
   B. The inability to see one's own or another's values, due to ethnocentricity.
   C. The practice of forcing one's own beliefs and practices on another.
   D. The acclimation of a culturally specific group to an environment that is not culturally sensitive.

10. Which of the following are likely to occur when the nurse and patient are culturally different?

    A. Anxiety.
    B. Conflict of values.
    C. Cultural shock.
    D. Cultural relativity.

11. Which of the following aspects of care vary significantly from culture to culture?

    A. Response to suffering.
    B. Definition of the sick role.
    C. Willingness to express needs.
    D. Rules of personal hygiene.

12. The nurse must be sensitive to ethnic customs and practices to prevent which of the following barriers to health care?

    A. Language problems resulting in embarrassing or frustrating situations.
    B. Belief that older children will inadvertently be exposed to disease in the health care facility.
    C. Differences in schedules and time values causing missed appointments.
    D. Expectation that pain is endured in silence, causing delays in seeking medical care.

13. Which of the following are examples of maintaining balance in various cultures?

    A. Maintaining harmony of body, mind, and spirit.
    B. Eating a prescribed combination of hot and cold foods.
    C. Following rules about keeping warm and dry after birth.
    D. Using Yin and Yang.

14. A cultural assessment includes obtaining information on:

    A. Whether the patient sees the condition as good or bad.
    B. What the person is doing for the presenting condition.
    C. What family and friends do for this condition.
    D. Style of communication appropriate to the culture.

15. Which of the following guidelines are beneficial for culture-specific caregiving?

    A. Use a straightforward, direct approach.
    B. Avoid pointing out when the individual is wrong.
    C. Incorporate customs into care plans.
    D. Teach patients in a one-to-one situation.

16. Goals of ethical, culturally sensitive care include:

    A. Maintain as many of the cultural ways as possible.
    B. Categorize patients based on culture-specific assessments.
    C. Make accommodations as necessary so customs can be continued.
    D. Restructure only those practices harmful to the person's health.

APPENDIX D • CULTURALLY COMPETENT CAREGIVING TOOLS

ANSWERS:

1. B

2. B.

3. A,B,C,D

4. A,B,C

5. A,B,C

6. B,C,D

7. A,B,C

8. D

9. A

10. A,B,C,

11. A,B,C,D

12. A,C,D

13. A,B,C,D

14. A,B,C,D

15. B,C,D

16. A,C,D

Source: Ramer, L. (1992). <u>Culturally Sensitive Caregiving and Childbearing Families</u>, White Plains, New York: March of Dimes Birth Defects Foundation.

Age Specific, Neonate
Clinical: Professional

AGE SPECIFIC, NEONATE
Clinical: Professional

CRITICAL ELEMENTS	MET	NOT MET
1. Introduce self to parents.		
2. Insure infant warmth due to immature heat regulations.		
3. Involve parents in care by explaining treatments.		
4. Provide protective environment and keep rails up after completing therapy.		
5. Handle gently and with care.		
6. Use equipment and parameters specific to size of neonate.		
7. Involve the parent(s) in education and planning for outpatients.		
8. Cuddle and hug as appropriate.		
9. Use distraction (pacifier and bottle).		
10. Follow department standards regarding venous heal sticks or venipunctures.		
11. Prepare medication is based on weight, or standards specified in department standards for neonates.		

[ ] PASSED   [ ] NEEDS TO REPEAT

VALIDATED BY: _____   DATE: _____

APPENDIX E • AGE-SPECIFIC CARE–COMPETENCE ASSESSMENT TOOLS

Age Specific, Adolescent
Clinical: Professional

AGE SPECIFIC, ADOLESCENT
Clinical: Professional

CRITICAL ELEMENTS	MET	NOT MET
1. Introduce self to parents and adolescent.		
2. Explain procedures to adolescent and parents in accurate and familiar terms.		
3. Encourage questions and expression of "fears".		
4. Explain all procedures and use of equipment.		
5. Provide for privacy.		
6. Involve in the decision making and planning of all aspects of care.		
7. Allow for and use relaxation techniques during procedures (asks for adolescent input).		
8. See independence as a need and encourage it as able to increase involvement and compliance.		
9. Allow adolescent to have as much control as can be safely given.		
10. Allow for elimination needs in planning care and procedures.		
11. Use equipment and parameters specific to size and age of adolescent, as defined in unit standards.		
12. Provide for communication based on individual disability or if normal channels are unavailable.		
13. Involve adolescent in food selections as able.		
14. Involve adolescent and parents as appropriate in all education.		
15. Provide discharge plan that is patient centered and include understanding of patient's home physical environment, as well as physical and emotional needs.		
16. Provide information regarding community services to parents and adolescent as requested or needed.		
17. Demonstrate accurate medication preparation and administration based on weight, age or unit standards.		

[ ] PASSED [ ] NEEDS TO REPEAT

VALIDATED BY: _____ DATE: _____

APPENDIX E • AGE-SPECIFIC CARE–COMPETENCE ASSESSMENT TOOLS

Age Specific, Adult
Clinical: Professional

AGE SPECIFIC, ADULT
Clinical: Professional

CRITICAL ELEMENTS	MET	NOT MET
1. Introduce self to patient and significant other(s).		
2. Provide education to patient and./or significant other based on learner's needs and readiness.		
3. Explain all procedures and the use of all equipment.		
4. Provide for mobility of patient.		
5. Provide privacy and insure confidentiality as able.		
6. Provides information on community support services.		
7. Promote and encourage patient decision making and planning of treatments and cares.		
8. Use equipment that is specific for size of adult.		
9. Provide discharge plan that is patient centered and include understanding of patient's home physical environment, as well as physical and emotional needs.		
10. Discharge plans may include having functional needs met for patient to return home/work.		
11. Demonstrate cultural and religious sensitivity in providing cares and seek to provide for special requests.		
12. Allows for elimination needs in planning cares and procedures.		
13. Identify mutual goals as able following assessment of physical, functional, emotional, and spiritual assessment.		
14. Provide for communication needs if normal channels are unavailable or patient unable.		
15. Incorporate social activities and financial needs in discharge plans.		

[ ] PASSED   [ ] NEEDS TO REPEAT

VALIDATED BY: _____ DATE: _____

APPENDIX E • AGE-SPECIFIC CARE–COMPETENCE ASSESSMENT TOOLS

Age Specific, Geriatirc
Clinical: Professional

AGE SPECIFIC, GERIATRIC
Clinical: Professional

CRITICAL ELEMENTS	MET	NOT MET
1. Introduce self to patient and significant other(s).		
2. Provide information based on assessment of learning ability/disability.		
3. Slow pace of learning activity to accommodate changes in how learning takes place in the older adult.		
4. Take frequent breaks, as needed due to fatigue and decreased muscle tone.		
5. Change positions slowly due to interactive physical changes of aging.		
6. Allow for bathroom breaks.		
7. Ensure proper room temperature due to decreased heat regulation.		
8. Perform procedures with caution due to fragile nature of skin.		
9. Provide for safety as determined by assessment of individual and surrounding environment.		
10. Use equipment that is parameter specific to size and age of geriatric patient.		
11. Involve patient/significant others in all decisions (as able) regarding cares.		
12. Assess patient self-care abilities and plan accordingly.		
13. Speak clearly, slowly and directly at patient to assist in patient's ability to discriminate sounds.		
14. Ensure adequate room lighting without causing excessive shadows or glare.		
15. Involve family members (significant others) in discharge planning and instructions.		
16. Provide for communication of needs if normal channels are bypassed.		
17. Demonstrate accurate preparation and distribution of medications based on patient's ability to swallow and his physical condition. Determine collaboratively alternative routes and medications if unable to tolerate medication route originally ordered.		

[ ] PASSED [ ] NEEDS TO REPEAT

VALIDATED BY: _____ DATE: _____

HealthEast Competency Program

AGE SPECIFIC CONSIDERATION RESOURCE PACKET

CREATED BY:
Bette-Jo Taylor, BSN, RNC, HealthEast Clinical Competency Project Manager
Dannelle Paulson, BSN, CCRN, HealthEast Life Support Coordinator
Donna Wilken, MA, RN, HealthEast Patient Education Specialist
Cindy O'Donovan, HealthEast Human Resources Special Projects

Copyrighted by HealthEast, September 1997
Bette-Jo Taylor, RNC, BSN
HealthEast Competency Project Manager
River Heights Professional Building, Suite 219
710 19th Ave. No., South St. Paul, MN 55075
1-612-232-6432

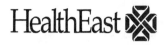

AGE SPECIFIC CONSIDERATION RESOURCE PACKET

CONTENTS:

Samples of HealthEast's
1. Algorithm for determining need of age specific validation tool
2. Checklist for compliance with age specific validation
   (includes how to tailor generic age specific validation tool for specific positions)
3. Generic Age Specific Validation Tool
   (Self-assessment, return demonstration, post-test)
4. Answer Key to Post-test
   (was only given to validators after they had been validated)
5. Age Specific Awareness Tool

NOTE: *Ongoing Education is very important. Here are a few resources we have found helpful.*

1. Growing Up With Us..., Inc., Mary Dunlap, 1-919-489-1238
2. Elderly Update, Pat Gault, 1-888-267-4833 Code #3037

BIBLIOGRAPHY:

1. Human Resources Management : Staff Education, Training , and Competency Appraisal for Hospitals,
2. Age Specific Competencies: Strategies for Implementation, Nursing Staff Development Insider, Volume 4, Issue 3, Pamela Brown-Stewart, RN, MSN, CCRN, May/June 1995
3. Age-Specific Criteria-Based Performance Appraisal, Briefings on JCAHO, February 1996
4. Type I of the Month: Age-Specific Competencies, Briefings on JCAHO, October 1996
5. A Framework for Assessing Age-Related Competency, National Nursing Staff Development Organization, 1996 Annual Convention
6. Management of Human Resources: The Organizational Approach to Education, Training, and Measurement of Current Competency, JOINT COMMISSION on Accreditation of Health Care Organizations, Education Program, 1996
7. Meeting JCAHO Standards: A Manual for HR Managers in Health Care, American Society for Health Care, Human Resources Administration, American Hospital Association, 1996
8. Age Specific Competencies; The Human Resources Challenge, JCAHO Workshop Handbook, 1996
9. Management of Human Resources in Hospitals and Examples of Compliance, 1997 Joint Commission in Accreditation of HealthCare Organizations

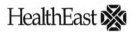

ALGORITHM FOR DETERMINING NEED OF AGE SPECIFIC VALIDATION TOOL

Answer yes or no to the following questions.

1. Do you or your area/s of responsibility provide direct patient/client care?

    Example: Physical therapist

2. Do you or your area/s of responsibility have patient/client contact?

    Example: Housekeeping

3. Do you or your area/s of responsibility work in areas where they may interact with patients/clients?

    Example: Painters

4. Do the services you or your areas of responsibility change or vary in anyway because of the age of a patient/client?

    Example: Pharmacy

IF YOU ANSWERED YES TO ANY OF THESE QUESTIONS, YOU NEED TO READ AND COMPLETE THE REST OF THIS PACKET.

IF YOU ANSWERED NO TO ALL OF THESE QUESTIONS, PLEASE MAKE SURE THIS ALGORITHM IS RETURNED TO CINDY O'DONOVAN, RIVER HEIGHTS, SUITE 314.

Manager_____   Dept/Work site_____

SBU_____   Phone number _____

APPENDIX E • AGE-SPECIFIC CARE–COMPETENCE ASSESSMENT TOOLS

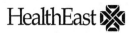

CHECKLIST FOR COMPLIANCE WITH AGE SPECIFIC VALIDATION

_____ 1. Review the attached validation tool and awareness tool.

_____ 2. Fill in the work area on the Validation tool and check each age category that applies for that work area. Make multiple copies if you manage multiple areas with different expectations.

_____ 3. Optional Step -- Fill in the Position Title for each position you supervise that need age specific competency assessment and identify what aspects of care are not applicable. If you do not do this step, you will need to review it carefully for accuracy after your staff has completed it.

_____ 4. Identify Department/Service/Unit specific policies or resources you have that you want your staff to be familiar with.

_____ 5. Complete the validation for yourself. You may chose to validate all of your staff, or you may identify select staff that you will validate and than have them validate everyone else. The individual/s validating others should be instructed to date and initial the appropriate boxes for completing learning module, discussed or review policy, performed independently, etc. The validator must check the answers on the post-test/s and provide feedback to the individual. The validator/s must sign the "validator" line on the bottom of the first page. If you delegate this to someone else, you must also sign the "Manager" line on the bottom of the first page of the validation tool after reviewing for completeness.

_____ 6. Make copies of the validation and awareness tools to distribute to all of your staff as appropriate.

_____ 7. Keep an attendance record of all staff completing the age specific validation.

_____ 8. Add Age Specific Validation to your 96/97 Mandatory Education Record and document date of completion.

_____ 9. Each staff person, should also record this on their Individual Education Record.

_____ 10. File the completed validation tools in the individual records on the unit.

_____ 11. When your staff has reached 100% compliance, file a copy of the attendance sheets in the usual manner and forward a copy to Cindy O'Donovan at Midway Hospital, 7th Floor.

Checklist for Compliance with Age Specific Validation
Page 2

_____ 12. By no later than June 1, 1997 you should have completed the validation process for **ALL** staff. This information should be recorded on your Mandatory Education Records and a copy forwarded to your site educator or the individual responsible for tracking facility/service compliance.

_____ 13. Remember to include this in all of your new employee's orientations.

NOTE: As the CBO/E process is completed each team will need to address more specific needs and resources to address the age specific issue, but this is where we will start for 1997.

NOTE: Resources may include: Age Specific Awareness Tool, HENSA Policies, HEPN Policies, Unit/Service Line Policies, Procedure cards, Learning Modules, Standards of Care, The HELP Program, Operation Manuals, etc.

APPENDIX E • AGE-SPECIFIC CARE–COMPETENCE ASSESSMENT TOOLS

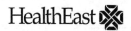

1/16/97

AGE SPECIFIC VALIDATION TOOL

NAME:_____ POSITION TITLE: Staff RN   SITE:_____

DIRECTIONS: It is required that **ALL** staff members who assess, treat, and otherwise manage OR work in areas that directly impact on patients must validate that they have the appropriate skills for providing care based on physical, psychosocial, educational, safety, and related criteria appropriate to the age of the patient.

1. Complete self-assessment.

2. Review HealthEast and unit learning resources and policies.

3. If you indicate you routinely perform this independently:
   Your manager or staff person who has been previously validated, needs to document observation of your successful ability to perform independently and you must correctly answer the post-test questions.

   If you RARELY care for this age group:
   You need to review the awareness tool/learning resources and successfully answer the post-test questions.

   If you NEVER and would never be expected to care for this age group of patients/ clients you do not need to do anything except check the "Have no interaction".

   If you provide care for the specified age group, but not the aspect of care identified, write "NA" for not applicable in the self-assessment column.

   If you are unable to correctly answer the post-test questions as appropriate for your job responsibilities, review the Age Specific Awareness tool and retake the post-test.

4. Your manager or designated staff need to verify that the self assessment accurately reflects the care you are expected to provide and that the expectations are met. (Signature at bottom of validation tool)

5. Sign the bottom employee signature block.

6. Return this completed validation tool to your manager for their review, signature and tracking.

Age categories in the scope of care for __Maternity Care__ (work area) are:
   _x_ 1. Neonates (0-29 days of age)
   ____ 2. Pediatrics (30 days to 14 years)
   _x_ 3. Adolescent (14 to 18 years)
   _x_ 4. Adult (19 to 70 years)
   ____ 5. Geriatric (71 years and older)

APPENDIX E • AGE-SPECIFIC CARE–COMPETENCE ASSESSMENT TOOLS

POSITION COMPETENCIES		SELF-ASSESSMENT			EXPECTATIONS/ ACTION PLAN					COMMENTS/ RESOURCES
		Routinely Perform Independently	Occasional Interaction/ Perform Independently	Need Review	Class or Learning Module	Discussed Information or Reviewed Policy	Assisted or Observed	Return Demonstration	Performed Independently	
___ HAVE NO INTERACTION WITH NEONATES										
1. Neonates (0-29 days of age)										Age Specific Awareness Tool
	a. Communication: Uses appropriate Language, includes parents/family/ significant other as appropriate.									
	b. Diagnostic testing: Recognizes and implements differences needed for testing based on age specifications.									
	c. Medication prep and administration: Provides proper dosages, uses the appropriate route, and is alert to response of medication that may vary depending on age.									HealthEast Pharmacy and Nursing Policy Book
	d. Equipment: Recognizes and safely uses various equipment as appropriate for age specifications.									Operation Manual
	e. Psycho-social: Provides appropriate emotional support, encourages questions and answers questions appropriately for age, encourages family support.									
	f. Growth and Development: Demonstrates understanding and adjusts cares to growth and development needs.									
	g. Appropriate food/nutrition needs: Demonstrates understanding of needs, provides foods that meet those needs, prepares foods so they can be easily ingested and digested taking into account personal preferences and age considerations.									
	h. Physical assessment: Demonstrates knowledge of physical assessment differences and norms for age and incorporates that information in the plan of care.									
	I. Education: Demonstrates understanding of the process of patient/client education. Provides education in a manner that accounts for age specific needs.									

NEONATE POST TEST

1. A neonate breaths only through it's _____.

2. Physical assessment of the healthy neonate includes:

    ____ a. fontanels closed

    ____ b. fontanels sunken

    ____ c. fontanels soft, but not sunken or bulging

3. Education should be directed at _____.

4. True or False (Circle)

    A bulb syringe should always be readily available in case there is a need for suctioning.

5. True or False (Circle)

    Infant weight is required to determine proper dosages of medications.

APPENDIX E • AGE-SPECIFIC CARE–COMPETENCE ASSESSMENT TOOLS

POSITION COMPETENCIES	SELF-ASSESSMENT			EXPECTATIONS/ ACTION PLAN					COMMENTS/ RESOURCES
	Routinely Perform Independently	Occasional Interaction/ Perform Independently	Need Review	Class or Learning Module	Discussed Information or Reviewed Policy	Assisted or Observed	Return Demonstration	Performed Independently	
____ HAVE NO INTERACTION WITH ADOLESCENTS									
1. Adolescent (14-18 years)									Age Specific Awareness Tool
a. Communication: Uses appropriate Language, includes parents/family/ significant other as appropriate.									
b. Diagnostic testing: Recognizes and implements differences needed for testing based on age specifications.									
c. Medication prep and administration: Provides proper dosages, uses the appropriate route, and is alert to response of medication that may vary depending on age.									HealthEast Pharmacy and Nursing Policy Book
d. Equipment: Recognizes and safely uses various equipment as appropriate for age specifications.									Operation Manual
e. Psycho-social: Provides appropriate emotional support, encourages questions and answers questions appropriately for age, encourages family support.									
f. Growth and Development: Demonstrates understanding and adjusts cares to growth and development needs.									
g. Appropriate food/nutrition needs: Demonstrates understanding of needs, provides foods that meet those needs, prepares foods so they can be easily ingested and digested taking into account personal preferences and age considerations.									
h. Physical assessment: Demonstrates knowledge of physical assessment differences and norms for age and incorporates that information in the plan of care.									
I. Education: Demonstrates understanding of the process of patient/client education. Provides education in a manner that accounts for age specific needs.									

APPENDIX E • AGE-SPECIFIC CARE–COMPETENCE ASSESSMENT TOOLS

ADOLESCENT POST TEST

1. True or False (Circle)

   An adolescent patient/client's physical assessment norms will be more consistent with the adult, with the exception of rapid growth and maturation of the reproductive system and sexual characteristics.

2. True or False (Circle)

   An adolescent is often critical of their own features and their identity may be threatened by hospitalization.

3. True or False (Circle)

   When it is possible, the plan of care should allow the teenager to make as many choices as possible. When it is not possible, it is important to explain why.

4. True or False (Circle)

   Adolescents have unlimited amounts of energy and do not require much sleep.

5. Education should **NOT** include:

   ____ a. parent/caregiver, but focus on the adolescent.

   ____ b. technical information and rationales.

   ____ c. information about immediate benefits and consequences.

   ____ d. minimizing concerns as not important.

APPENDIX E • AGE-SPECIFIC CARE–COMPETENCE ASSESSMENT TOOLS

POSITION COMPETENCIES	SELF-ASSESSMENT			EXPECTATIONS/ ACTION PLAN					COMMENTS/ RESOURCES
____ HAVE NO INTERACTION WITH ADULTS	Routinely Perform Independently	Occasional Interaction/ Perform Independently	Need Review	Class or Learning Module	Discussed Information or Reviewed Policy	Assisted or Observed	Return Demonstration	Performed Independently	
1. **Adults (19-70 years)**									Age Specific Awareness Tool
a. Communication: Uses appropriate Language, includes parents/family/ significant other as appropriate.									
b. Diagnostic testing: Recognizes and implements differences needed for testing based on age specifications.									
c. Medication prep and administration: Provides proper dosages, uses the appropriate route, and is alert to response of medication that may vary depending on age.									HealthEast Pharmacy and Nursing Policy Book
d. Equipment: Recognizes and safely uses various equipment as appropriate for age specifications.									Operation Manual
e. Psycho-social: Provides appropriate emotional support, encourages questions and answers questions appropriately for age, encourages family support.									
f. Growth and Development: Demonstrates understanding and adjusts cares to growth and development needs.									
g. Appropriate food/nutrition needs: Demonstrates understanding of needs, provides foods that meet those needs, prepares foods so they can be easily ingested and digested taking into account personal preferences and age considerations.									
h. Physical assessment: Demonstrates knowledge of physical assessment differences and norms for age and incorporates that information in the plan of care.									
I. Education: Demonstrates understanding of the process of patient/client education. Provides education in a manner that accounts for age specific needs.									

APPENDIX E • AGE-SPECIFIC CARE–COMPETENCE ASSESSMENT TOOLS

ADULT POST TEST

1. True or False (Circle)

   Muscular efficiency, skeletal growth, and GI system are at their peak between 20 to 30 years of age.

2. True or False (Circle)

   An adult is more achievement oriented; working up the career ladder, is moving from dependency to responsibility (increasing responsibility for children and parents.

3. True or False (Circle)

   When it is possible, the plan of care should allow the adult to make as many choices as possible.

4. True or False (Circle)

   Adults have no need for patient education, they already know everything or they will ask for any information they need.

5. True or False (Circle)

   Mid-life crisis is only an excuse to behave unresponsibly.

ANSWERS FOR POST TEST QUESTIONS

NEONATE

1. Nose.
2. C.
3. The parents.
4. True
5. True

ADOLESCENT

1. True
2. True
3. True
4. False (Adolescents require extra sleep, due to their rapid growth.)
5. D.

ADULT

1. True
2. True
3. True
4. False (Adults need patient education and to be encouraged to ask questions.)
5. False (Mid-Life crisis is real and may require emotional support.)

APPENDIX E • AGE-SPECIFIC CARE–COMPETENCE ASSESSMENT TOOLS

HealthEast — Age-Specific Awareness Tool

PHYSICAL	MOTOR/SENSORY ADAPTATION	COGNITIVE	PSYCHOSOCIAL	INTERVENTIONS
♦ Neonates temperature stabilizes within four hours after birth ♦ Heart rate often irregular, murmur may be present. Femoral pulses readily palpable. ♦ Obligate nose-breathers. ♦ Temperature: 97.9° - 98.6° F ♦ HR: apical = 120 – 140 beats/min. Listen one full minute. ♦ Respirations: 30-60 breaths/min. ♦ BP: Weight Systolic Diastolic 3 kg 60-80 35-55 2-3 kg 50-70 27-45 1-2 kg 40-60 20-35	♦ Mature newborns demonstrate general neuromuscular function by moving their extremities and attempting head control. ♦ Occasional twitching or flailing movements is normal. ♦ Cry tearlessly. ♦ Limpness or total absence of muscular response is _never_ normal. ♦ Responds to light (blink reflex). ♦ Responds to sound (moro reflex). ♦ Will grasp an object placed in their palm (palmar grasp reflex). ♦ When cheek touched, child will turn head in that direction (rooting reflex). ♦ When lips touched, baby makes a sucking motion. ♦ When sole of foot at base of toes touched, the toes grasp in the same manner as fingers do. ♦ When on their backs, the baby head usually turns to one side or the other. The arm and leg on the side to which the head is turned extends, and the opposite arm and leg contract (tonic neck reflex).	♦ Recognize mothers voice ♦ Response to odors ♦ Focus best on black and white objects at a distance of 9-12 inches **Patient/Family Education:** ♦ Aimed at parents.	♦ A newborn usually responds to being held closely by cuddling. ♦ Significant persons are the parents or primary caregivers.	♦ Involve parents in procedures. Encourage parents to assist with care. ♦ Keep parent in infant's line of vision. ♦ Limit the number of caregivers caring for the infant. Limit time of treatment. ♦ Minimize noise. ♦ Keep newborn warm. Undress only the body part being examined. ♦ Have bulb syringe available in case there is a need for suctioning. ♦ Keep crib siderails up at all times. ♦ Cuddle and hug the infant. ♦ Make sure toys are age appropriate. No removable parts and check for safety approval. ♦ Assess for and provide support in managing pain. ♦ Assess respiratory rate and heart rate before infant cries; then follow head-to-toe procedure.

INFANCY: Birth to 29 Days

Every minority and non-minority group has unique characteristics based on common values, beliefs, practices, race ethnicity country or origin and language.
Care givers need to acquire a basic understanding of their patients culture and background and give the time and attention needed to ensure accurate and smooth communication.

APPENDIX E • AGE-SPECIFIC CARE–COMPETENCE ASSESSMENT TOOLS

HealthEast — Age-Specific Awareness Tool

PHYSICAL	MOTOR/SENSORY ADAPTATION	COGNITIVE	PSYCHOSOCIAL	INTERVENTIONS
◆ Gains weight/height rapidly (doubles weight/height by 50% in six months). ◆ Starts as a nose breather (2-4 months). ◆ Towards the end of the first year: - Primitive reflexes diminish - Fontanel closes, anterior 12-18 months; posterior 2 months. - Regular bladder and bowel pattern develops. ◆ Temperature: 99.4° - 99.7° F ◆ HR: apical = 110-130 beats/min. ◆ Respirations: 30-40 breaths/min. ◆ BP = 95 - 110 mmHg systolic and 50 - 60 mmHg diastolic.	◆ Brings hand to mouth. ◆ Responds to light and sound. ◆ Towards the middle of the year, progresses to raising head, turning, rolling over, and bringing hand to mouth. ◆ Towards the end of the year, progresses to crawling, standing alone, walking with assistance and grasping strongly. ◆ Repeats actions to fine tune learning. ◆ Begins to develop a sense of object permanence. ◆ Reactions move from reflexive to intentional.	◆ Manipulates objects in the environment. ◆ Recognizes bright objects and progresses to recognizing familiar objects and persons. ◆ Towards the end of the year, speaks two words, mimics sounds. ◆ Obeys simple commands and understands meaning of several words. ◆ Seeks novel experiences. ◆ Learns by imitation. **Patient/Family Education:** ◆ Assess both parent and child for learning needs. Teaching is aimed at parents. ◆ Tell child why, and what to expect. ◆ Be positive and honest. ◆ Use language consistent with what child's family uses. ◆ Children cannot imagine what they have not experienced - explain what the child will taste, hear, see, feel and touch.	◆ Significant persons are the parents or primary caregivers. ◆ Develops a sense of trust and security if needs are met consistently and with a degree of predictability. ◆ Fears unfamiliar situations. Copes by using self-comforting measures. ◆ Smiles, repeats actions that elicit response from others, i.e., waves goodbye, plays pat-a-cake. ◆ Seven to eight months: fear of strangers. ◆ Nine to ten months: separation anxiety.	◆ Involve parents to assist with care and/or in procedures. ◆ Keep parent in infant's line of vision. ◆ Limit the number of caregivers caring for the infant. Limit time of treatment. ◆ Give familiar objects to the infant. ◆ Cuddle and hug the infant. ◆ Minimize noise. ◆ Use distraction (pacifier, bottle, tongue blade, etc.). ◆ Keep crib siderails up at all times. ◆ Make sure toys are age appropriate. No removable parts and check for safety approval. ◆ Have bulb syringe available in case there is a need for suctioning. ◆ Ask parents about immunization history. ◆ Assess for and provide support in managing pain. ◆ Begin examination with heart rate and respiratory assessment; then head-to-toe.

PEDIATRIC: 30 Days to 14 Years
(Infant: 1 month to 1 year)

Every minority and non-minority group has unique characteristics based on common values, beliefs, practices, race ethnicity country or origin and language.
Care givers need to acquire a basic understanding of their patients culture and background and give the time and attention needed to ensure accurate and smooth communication.

APPENDIX E • AGE-SPECIFIC CARE–COMPETENCE ASSESSMENT TOOLS

HealthEast

Age-Specific Awareness Tool

PHYSICAL	MOTOR/SENSORY ADAPTATION	COGNITIVE	PSYCHOSOCIAL	INTERVENTIONS
◆ Learning bladder and bowel control. ◆ Abdomen protrudes. ◆ Decreased appetite and growth. ◆ Temporary teeth erupt; all 20 deciduous teeth by 2 ½ - 3 years. ◆ Grows 2 - 2 ½ inches and 4 - 6 lbs. yearly. ◆ Elimination: 18 months bowel control; 2 - 3 years daytime bladder control. ◆ Temperature = 99° F ◆ Pulse = 90 - 140 min. ◆ Respirations = 20 - 35/min. ◆ BP = 80 - 100 mmHg systolic and 50 - 80 mmHg diastolic.	◆ Responds better to visual rather than spoken cues. ◆ Walks independently, progressing to running, jumping and climbing. ◆ Feeds self. ◆ Loves to experiment. ◆ Fully formed sense of object permanence. ◆ Body language and actions match. **Patient/Family Education:** ◆ Assess both parent and child for learning needs. Teaching is aimed at parents. ◆ Tell child why, and what to expect. ◆ Be positive and honest. ◆ Use language consistent with what child's family uses. ◆ Children cannot imagine what they have not experienced - explain what the child will taste, hear, see, feel and touch. ◆ Explain procedure to child shortly before it happens. ◆ Some children think they are being punished - they need reassurance that it was nothing they did.	◆ Develops concepts by use of language. Constructs 3 - 4 word sentences. ◆ Sees things only from own point of view (egocentric). ◆ Able to group similar items. ◆ Has a short attention span. Beginning memory. ◆ Ties words to actions, can understand simple directions and requests. ◆ Ability to make themself understood is limited.	◆ Significant persons are parents. ◆ Discovers ability to explore and manipulate environment. ◆ Asserts independence (autonomy) and develops a sense of will, has temper tantrums. ◆ Understands ownership ("mine"). ◆ Attached to security objects and toys. ◆ Knows own gender and differences of gender. ◆ Able to put toys away. ◆ Plays simple games, enjoys being read to, plays alone. ◆ Skills may regress due to illness/hospitalization.	◆ Use firm, direct approach. Give one direction at a time. ◆ Use distraction techniques. May use age appropriate toys. ◆ Prepare child shortly before a procedure. Allow child to handle equipment. ◆ Allow choices when possible. ◆ Emphasize those aspects that require the child's cooperation. ◆ Provide favorite, age-specific foods when applicable. ◆ Allow for rest periods after eating based on home routines to the degree possible. ◆ Emphasize the importance of mother (parent) staying with child at night. ◆ Set limits. ◆ Give permission to express feelings. ◆ Maintain safety at all times. ◆ Assess for and provide support in managing pain. ◆ Use head-to-toe procedures for physical exam; leave uncomfortable procedure(s) for last.

PEDIATRIC: 30 Days to 14 Years
(Toddler: 1 - 3 years)

Every minority and non-minority group has unique characteristics based on common values, beliefs, practices, race ethnicity country or origin and language.
Care givers need to acquire a basic understanding of their patients culture and background and give the time and attention needed to ensure accurate and smooth communication.

APPENDIX E • AGE-SPECIFIC CARE–COMPETENCE ASSESSMENT TOOLS

HealthEast — Age-Specific Awareness Tool

PHYSICAL	MOTOR/SENSORY ADAPTATION	COGNITIVE	PSYCHOSOCIAL	INTERVENTIONS

◆ Gains weight and grows in height 2 - 2 ½ inches a year.
◆ Temperature = 98.6° +/- 1 F.
◆ Pulse = 80 - 100/min.
◆ Respirations = 30/min +/- 5.
◆ BP = 80 - 110 mmHg systolic and 50 - 78 mmHg diastolic.
	◆ Skips, hops, roller skates, and jumps rope.
	◆ Dresses/undresses independently.
	◆ Prints first name. Draws person with six major parts.
		◆ Remains egocentric.
		◆ Major cognitive skills is conversation.
		◆ Understands that the amount of something is the same irregardless of shape or number of pieces.
		◆ Able to classify objects, enjoys doing puzzles.
		◆ Understands numbers, can count.
		◆ Constructs sentences, questions things "why?".
		◆ Knows own phone number and address.
		◆ Attention span is short.
		◆ Ritualistic.
		◆ Magical thinking.
			◆ Significant persons are parents, siblings, peers.
			◆ Increasing independence and beginning to assert self, likes to boast and tattle.
			◆ Masters new tasks and acquires new skills.
			◆ Behavior is modified by rewards and punishment.
			◆ Plays cooperatively, able to live by rules, capable of sharing.
			◆ May be physically aggressive.
			◆ Learns appropriate social manners.
			◆ Five year old: uses sentences, knows colors, numbers, alphabet.
			◆ Become fearful about procedures performed on a part of the body they cannot see or one that may be uncomfortable.
				◆ Explain procedures, unfamiliar objects.
				◆ Demonstrate use of equipment.
				◆ Encourage child to verbalize. Give permission to express feelings.
				◆ Use doll/puppets for explanations when performing procedures.
				◆ Involve the child whenever possible. Praise for good behavior.
				◆ Maintain safety at all times.
				◆ Provide rest periods.
				◆ Assess for and prove support in managing pain:
				  - Offer distractions, e.g., count to 20.
				  - Offer a badge of courage (stickers, etc.).
				◆ Focus on one thing at a time.
				◆ Limit movement restrictions.
				◆ Use head-to-toe procedures for physical exam; leave genitalia for last.

Patient/Family Education:

◆ Assess both parent and child for learning needs. Teaching is aimed at parents.
◆ Tell child why, and what to expect.
◆ Be positive and honest.
◆ Use language consistent with what child's family uses.
◆ Children cannot imagine what they have not experienced - explain what the child will taste, hear, see, feel and touch.
◆ Explain procedure to child shortly before it happens.
◆ Children learn best from short frequent teaching sessions. Group learning may be effective.
◆ If using learning aids such as video, written material or computer, be sure it is age appropriate.
◆ Some children think they are being punished - they need reassurance that it was nothing they did.
◆ Children unable to attend school need to have arrangements made for continuation of class work.

PEDIATRIC: 30 Days to 14 Years
(Preschool: 3 - 5 years)

Every minority and non-minority group has unique characteristics based on common values, beliefs, practices, race ethnicity country or origin and language.
Care givers need to acquire a basic understanding of their patients culture and background and give the time and attention needed to ensure accurate and smooth communication.

APPENDIX E • AGE-SPECIFIC CARE–COMPETENCE ASSESSMENT TOOLS

HealthEast

Age-Specific Awareness Tool

PHYSICAL	MOTOR/SENSORY ADAPTATION	COGNITIVE	PSYCHOSOCIAL	INTERVENTIONS
◆ Permanent teeth erupt. ◆ Starts pubescent changes. ◆ Growth is slow and regular. ◆ May experience "growing" pains because of stretching of muscles with growth of long bones. ◆ Temperature = 98.6° F +/- 1° F. ◆ Pulse = 60 - 100/min. ◆ Respirations = 18 - 20/min. ◆ BP = 84 - 120 mmHg systolic and 56 - 80 mmHg diastolic.	◆ Uses knife, common utensils and tools. ◆ Cares for pets. ◆ Draws, paints. ◆ Makes useful articles. ◆ Assists in household chores. ◆ Likes quiet as well as active games. ◆ Inquisitive	◆ Increased attention span and cognitive skills. ◆ Capable of logical operation with concrete things. ◆ Comprehends and can tell time. Functions in the present. ◆ Starts to think abstractly and to reason, can handle and classify problems, able to test hypotheses. ◆ Proud of school accomplishments. ◆ Enjoys reading. ◆ Starts to view things from different perspectives. ◆ Rule bound.	◆ Significant persons are peers, family, teachers. ◆ Prefers friends to family. Belonging and gaining approval of peer group is important. ◆ Works hard to be successful in what he/she does. ◆ Behavior is controlled by expectations, regulations and anticipation of praise or blame. ◆ Intention is considered when judging behavior. ◆ Likes to explore. ◆ Uses phone. ◆ Plays games with rules.	◆ Explain "why" and "how's" of procedures. ◆ Allow child to have some control. Major fear is loss of control. ◆ Provide privacy. Ask whether child wants parent present or not. ◆ Assess response after and prior to next dose. ◆ Promote independence. ◆ Clearly define and reinforce behavior limits. ◆ Use visual aids; be concrete and specific. ◆ Relate to child's abilities. ◆ Assess for and provide support in managing pain. ◆ Use head-to-toe procedures on physical exam; leave genitalia for last.

Patient/Family Education:
◆ Assess both parent and child for learning needs. Teaching is aimed at parents.
◆ Teach the child according to how he or she is functioning at the time, not chronological age.
◆ Tell child why, and what to expect.
◆ Be positive and honest.
◆ Children don't have enough experience to understand common medical terms. Use language consistent with what child's family uses.
◆ Children cannot imagine what they have not experienced - explain what the child will taste, hear, see, feel and touch.
◆ Explain procedure to child shortly before it happens.
◆ Children learn best from short frequent teaching sessions. Group learning may be effective.
◆ If using learning aids such as video, written material or computer, be sure it is age appropriate.
◆ Some children think they are being punished - they need reassurance that it was nothing they did.
◆ Children unable to attend school need to have arrangements made for continuation of class work.

PEDIATRIC: 30 Days to 14 Years
(School Age: 6 - 14 years)

Every minority and non-minority group has unique characteristics based on common values, beliefs, practices, race ethnicity country or origin and language.
Care givers need to acquire a basic understanding of their patients culture and background and give the time and attention needed to ensure accurate and smooth communication.

APPENDIX E • AGE-SPECIFIC CARE–COMPETENCE ASSESSMENT TOOLS

HealthEast

Age-Specific Awareness Tool

PHYSICAL	MOTOR/SENSORY ADAPTATION	COGNITIVE	PSYCHOSOCIAL	INTERVENTIONS
◆ Rapid growth of skeletal size, muscle mass, adipose tissue and skin. ◆ Maturation of the reproductive system; development of primary and secondary sexual characteristics. ◆ Onset of menarche in girls and nocturnal emissions in boys. ◆ Vital signs approximate those of the adult. ◆ Pulse = 60 - 90/min. ◆ Respirations = 12 - 16/min. ◆ BP = 94 - 140 mmHg systolic and 60 - 90 mmHg diastolic.	◆ Awkward in gross motor activity. ◆ Easily fatigued, may need more rest and sleep. ◆ Fine motor skills are improving.	◆ Increased ability to use abstract thought and logic. ◆ Able to handle hypothetical situations or thought. ◆ Ability to use introspection. ◆ Develops more internal growth of self-esteem. ◆ Beginning development of occupational identify (what I want to be). ◆ Authority viewed with skepticism.	◆ Self-conscious. ◆ Interested and confused by own development. ◆ Often critical of own features and concerned with physical appearance. ◆ Belonging to peer groups are important and valued; may criticize parents. ◆ Interested in the opposite sex. ◆ Accepts criticism or advice reluctantly. ◆ Longs for independence but also desires dependence. ◆ Identity is threatened by hospitalization as adolescents are concerned about bodily changes and appearances. ◆ Health recommendations are viewed as interference with their independence.	◆ Supplement explanations with rationale. ◆ Encourage questions regarding fears. ◆ Provide privacy. Ask if they want parent present or not. ◆ Involve in planning and decision-making. Allow adolescent to maintain control. ◆ Do not talk about the individual in front of the individual. ◆ Assess and manage pain based on patient's needs and response. ◆ Use head-to-toe procedure for physical exam; leave genitalia for last.

Patient/Family Education:
- Talk to adolescent, not over them to parents.
- They need to know why something is being done. In language they understand.
- They may not ask questions, so you may need to anticipate questions they may have.
- Be positive and honest.
- Want more technical information, they understand more detailed information and abstract concepts.
- Need to know how their independence and appearance will change.
- If using learning aids such as video, written material or computer, be sure it is age appropriate.
- Focus on immediate benefits and consequences.
- Help the adolescent be responsible and successful.
- Involve parents int he care while maintaining focus on adolescent.
- Adolescents who are unable to attend school need to have arrangements made for continuation of class work.

ADOLESCENCE: 14 - 18 Years

Every minority and non-minority group has unique characteristics based on common values, beliefs, practices, race ethnicity country or origin and language. Care givers need to acquire a basic understanding of their patients culture and background and give the time and attention needed to ensure accurate and smooth communication.

APPENDIX E • AGE-SPECIFIC CARE–COMPETENCE ASSESSMENT TOOLS

HealthEast

Age-Specific Awareness Tool

PHYSICAL	MOTOR/SENSORY ADAPTATION	COGNITIVE	PSYCHOSOCIAL	INTERVENTIONS
Age 19 - 45: ◆ Growth of skeletal systems continue until age 30, then bone mass begins to decrease. ◆ Skin begins to lose moisture. Loss of skin elasticity and increased appearance of wrinkles. ◆ Muscular efficiency is at its peak between 20 - 30 years, then decreases if not used. ◆ GI system decreases secretions after age 30. **Age 40 - 65:** ◆ Bone mass beings to decrease. ◆ Loss of skeletal height; calcium loss especially after menopause. ◆ Decreased muscle strength and mass if not used, endurance declines. ◆ Loss of skin elasticity, dry skin, increased appearance of wrinkles. ◆ Decreased renal functioning, metabolic rate, heat/cold tolerance, prone to infection. ◆ Receding hair line in males, more facial hair in females.	◆ Visual changes in accommodation and convergence. ◆ Some loss in hearing, especially high tones. **Age 40 - 65:** ◆ Slowing of reflexes. ◆ Muscle activity may increase or decrease. ◆ Visual changes especially farsightedness. ◆ Noticeable loss of hearing and taste. ◆ Muscles and joints respond more slowly. ◆ Decreased balance and coordination. ◆ More prolonged response to stress.	◆ Mental abilities reach their peak during the twenties (reasoning, creative imagination, information recall and verbal skills) followed by gradual decrease. ◆ Re-evaluation of current life style and value system. ◆ Gradual decrease in mental performance speed.	◆ Searching for and finding a place for self in society. ◆ Initiating a career, finding a mate, developing loving relationships, marriage, establishing a family, parenting. ◆ Achievement oriented; working up the career ladder. ◆ Moves from dependency to responsibility. Responsible for children and aging parents. ◆ Mid-life crisis. ◆ May experience empty nest syndrome.	◆ Involve individual/significant other in plan of care. ◆ Explore impact of illness/hospitalization to work/job, family, children. ◆ Watch for body language as a cue for feelings. Assess for potential stresses related to multiple roles. ◆ Allow for as much decision-making as possible. ◆ Assess and manage pain based on patient needs and response. ◆ Provide information on pain control methods, assessment scale, schedule for pain medication as soon as pain begins, providing information of degree of pain relief, types of pain.
Patient/Family Education: ◆ Use open ended questions to learn about the patients beliefs, practices, community and cultural influences. Because health behaviors are often culturally based, sensitivity to these issues is crucial in a successful health program. Observe body language. ◆ Careful assessment of learning needs and abilities. Identify barriers and develop plan. Use adult learning principles (see principles) ◆ Assess ability to speak and read English. Identify other family members who can ready and interpret for the patient. Make provisions for those who do not speak English. ◆ Address people formally, unless patient says otherwise. Convey respect. ◆ Provide education materials and visual aids in a language and reading level patients can read. Identify key points in the materials. Evaluate learning, plan for needed follow-up if needed. ◆ Be non-judgmental. Do not make assumptions. ◆ Keep explanations simple and clear by using concrete directions and examples, rather than abstract statements. ◆ Give person time to absorb what you have said and encourage to ask questions. ◆ Incorporate resources to provide person with the ability to use the new knowledge or change to healthier behaviors.				**Adult Learning Principles:** ◆ Adults want to participate in an interactive process. They bring past experiences into learning. ◆ Adults use learning to satisfy a need. ◆ Adults learn well in groups and from peers. ◆ Learning needs to be applied immediately. ◆ Learning must be reinforced. ◆ Relate new learning to what is already known. ◆ Accommodate different learning styles. ◆ Inform learning of progress and reward desired learning. ◆ Material to be learned needs to "make sense to the learner".

ADULTHOOD: 19 - 70 Years

Every minority and non-minority group has unique characteristics based on common values, beliefs, practices, race ethnicity country or origin and language.
Care givers need to acquire a basic understanding of their patients culture and background and give the time and attention needed to ensure accurate and smooth communication.

APPENDIX E • AGE-SPECIFIC CARE–COMPETENCE ASSESSMENT TOOLS

HealthEast — Age-Specific Awareness Tool

PHYSICAL	MOTOR/SENSORY ADAPTATION	COGNITIVE	PSYCHOSOCIAL	INTERVENTIONS
♦ Decreased tolerance to heat/cold. ♦ Decreased peripheral circulation. ♦ Declining cardiac/renal function. ♦ Decreased response to stress and sensory stimuli. ♦ Atrophy of reproductive organs. ♦ Loss of teeth leading to changes in food intake. ♦ More skeletal changes, including shrinkage in intervertebral disc. ♦ Increase wrinkles. ♦ Gradual loss of fat layers on limbs and face with age.	♦ Decreased visual acuity. ♦ Decreased mobility. ♦ Hearing loss continues. ♦ Decreased sensitivity of taste buds and smell. ♦ Decreased tolerance to pain. ♦ Hesitant to respond; skills declining. ♦ Paresthesia common.	♦ Decline depends upon earlier cognitive abilities, general health and involvement in society. ♦ Sharing wisdom with others. ♦ Decrease in memory, slowing of mental functions. ♦ Drop in performance.	♦ Retirement. ♦ Death of spouse and friends; acceptance of death. ♦ Adapting to change of social role. Introspection and life review. ♦ Developing supportive relationships. ♦ Pursuing second career, interest, hobbies, community activities, leisure activities. ♦ Coming to terms with accomplishments. ♦ Children leave home; reestablished as couple; grand parenthood. ♦ Concern for health increases. ♦ Decrease authority and mobility.	♦ Encourage self care. ♦ Explore individual's support system. Involve family with care. ♦ Explore related existing conditions. ♦ Provide adequate nutrition. May need smaller, more frequent meals. ♦ Keep environment safe, e.g., SR ↑ bed ↓ wheels locked, turn/assist q 2 hours. ♦ Assess skin integrity frequently. Use tape sparingly on fragile skin. Apply lotion to skin immediately after bathing. ♦ Monitor bowel elimination q 24 hours. ♦ Assess for and provide support for pain management every 2 - 4 hours. This age group is more susceptible to side effects of any medication. ♦ Be aware of possible need for warmer environment (room temperature, need for an extra blanket). ♦ Assess resources for discharge.
Patient/Family Education: • Use open ended questions to learn about the patients beliefs, practices, community and cultural influences. Because health behaviors are often culturally based, sensitivity to these issues is crucial in a successful health program. Observe body language. • Assess if the person is physically and emotionally ready to learn. Identify other family members or friends who need learning to provide ongoing care. • Carefully assess ability to see, hear and pick up or use objects, Remember, some people deny any disabilities. • Elderly are motivated to learn by a desire to stay independent. So the learning plan needs to help work toward that goal. • Determine best time of day for concentration. Teach in quiet well lighted area free from distraction. • Encourage use of visual or hearing aids - glasses, magnifying glass, hearing aids. Speak in regular voice, face person at eye level, and use short sentences. • Use oversized teaching aids, if appropriate with large type. Contrasting colors such as red and yellow enhance visibility. • Keep explanations simple and clear by using concrete directions and examples, rather than abstract statements. • Give person time to absorb what you have said and encourage to ask questions. • Incorporate resources to provide person with the ability to use the new knowledge or change to healthier behaviors.				

GERIATRICS: 70+ Years

Every minority and non-minority group has unique characteristics based on common values, beliefs, practices, race ethnicity country or origin and language. Care givers need to acquire a basic understanding of their patients culture and background and give the time and attention needed to ensure accurate and smooth communication.

APPENDIX F • INTERPERSONAL SKILLS–ASSESSMENT TOOLS

St. Joseph's Hospital **HOSPITAL STAFF**
Breese, Illinois
                          Name _____

SKILLS VALIDATION
                                   Date _____

TOPIC: INTERPERSONAL SKILLS/CUSTOMER SERVICE

OBJECTIVE: After completion of this skill the participant will be knowledgeable in Interpersonal Skills and Customer Service.

LEVEL 1:   Orientation period when practitioner is dependent on others to meet practice specifications. *With supervision uses practice standards on providing service. *Action plan required with target date for improvement.

LEVEL 2:   Characterized by independence in practice. *Independently uses practice standards in providing service.

LEVEL 3:   Practitioner has mastered competencies and can fulfill resource and consultative role. *Assists others in the application of practice standards in providing service.

		Level 1	Level 2	Level 3
1.	Provides cooperative and courteous service to patients, physicians, visitors and/or co-workers.			
2.	Maintains positive attitude and commitment to interpersonal service towards patients, physicians, visitors, and/or co-workers demonstrated by routine helpfulness, initiative in assisting others. Is consistently polite to all of the above and refers them to appropriate sources for assistance.			
3.	Promotes effective working relationships and works effectively as a part of the department team.			
4.	Communicates effectively with peers, health team members and Managers.			
5.	Interacts effectively with patients, families, and significant others.			
6.	Adapts to changes in a positive, professional manner.			
7.	Cooperates well with staff, physicians, managers, and other departments.			
8.	Resolves problems. Supports problem solving approach to both department and patient need.			
9.	Follows through on problems that may compromise patient care by using the appropriate chain of command.			

Action Plan & Date

_____
_____
_____

                     Validator's Signature: _____

PATIENT FEEDBACK INTERVIEW GUIDE

- Would you like to tell me about your labor and birth experience?
- Do you remember the name/s of the nurses who cared for you during your labor and delivery?
- Were you satisfied with the nursing care you received?
- Is there anything you feel we could have done that would have made your experience better?
- Do you have suggestions for the nurses who cared for you that could help them in caring for other women in labor?
- Were your support persons/family members welcomed as participants in your childbirth experience?
- Would you choose our hospital in the future if you plan another pregnancy?

This type of interview guide can be used to solicit feedback from women during the immediate postpartum period before discharge or by telephone at home during the first week postpartum. The interpersonal aspects of clinical nursing skills can be evaluated based on patient and family feedback. Some women will provide data about all issues of interest in their response to the first question. Valuable information about nursing care during the intrapartum period can be gathered by talking with the woman and her family. Suggestions can be used to improve overall quality of care and patient satisfaction.

Another important benefit of this approach is the ability to share with nurses positive remarks about their individual contributions to the patient's childbearing experience. Often women will take the time to provide indepth comments about the nurses who cared for them during labor and delivery. While many times perinatal nurses feel rushed to accomplish all there is to do related to documentation and the technical aspects of intrapartum care, it is gratifying to know we can still make a significant difference. Conversely, comments about nurses who could use some improvement in clinical and/or interpersonal skills, are also valuable because they allow those nurses to see how they are perceived by patients and family members, and this can lead to appropriate behavior changes.

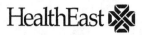

CRITICAL THINKING

Critical Thinking is a method of problem solving and it supports learning.

Challenges: Can appear threatening to the individual.

The steps of the Critical Thinking Process include:

    Identify Assumptions

    Check Accuracy and Validity of Assumptions

    Take Alternative Perspectives

    Take Informed Actions

Note: By using the Critical Thinking Process you may have two individuals come up with two different correct answers. The important assessment is can the individual explain how they arrived at their answer.

There are three different types of Assumptions:

    PARADIGMATIC (Framing/Structuring)
    What we believe to be always true. Shapes the rest of our thinking. Would never question these assumptions without outside influence. Very difficult to change.

        Example: Germs cause disease. Dirty hands pass germs along.

    PRESCRIPTIVE (What should happen)
    Based on what we "know" to be true this is what should happen.

        Example: Everyone should wash their hands.

    CAUSAL (What does happen)
    If you do this, this will happen. If this happens, this will follow.

        Example: If everyone washed their hands, no one would get sick.

Note: Assumptions are built from our experiences. To be open to the "full" truth and to learn, we must be willing to examine our assumptions.

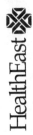

CRITICAL THINKING VALIDATION

Name: _____ **Site:** _____ **Position:** _____

Describe a situation where you utilized the critical thinking process or respond to the provided scenario.

List 3-5 assumptions:

1. _____
2. _____
3. _____
4. _____
5. _____

Identify type of assumption:
(Paradigmatic, prescriptive, causal)

_____
_____
_____
_____
_____

Describe how you verified the accuracy or inaccuracy of your assumptions:

_____
_____
_____
_____
_____
_____
_____
_____
_____

Critical Thinking Validation

List the potential actions you could have taken and the probable outcomes.

1. _____
2. _____
3. _____
4. _____

Identify what information you used to take an informed action and describe that action.

_____
_____

What was the outcome of your informed action?

_____
_____

What was your key learning from this experience? Would you do anything differently if presented with the same situation in the future?

_____
_____
_____

Signature of Validator: _____ Date: _____

APPENDIX H • ANTEPARTUM/INTRAPARTUM COMPETENCE– ASSESSMENT TOOLS AND SKILLS CHECKLISTS

PALOS COMMUNITY HOSPITAL

COMPETENCE-BASED CHECKLIST
ANTEPARTUM/INTRAPARTUM REGISTERED NURSE

EMPLOYEE _____

DATE CHECKLIST STARTED _____

DATE CHECKLIST COMPLETED _____

Dates are placed in boxes as skills are completed.

	Observed Skill Performed by Preceptor	Skill Performed With Supervision	Skill Performed Independently	Preceptor's Signature
I. Completes admission process for patient in labor				
II. Perform vaginal exam for: A. Presentation				
B. Station				
C. Dilatation				
D. Effacement				
III. Perform nitrazine test				
IV. Assess deep tendon reflexes				
V. Assess patient for edema				
VI. Prep perineum				
VII. Monitor uterine contractions via palpation				
VIII. Performs Leopold's Maneuvers				
IX. Obtain fetal heart tones with doppler				
X. Operate electronic fetal monitoring equipment safely: A. Assemble and apply external fetal monitor				
B. Assist with the application of fetal scalp electrode				
C. Assist with the application of IUPC				
D. Conduct NST				

APPENDIX H • ANTEPARTUM/INTRAPARTUM COMPETENCE–ASSESSMENT TOOLS AND SKILLS CHECKLISTS

	Observed Skill Performed by Preceptor	Skill Performed With Supervision	Skill Performed Independently	Preceptor's Signature
E. Change time and date on monitor paper				
F. Enter patient into central fetal monitoring system				
G. Utilize telemetry unit				
XI. Demonstrate an understanding of nursing management of patients in the following situations: A. Receiving Pitocin to induce labor				
B. Receiving Pitocin to augment labor				
C. Receiving tocolytics to arrest labor				
D. During recovery after NSVD				
E. During recovery after Cesarean Section				
F. Receiving MgSO4 for preeclampsia				
G. Receiving epidural anesthesia during labor				
H. Receiving amniofusion				
XII. Perform sterile scrub				
XIII. Perform function of circulating nurse during NSVD				
XIV. Cesarean Section: A. Pre-op preparation				
B. Notify appropriate resource people				
C. Function as circulating nurse				
XV. Maintain safety principles related to needle, sponge, and instrument count				
XVI. Obtain cord blood for PH and gases				
XVII. Understand the process for notifying neonatology for high risk delivery				
XVIII. Locate supplies/equipment and prepare: A. Birthing Room for NSVD				

APPENDIX H • ANTEPARTUM/INTRAPARTUM COMPETENCE– ASSESSMENT TOOLS AND SKILLS CHECKLISTS

	Observed Skill Performed by Preceptor	Skill Performed With Supervision	Skill Performed Independently	Preceptor's Signature
XIX Operate the following equipment safety: A. Vacuum extractor (electric)				
B. Hand-held vacuum extractor				
C. Birthing bed				
D. Infant warmer				
E. Infant transporter				
F. Delivery Room/or table				
G. Dinamap				
H. Cardiac monitor				
I. Electrocautery				
J. Wall suction				
K. Infusion pump				
L. Neonatal stabilizing unit				
XX. Locate and be familiar with the contents of: A. Trach tray				
B. Hyperthermia tray				
C. Preeclampsia Tray				
D. Infant resuscitation equipment				
1. Birthing Room				
2. OR/DR				
XXI. Organize and document pertinent information using the following: A. Antepartum Admission Assessment				
B. Labor & Delivery Summary				
C. Labor Flow Sheet				
D. Newborn Identification				

APPENDIX H • ANTEPARTUM/INTRAPARTUM COMPETENCE– ASSESSMENT TOOLS AND SKILLS CHECKLISTS

	Observed Skill Performed by Preceptor	Skill Performed With Supervision	Skill Performed Independently	Preceptor's Signature
E. Consent Forms				
XXII. Initiate IV using an angiocath				
1.				
2.				
3.				
				Date
XXIII. Begin certification process for application of Fetal Scalp Electrodes				
XXIV. View the following video tapes: A. OR Procedures: Preparing and Maintaining the Sterile Field				
B. Application of the Spiral Electrode				
C. Introduction to Soft Cup V.E.				
D. Electrocautery Unit				
E. Understanding Preterm Labor				

F. AWHONN Electronic Fetal Monitoring (2nd edition)
        • Instrumentation
        • Pattern Interpretation
        • Clinical Applications				

G. AWHONN Critical concepts in Fetal Heart Rate Monitoring (2nd edition)
        • Antepartum Fetal Surveillance
        • The Fetal Response
        • Systematic Analysis
        • Advanced Clinical Applications
        • Fetal Blood Sampling				

H. AWHONN Critical Care Obstetrics
        • Preeclampsia/HELLP
        • EKG Interpretation				

I. Venipuncture Technique & Complications				
J. IV Therapy Problems				
K. AWHONN Cross Training for OB Nursing Staff				
1. Antepartum Care				

APPENDIX H • ANTEPARTUM/INTRAPARTUM COMPETENCE– ASSESSMENT TOOLS AND SKILLS CHECKLISTS

		Observed Skill Performed by Preceptor	Skill Performed With Supervision	Skill Performed Independently	Preceptor's Signature
	2. Intrapartum Care				
	L. Duraprep				
XXV.	Review the Maternity Policy & Procedure Manual for policies referred to in the checklist				
XXVI.	Review the Newborn Policy & Procedure Manual				
XXVII.	Review the policies for the following infrequently occurring procedures				
	A. Fetal Scalp Blood Sampling				
	B. Hyperstimulation				
	C. Administration of Blood & Blood Products (Med/Surg. Manual)				
	D. Protocol for Use of Prostaglandin E2 Vaginal Suppository				
	E. Guidelines for Use of Prostin 15M (Hemabate)				
	F. Oxytocin Challenge Test				
	G. Dilatation and Uterine Evacuation in OB				
	H. Neonatal Resuscitation				

APPENDIX H • ANTEPARTUM/INTRAPARTUM COMPETENCE–ASSESSMENT TOOLS AND SKILLS CHECKLISTS

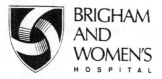
BRIGHAM AND WOMEN'S HOSPITAL

75 Francis Street
Boston, Massachusetts 02115

Phone:

I certify at this point and time the competence of

_____

to practice in <u>Center for Labor & Birth</u> according to unit based standards and performance criteria.

_____
Nurse Manager   **Date**

A Teaching Affiliate of Harvard Medical School

APPENDIX H • ANTEPARTUM/INTRAPARTUM COMPETENCE–ASSESSMENT TOOLS AND SKILLS CHECKLISTS

STANDARDS	PERFORMANCE CRITERIA	MEETS CRITERIA
STANDARD I		YES NO
Nursing care will be planned, coordinated and evaluated within a primary nursing system.	1. All RN's working on CLB will assume the responsibility for being a primary nurse.	
	2. Each RN demonstrates their responsibility for planning and coordinating their primary patient's/family's care by documenting the following: A) patient's concerns/desires B) communication with obstetric care provider (OBCP) including the interdisciplinary plan of care C) appropriate nursing diagnosis D) evaluation of plan of care and revisions	
	3. Each primary nurse is responsible for identifying her/himself and his/her role to the patient. They should also make the patient aware of the primary team nurse coverage.	
STANDARD II		YES NO
Nursing care will be provided on the basis of an individualized assessment, diagnosis, mutually established goals and plan of care, and ongoing evaluation.	1. An initial assessment is performed by an RN within 15 minutes of a patient presenting to CLB.	
	2. The patient's health history will be obtained by the primary nurse utilizing: ~ patient interview and physical assessment ~ Nursing History Questionnaire (obstetrical) ~ support person	
	3. Mutually established goals will be identified, developed and evaluated based on the patient's identified needs by the primary RN and will be documented in the nursing record.	

APPENDIX H • ANTEPARTUM/INTRAPARTUM COMPETENCE-ASSESSMENT TOOLS AND SKILLS CHECKLISTS

STANDARD III			YES	NO

Nursing care will be provided in a safe and effective manner in accordance with appropriate polices, procedures, guidelines and protocols (PPG's)

1. All CLB RN's maintain an updated Nursing Education Record in the Education Notebook which documents the following:
   A) mandatory annual inservices/videos
   B) equipment competencies
   C) inservices of new equipment
   D) staff meeting attendance/reading minutes.

2. All CLB RN's will utilize the established PPG's in meeting the nursing needs of their patients.

STANDARD IV			YES	NO

The patient's physiologic/functional status will be monitored as required by acuity and nursing interventions will be instituted to meet physiologic/functional needs.

1. All CLB RN's will evaluate the maternal/fetal neonatal physiologic status in accordance with established PPG's and will institute the appropriate nursing interventions.

STANDARD V			YES	NO

Nursing care will be provided holistically with compassion, respect and empathy taking into account the patient's family's culture, developmental stage, strengths/resources and unmet physical and psychosocial needs.

1. Each CLB RN will encourage and assist family and/or significant others to be supportive of the patient.

2. When parents and infant are separated each CLB RN will maintain communication with the infant's care providers. Visitation will be encouraged and facilitated when feasible.

3. Each CLB RN will utilize the available services to assist with meeting their primary patient's needs which include:

   A) social service
   B) NICU
   C) interpretive services
   D) chaplaincy services

235

APPENDIX H • ANTEPARTUM/INTRAPARTUM COMPETENCE–ASSESSMENT TOOLS AND SKILLS CHECKLISTS

STANDARD VI		YES NO

The patient and family will participate in education needed to manage heath priorities throughout the hospital stay and in preparation for discharge.

1. The primary RN will provide the patient discharged home from CLB with a discharge instruction sheet which has individualized to meet their needs.

2. The primary RN will provide educational instruction for their patient and family/significant other individualized to their needs.

STANDARD VII		YES NO

Nursing care and services needed post-discharge will be assessed and arranged for in collaboration with the patient and family.

1. The primary RN will assess the patient's support systems, psychosocial needs, role and responsibilities at home.

2. The primary RN will collaborate with all of the patient's health care providers and the patient and her family in planning her discharge from CLB. discharge from CLB.

STANDARD VIII		YES NO

Documentation of nursing care will reflect the patient's status and response to interventions, and will be recorded in accordance with established departmental and unit based standards.

1. The primary RN will complete a comprehensive health assessment, including VS and FH check when appropriate, and document these on appropriate form.

2. When patient care is transferred from one CLB RN to another a note will be written by the transferring RN stating the name of the accepting RN and the time of transfer of care.

3. Each CLB RN will document patient's status, education regarding interventions, plan for implementation and response which may include:
   ~ VS
   ~ FHR
   ~ contractions
   ~ patient's stated comfort level
   ~ other physical measurements related to the medication/intervention.
   ~ presence/absence of side effects or allergic reactions.

APPENDIX H • ANTEPARTUM/INTRAPARTUM COMPETENCE–ASSESSMENT TOOLS AND SKILLS CHECKLISTS

STANDARD IX			YES	NO
Nursing care will be provided in a manner which respects patient's antomony, privacy confidentiality and the right of self determination.	1.	On admission a CLB RN will interview the patient alone to provide privacy and confidentiality whenever feasible.		
	2.	The patient's primary RN will give the patient the opportunity to participate in the development of the plan of care.		

APPENDIX I • COMPETENCE ASSESSMENT TOOL FOR NURSES PROVIDING CARE TO CRITICALLY ILL PREGNANT WOMEN

**Brigham and Women's Hospital
Performance Competency***
**Labor and Delivery Critical Care Course II
Clinical Experience**

NAME: _____
UNIT: _____ UNIT: _____
PRECEPTOR: _____ PRECEPTOR: _____
DATES: _____ DATES: _____

OBJECTIVE	EVALUATION CRITERIA	METHODS	DATE COMPLETED	SUPERVISED BY:
1. Utilize the nursing process and patient care documentation system.	I. The orientee will demonstrate the ability to: A. Formulate and maintain an individual nursing care plan for a critically ill patient. 1. Complete and document a biopsychosocial nursing assessment or admission using the functional health pattern 2. Complete a patient problem list 3. Prescribe nursing interventions 4. Identify expected outcomes 5. Complete a SOAP note at appropriate interval B. Document pertinent information on flow sheets and in the nursing progress notes. C. Demonstrate ability to write a transfer note.	A. Review with preceptor and submit examples of nursing assessment problem. List and SOAP note from 2 patients. B. Review with preceptor. C. Review with preceptor and submit examples from 2 patients.*	A. Patient #1 Patient #2	

APPENDIX I • COMPETENCE ASSESSMENT TOOL FOR NURSES PROVIDING CARE TO CRITICALLY ILL PREGNANT WOMEN

OBJECTIVE	EVALUATION CRITERIA	METHODS	DATE COMPLETED	SUPERVISED BY:
		* If unable to obtain experience, the nurse is to write a transfer note on 2 of the patients cared for.	C. Patient #1 ___ Patient #2 ___	
Demonstrate a working knowledge of the equipment commonly used on the unit.	2. The orientee will demonstrate a working knowledge of the following pieces of equipment: A. Wall suction B. Gomco suction C. Defibrillator D. O$_2$ flow meters E. infusion pump/controller F. Hypo/Hyperthermia blanket G. Invasive hemodynamic monitoring equipment Specify Brand _____ H. Periferal O$_2$ Saturation I. Marquette EKG machine	Review applicable procedures. Review and demonstrate use. (Can be done in mock setting if no patient is available.)	A. ___ B. ___ C. ___ D. ___ E. ___ F. ___ G. ___ H. ___ I. ___	
3. Demonstrate the ability to locate all items on the crash cart.	3. The orientee will check the crash cart × 5 and demonstrate the ability to locate and describe the use of the following: A. Medications B. Respiratory support equipment C. IV therapy equipment D. Central line equipment E. Cardiac monitoring equipment	3. Self-review of L & D crash cart × 3. Joint review with preceptor of ICU crash cart × 2.	A. ___ B. ___ C. ___ D. ___ E. ___	
4. Demonstrate the ability to care for a patient who has an actual or potential alteration in cardiac output.	4. The orientee will demonstrate the ability to: A. Perform a cardiovascular nursing assessment on a patient with a cardiovascular problem, including:	4. A. Self-review of ICU consortia course content.	A. ___	

APPENDIX I • COMPETENCE ASSESSMENT TOOL FOR NURSES PROVIDING CARE TO CRITICALLY ILL PREGNANT WOMEN

OBJECTIVE	EVALUATION CRITERIA	METHODS	DATE COMPLETED	SUPERVISED BY:
	1. Assess:	B. Review standards discussion with preceptor.	B.	
	a. Quality of peripheral pulses	C. Perform 1 assessment on a normal individual.	C.	
	b. Skin color			
	c. Skin temperature	Submission of 1 cardiovascular nursing assessment on nursing progress note.		
	d. Capillary filling			
	e. Presence/absence			
	f. Blood pressure			
	g. Pulse			
	—quality			
	—rhythm			
	h. Presence or absence jugular venous distention (JVD)			
	2. Document assessment on Nursing progress note			
	B. Care for a patient on a cardiac monitor:	B. Review procedure: Application of Cardiac Monitor Leads Demonstration #'s 1-11		
	1. Prepare skin sites for lead placement			
	a. shave site (if necessary)			
	b. clean areas with alcohol prep pad			
	2. Apply electrodes to skin sites			
	a. Connect electrode to lead wire			
	b. Apply electrode to predetermined site			
	3. Position cable to avoid damage			
	4. Set rate alarms on monitor			
	5. Adjust complex position on scope			
	6. Turn lead section to obtain best training			
	7. Check gain/size switch for height			
	8. Adjust beat loudness			
	9. Document rhythm strip			
	10. Change ECG paper			
	11. Verbalize methods to be used in checking sources of false alarm triggering			
	a. high rate alarm			
	b. low rate alarm			

APPENDIX I • COMPETENCE ASSESSMENT TOOL FOR NURSES PROVIDING CARE TO CRITICALLY ILL PREGNANT WOMEN

OBJECTIVE	EVALUATION CRITERIA	METHODS	DATE COMPLETED	SUPERVISED BY:
	12. Identify alterations in ECG monitor recordings and state the significance and appropriate intervention of each:	12.	12.	
	a. dysrhythmia recognition	A. Heartsim session	A. _____	_____
		B. Strip review with preceptor on assigned patients	B. _____	_____
	1. NSR		1. _____	_____
	2. Sinus Bradycardia		2. _____	_____
	3. Sinus Tachycardia		3. _____	_____
	4. Atrial Ectopy		4. _____	_____
	5. Ventricular ectopy		5. _____	_____
	6. Atrial Fibrillation		6. _____	_____
	7. Ventricular Tachycardia		7. _____	_____
	8. Ventricular Fibrillation		8. _____	_____
	9. First Degree Block		9. _____	_____
	10. Second Degree Block, Type I		10. _____	_____
	11. Second Degree Block Type II		11. _____	_____
	12. Third Degree Block		12. _____	_____
	13. Junctional Rhythm		13. _____	_____
	14. Premature Junctional Beats		14. _____	_____
	b. excessive artifact			
	c. electrical interference			
	d. low/high QRS voltage			
	C. Use of Transport Monitor			
	D. State the indication and actions of the following medications:	D. Review with preceptor and/or written examination		
	1. Apresoline		1. _____	_____
	2. Labetalol		2. _____	_____
	3. Dopamine		3. _____	_____
	4. Levophed		4. _____	_____
	5. Lidocaine		5. _____	_____
	6. Neosynephrine		6. _____	_____
	7. Nipride		7. _____	_____
	8. Albumin		8. _____	_____
	9. Dobutemine			
	10. Nitroglycerin			

APPENDIX I • COMPETENCE ASSESSMENT TOOL FOR NURSES PROVIDING CARE TO CRITICALLY ILL PREGNANT WOMEN

OBJECTIVE	EVALUATION CRITERIA	METHODS	DATE COMPLETED	SUPERVISED BY:
	E. Demonstrate the ability to care for a patient with an invasive hemodynamic monitoring line:	E. Demonstration except #9—verbalizes understanding of technique for obtaining cardiac output		

	1. Set up
	   a. identifies supplies
	      1. CVP
	      2. Arterial
	      3. PA
	   2. Machine calibration
	   3. Assist with insertion
		Review Procedures:
		Pulmonary Artery
			1. CVP _____
			   Arterial _____
			   PA _____
			2. _____
			3. CVP _____
			   Arterial _____
			   PA _____	

	4. Change dressing and tubing	Techniques arterial line dressing change
		Central venous catheter dressing change
			4. CVP _____
			   Arterial _____
			   PA _____	

	5. Readings
	   a. leveling points
	      1. line set-up
	      2. patient
	   b. zeroing
	   c. interpretation
	      1. identifies dampened wave form
		Blood sampling from an arterial line
		
		Measuring a cardiac output
		Removal of an arterial catheter
			5. _____	

	6. Removal
	7. Draw blood sample
	8. Wedging technique
	9. Cardiac output technique
	10. Monitor circulation of involved extremity and document same
	11. Document above appropriately
	12. State causes of problems and appropriate nursing interventions
	   a. Damped waveform i.e., air/blood in line, kinks, catheter against intima.
	   b. Spontaneous change in waveform i.e., system malfunction, catheter in improper position, gross change in patient pressures.
			6. Arterial _____
			7. CVP _____
			   Arterial _____
			8. PA _____
			9. PA _____
			10. _____
			11. _____
			12. _____	

APPENDIX I • COMPETENCE ASSESSMENT TOOL FOR NURSES PROVIDING CARE TO CRITICALLY ILL PREGNANT WOMEN

OBJECTIVE	EVALUATION CRITERIA	METHODS	DATE COMPLETED	SUPERVISED BY:
	c. Wedge unobtainable i.e., catheter in improper position inadequate balloon, balloon rupture. 1. Note specific caution when no resistance to wedging attempt and balloon rupture suspected. d. Permanent wedge i.e., improper catheter position.			
	13. Identify possible causes of catheter "whip" i.e., line set-up greater than 5 feet, high resonance due to mechanical ventilation or pulmonary hypertension, artifact.		13. _____	_____
	14. State potential dangers of arterial lines i.e., air/blood embolism, sepsis, hemorrhage, arterial occlusion.		14. _____	_____
	15. State potential dangers of pulmonary artery lines i.e., air/blood embolism, dysrhythmias pulmonary infarction, endocarditis, sepsis, pneumothorax.		15. _____	_____

	Identify the following Principles of Hemodynamics:
	 1. Describe cardiac anatomy including chambers and valves.
	 2. Define preload afterload cardiac output wedge.
	 3. State normal pressure values.
	   a. Right atrial pressure (RAP)
	   b. Right ventricular pressure (RVP)
	   c. Pulmonary artery pressure (PAP)
	   d. Pulmonary capillary wedge pressure (PCWP)
	   e. Left atrial pressure (LAP)
	   f. Cardiac output (CO)
	   g. Blood pressure (BP)
		Self-review of ICU consort content from ICU consortia course content
		
		 Written examination
		
		 Review with preceptor in context of assigned patients
			1. _____
			
			 2. _____
			
			 3. _____
				_____
				
				 _____
				
				 _____

APPENDIX I • COMPETENCE ASSESSMENT TOOL FOR NURSES PROVIDING CARE TO CRITICALLY ILL PREGNANT WOMEN

OBJECTIVE	EVALUATION CRITERIA	METHODS	DATE COMPLETED	SUPERVISED BY:
	4. State possible causes of elevated PCWP i.e., congestive heart failure, hypervolemia, pulmonary edema, pulmonary hypertension, valve problems.		4. _____	_____
	5. State possible causes of lowered PCWP i.e., hypovolemia.		5. _____	_____
	6. State significance of dicrotic notch in arterial and pulmonary artery waveforms.			
	7. Identify waveform progression from right atrium through pulmonary capillary wedge.	Self-review of ICU consortia course content		

5. Demonstrate the ability to care for a patient who has an actual or potential ineffective breathing pattern, impaired gas exchange, or ineffective airway clearance.	5. The orientee will demonstrate the ability to:
	 A. Perform a respiratory nursing assessment on a patient with an alteration in respiratory status including:
	   1. Inspection
	     a. Rate of breathing
	     b. Rhythm of breathing
	     c. Effort of breathing
	     d. Chest measurements
	       —symmetrical
	       —asymmetrical
	     e. Skin, mucous membrane and nailbed color
	   2. Auscultation
	   3. Document assessment on patient care flow sheet/nursing progress note
	 B. Safely operate and explain rationale for use of delivery equipment:
	   1. Nasal cannula
	   2. Face mask
	   3. Face tent
		A. Review standards
		 Discuss with Preceptor submission of one respiratory assessment on nursing progress note
		
		 B. Demonstration (Can be done in mock session if no patient available)
			A. _____
			
			 1. _____
			 2. _____
			 3. _____
				_____
				
				 _____
				 _____
				 _____

244

APPENDIX I • COMPETENCE ASSESSMENT TOOL FOR NURSES PROVIDING CARE TO CRITICALLY ILL PREGNANT WOMEN

OBJECTIVE	EVALUATION CRITERIA	METHODS	DATE COMPLETED	SUPERVISED BY:
	4. Venti mask 5. Heated mist 6. Cool Mist 7. Ambu bag 8. Portable oxygen tank	Self-review of ICU consortia course content	4. _____ 5. _____ 6. _____ 7. _____ 8. _____	

	C. Correctly interpret ABG's
	   1. Normal values
	   2. Respiratory acidosis
	   3. Metabolic acidosis
	   4. Respiratory alkalosis
	   5. Metabolic alkalosis
		C. Lab result review with preceptor (Focus on non-ventilated patients)	C. _____	

	D. Identify values indicating the need for mechanical ventilation			

6. Demonstrate the ability to care for a patient with an altered level of consciousness.	6. Demonstrate the ability to:
	   1. Perform a baseline neurological assessment.
	     a. Level of consciousness
	     b. Speech
	     c. Sensation
	     d. Motor movement, strength
	     e. Posture
	     f. Muscle tone
	     g. Pupil reaction
	     h. Orientation
	   2. Maintain a safe environment
	     a. Seizure precautions
	     b. Proper body alignment
	     c. Airway patency
	   3. State the nursing responsibilities during a seizure
		6. Self-review of ICU consortia course content	1. _____
			
			2. _____
			
			3. _____	

APPENDIX I • COMPETENCE ASSESSMENT TOOL FOR NURSES PROVIDING CARE TO CRITICALLY ILL PREGNANT WOMEN

Suggested patient diagnoses during clinical experience:
- hypovolemic shock
- septic shock
- cardiogenic shock
- multiple trauma
- aneurysms
- hypertensive emergencies
- coagulopathies
- CHF
- pulmonary edema
- pulmonary embolus
- cardiac arrest (highly suggested)
- cardiac valvular disease

*Competencies adapted from:
1. BWH—Orientation—Medical ICU 7/88
2. BWH Cardiac Monitoring Competency for the Acute and Intermediate Areas 10/88
3. BWH Respiratory Care Competency for the Acute and Intermediate Areas 12/88
4. BWH—Hemodynamic Monitoring Competency for the Acute and Intermediate Areas 12/88
5. Bartlett Surgical Unit (7BC) Orientation Objectives 11/88

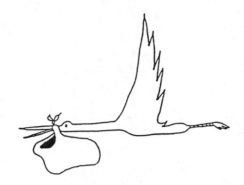

ELECTRONIC FETAL MONITORING

TRACING-OF-THE-MONTH CLUB

A Monthly Home Study Program

by

Cydney Afriat Menihan, CNM, MSN, RDMS

Perinatal Productions, Narragansett, Rhode Island

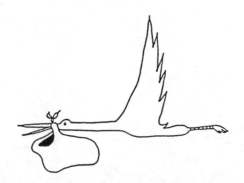

EFM TRACING-OF-THE MONTH CLUB

OBJECTIVES

By assessing each fetal monitoring tracing, the participant will be able to:

* Describe the maternal/fetal physiologic changes that may be responsible for periodic and baseline changes in fetal heart rate.

* Identify the nonreassuring components of each tracing.

* List the problems present on each tracing.

* List the possible causes of each problem.

* Describe all nonsurgical intervention that would be indicated to correct each of the problems.

* Determine if the pattern is reassuring or nonreassuring.
* List the possible causes of baseline and periodic changes

Perinatal Production, Narragansett, Rhode Island

EFM TRACING-OF-THE-MONTH
001

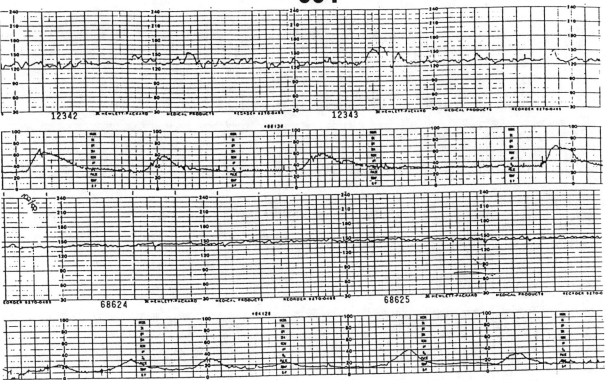

Patient Information:

Tracing Interpretation:
      Instrumentation for FHR_____ UA_____

Baseline FHR_____	Contraction Frequency_____
STV_____	Contraction Duration_____
Accelerations_____	Contraction Intensity_____
Decelerations_____	Resting Tone_____

Problem List: **Possible Causes:**   **Intervention:**

REASSURING_____ NONREASSURING TRACING_____
Perinatal Productions, Narragansett, RI

APPENDIX J • FETAL MONITORING RESOURCES

EFM TRACING-OF-THE-MONTH 002

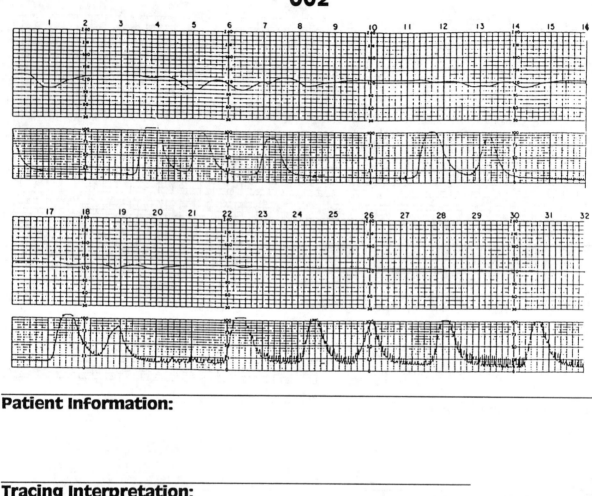

Patient Information:

Tracing Interpretation:
    Instrumentation for FHR_____ UA_____

Baseline FHR_____	**Contraction Frequency**_____
STV_____	**Contraction Duration**_____
Accelerations_____	**Contraction Intensity**_____
Decelerations_____	**Resting Tone**_____

Problem List: **Possible Causes:**   **Intervention:**

REASSURING_____ **NONREASSURING TRACING**_____
Perinatal Productions, Narragansett, RI

APPENDIX J • FETAL MONITORING RESOURCES

EFM TRACING-OF-THE-MONTH
003

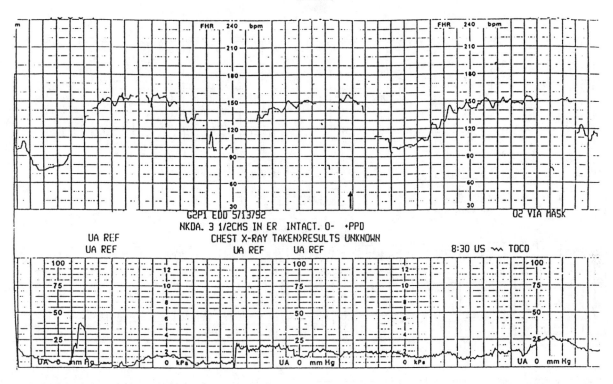

Patient Information:

_____

Tracing Interpretation:
      Instrumentation for FHR_____ **UA**_____

Baseline FHR_____ **Contraction Frequency**_____
STV_____ **Contraction Duration**_____
Accelerations_____ **Contraction Intensity**_____
Decelerations_____ **Resting Tone**_____

Problem List: **Possible Causes:**   **Intervention:**

REASSURING_____ **NONREASSURING TRACING**_____
Perinatal Productions, Narragansett, RI

APPENDIX J • FETAL MONITORING RESOURCES

EFM TRACING-OF-THE-MONTH
004

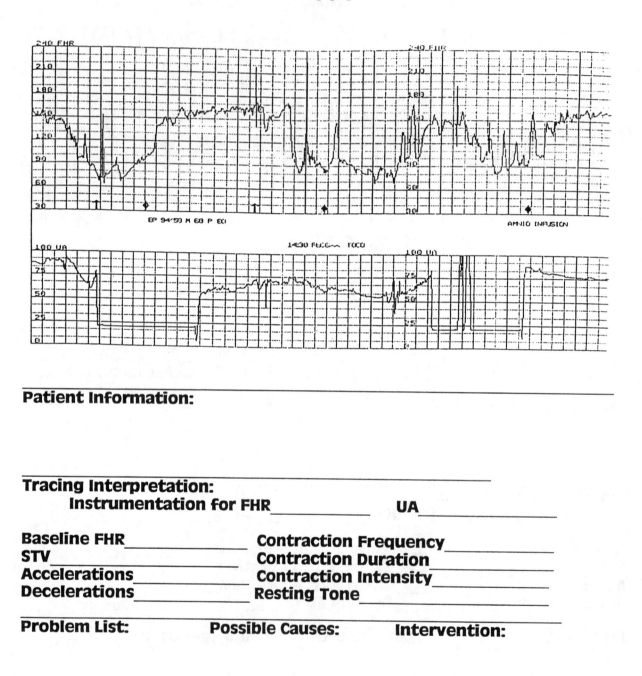

Patient Information:

Tracing Interpretation:
     Instrumentation for FHR_____ **UA**_____

Baseline FHR_____	**Contraction Frequency**_____
STV_____	**Contraction Duration**_____
Accelerations_____	**Contraction Intensity**_____
Decelerations_____	**Resting Tone**_____

Problem List: **Possible Causes:**   **Intervention:**

REASSURING_____ **NONREASSURING TRACING**
    Perinatal Productions, Narragansett, RI

APPENDIX J • FETAL MONITORING RESOURCES

EFM TRACING-OF-THE-MONTH 005

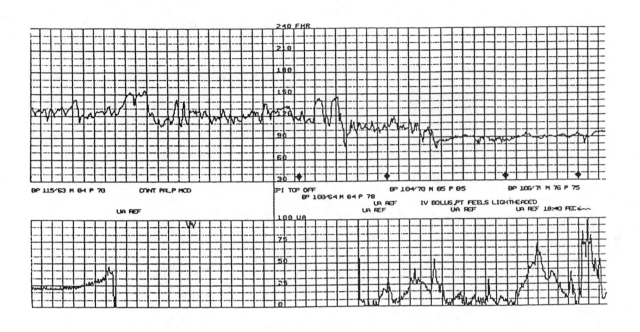

Patient Information:

Tracing Interpretation:
  Instrumentation for FHR_____ UA_____

Baseline FHR_____ **Contraction Frequency**_____
STV_____ **Contraction Duration**_____
Accelerations_____ **Contraction Intensity**_____
Decelerations_____ **Resting Tone**_____

Problem List: **Possible Causes:**   **Intervention:**

REASSURING_____ **NONREASSURING TRACING**_____
Perinatal Productions, Narragansett, RI

APPENDIX J • FETAL MONITORING RESOURCES

EFM TRACING-OF-THE-MONTH
006

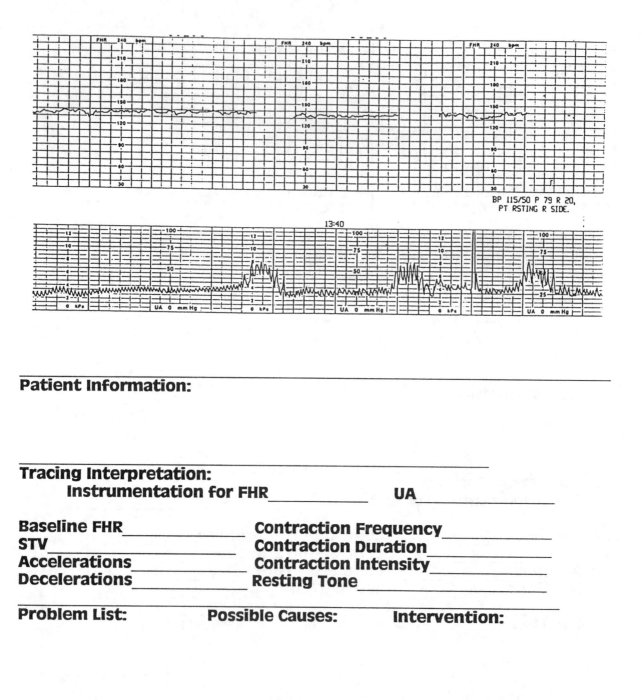

Patient Information: _____

Tracing Interpretation:
  Instrumentation for FHR _____   UA _____

Baseline FHR _____   **Contraction Frequency** _____
STV _____   **Contraction Duration** _____
Accelerations _____   **Contraction Intensity** _____
Decelerations _____   **Resting Tone** _____

Problem List: **Possible Causes:**   **Intervention:**

REASSURING _____ **NONREASSURING TRACING** _____
Perinatal Productions, Narragansett, RI

APPENDIX J • FETAL MONITORING RESOURCES

EFM TRACING-OF-THE-MONTH
007

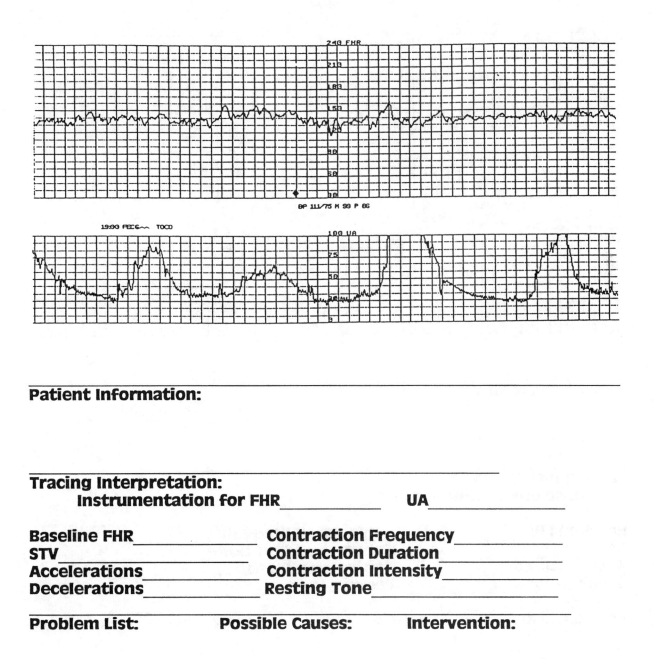

Patient Information:

Tracing Interpretation:
    Instrumentation for FHR_____ UA_____

Baseline FHR_____ Contraction Frequency_____
STV_____ Contraction Duration_____
Accelerations_____ Contraction Intensity_____
Decelerations_____ Resting Tone_____

Problem List: **Possible Causes:**   **Intervention:**

REASSURING_____ **NONREASSURING TRACING**_____
Perinatal Productions, Narragansett, RI

APPENDIX J • FETAL MONITORING RESOURCES

EFM TRACING-OF-THE-MONTH
008

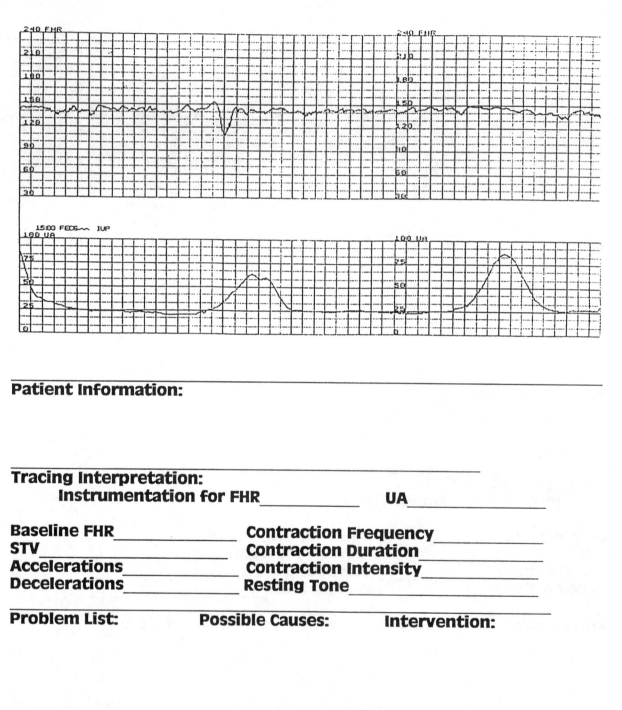

Patient Information:

Tracing Interpretation:
      Instrumentation for FHR_____ UA_____

Baseline FHR_____ Contraction Frequency_____
STV_____ Contraction Duration_____
Accelerations_____ Contraction Intensity_____
Decelerations_____ Resting Tone_____

Problem List: **Possible Causes:**   **Intervention:**

REASSURING_____**NONREASSURING TRACING**_____
      Perinatal Productions, Narragansett, RI

APPENDIX J • FETAL MONITORING RESOURCES

EFM TRACING-OF-THE-MONTH
009

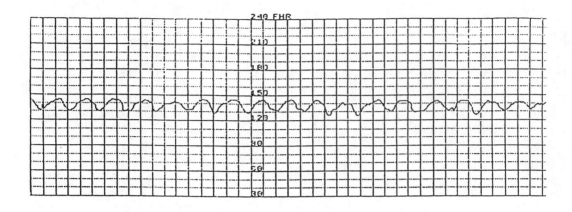

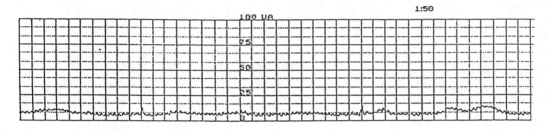

Patient Information:

Tracing Interpretation:
  Instrumentation for FHR_____ UA_____

Baseline FHR_____ Contraction Frequency_____
STV_____ Contraction Duration_____
Accelerations_____ Contraction Intensity_____
Decelerations_____ Resting Tone_____

Problem List: **Possible Causes:**   **Intervention:**

REASSURING_____ **NONREASSURING TRACING**_____
Perinatal Productions, Narragansett, RI

APPENDIX J • FETAL MONITORING RESOURCES

EFM TRACING-OF-THE-MONTH
010

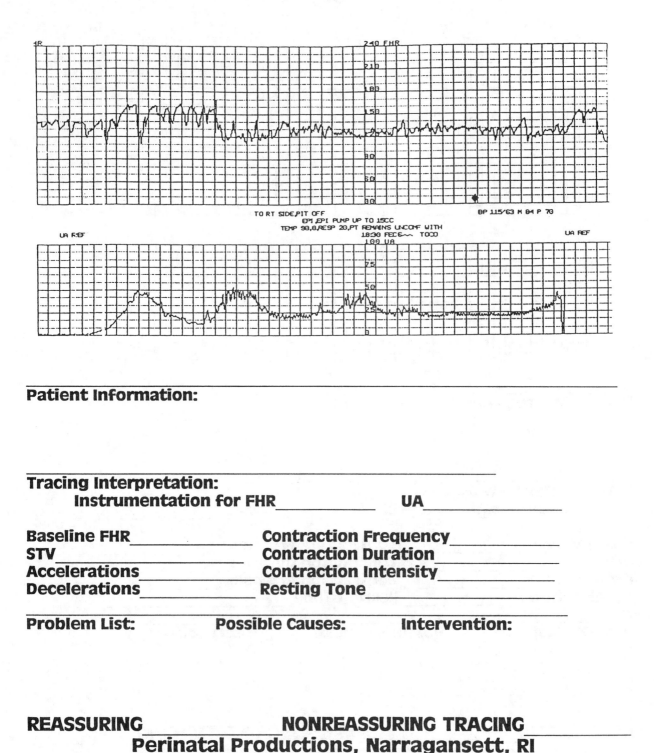

Patient Information:

Tracing Interpretation:
      Instrumentation for FHR_____ UA_____

Baseline FHR_____   **Contraction Frequency**_____
STV_____   **Contraction Duration**_____
Accelerations_____   **Contraction Intensity**_____
Decelerations_____   **Resting Tone**_____

Problem List: **Possible Causes:**   **Intervention:**

REASSURING_____   **NONREASSURING TRACING**_____
Perinatal Productions, Narragansett, RI

APPENDIX J • FETAL MONITORING RESOURCES

EFM TRACING-OF-THE-MONTH
001

Patient Information:

25 y.o. G3P2002 at 39 weeks' gestation who was admitted in early labor. At the end of the first panel, she was examined and found to be 5cm/100%/-2, vertex, intact. She has no prenatal, medical or surgical problems.

Tracing Interpretation:
Instrumentation for FHR External   **UA** External

Baseline FHR 130-140 bpm   **Contraction Frequency** q 2-4 min
STV N/A   **Contraction Duration** 30-50 sec.
Accelerations yes   **Contraction Intensity** n/a
Decelerations none   **Resting Tone** n/a

Problem List:	Possible Causes:	Intervention:
1. Loss of accelertions in panel B	Medication	none

REASSURING   x   **NONREASSURING TRACING**

Perinatal Productions, Narragansett, RI

EFM TRACING-OF-THE-MONTH
002

Patient Information:

32 y.o. G1P0 at 42 weeks' gestation who is being induced for post dates. At this stage of the tracing, she is 4cm/100%/-1, direct OA, with ruptured membranes revealing clear fluid. The pitocin is at 10 mU/min.

Tracing Interpretation:
Instrumentation for FHR scalp lead   **UA** external toco

Baseline FHR 130-120 bpm   **Contraction Frequency** q 2-4
STV absent   **Contraction Duration** 40-60 sec.
Accelerations none   **Contraction Intensity** n/a
Decelerations late   **Resting Tone** n/a

Problem List:	Possible Causes:	Intervention:
1. Late decelerations	1. Uterine hyperstim	1 discontinue pitocin
	2. Maternal supine position	2. turn to lateral position
	3. Uteroplacental insufficiency	3. Oxygen administration
		4. Notify MD or CNM
2. Absent STV	1. R/O medications	5. Record review
	2. Fetal hypoxia	6. Possible tocolysis

REASSURING   **NONREASSURINGTRACING**   x

Perinatal Productions, Narragansett, RI

APPENDIX J • FETAL MONITORING RESOURCES

EFM TRACING-OF-THE-MONTH
003

Patient Information:

17 y.o. G2P1 admitted in active labor with no prenatal care. Presents with active vaginal bleeding. This portion of the tracing was obtained immediately upon admission.

Tracing Interpretation:

Instrumentation for FHR ext   **UA** ext

Baseline FHR 150-160   **Contraction Frequency** ?
STV n/a   **Contraction Duration** ?
Accelerations none   **Contraction Intensity** n/a
Decelerations late   **Resting Tone** n/a

Problem List:	Possible Causes:	Intervention:
1. late decelerations	1. Uterine hyperstim	1. Possible tocolysis
2. no accelerations	2. Drug abuse	2. Drug history/urine screen
	3. Abruption	3. Start IV, give fluids
		4. Notify MD
		5. Place scalp lead
		6. Scalp stimulation to obtain an acceleration/or do fetal blood gas.

REASSURING _____   **NONREASSURING TRACING** x

Perinatal Productions, Narragansett, RI

EFM TRACING-OF-THE-MONTH
004

Patient Information:

G4P3 at 38 weeks' with no prenatal complications. At this point in the tracing, she is 7cm/100%/+1, LOA, membranes ruptured with thin meconium. She has the urge to push.

Tracing Interpretation:

Instrumentation for FHR direct   **UA** external

Baseline FHR 160-170 bpm   **Contraction Frequency** ?
STV average   **Contraction Duration** ?
Accelerations none   **Contraction Intensity** n/a
Decelerations variable   **Resting Tone** n/a

Problem List:	Possible Causes:	Intervention:
1. Variable decelerations	1. Cord Compression	1. Change maternal position
		2. Vaginal exam
		3. Have patent IV
		4. Possible oxygen administration
		5. Notify MD or CNM

REASSURING _____   **NONREASSURING TRACING** x

Perinatal Productions, Narragansett, RI

APPENDIX J • FETAL MONITORING RESOURCES

EFM TRACING-OF-THE-MONTH
005

Patient Information:

22 y.o. G1P0 at term who is in active labor. She had an epidural earlier in labor, but complained of increasing pain. The epidural was topped-off.

Tracing Interpretation:
   Instrumentation for FHR __direct lead__   UA __external__

Baseline FHR __120-130 bpm__   **Contraction Frequency** __q 2-3__
STV __average__   **Contraction Duration** __about 60 sec.__
Accelerations __present__   **Contraction Intensity** __n/a__
Decelerations __prolonged__   **Resting Tone** __n/a__

Problem List: **Possible Causes:**   **Intervention:**
1. Prolonged decelera-   1. Maternal hypotension   1. Change maternal position
   tions   to lateral.
                           2. Uterine hypertonus   2. Hydrate
                              (?)   3. Palpate the uterus
                                                          4. Consider tocolysis
                                                          5. Notify MD
                           2. Cord prolapse   6. Vaginal examination

REASSURING _____ **NONREASSURING TRACING** __x__

Perinatal Productions, Narragansett, RI

EFM TRACING-OF-THE-MONTH
006

Patient Information:

G3P2 at 37 weeks' gestation who presented with spontaneous ruputre of membranes, contractions every 5 minutes and complaining of decreased fetal movement for two days.

Tracing Interpretation:
   Instrumentation for FHR __ext__   UA __ext__

Baseline FHR __130 bpm__   **Contraction Frequency** __2-3 minutes__
STV __n/a__   **Contraction Duration** __45-60 sec.__
Accelerations __none__   **Contraction Intensity** __n/a__
Decelerations __none__   **Resting Tone** __n/a__

Problem List: **Possible Causes:**   **Intervention:**
1. No accelerations   1. Fetal sleep   1. Abdominal palpation/stimulation
                           2. Medication effect   2. Review maternal history
                           3. Hypoxia   3. Fetal scalp stimulation
                                                          4. Apply scalp electrode
                                                          5. Consider fetal blood gas
                                                          6. Notify MD or CNM
                                                          7. Hydrate
                                                          8. Oxygen

REASSURING _____ **NONREASSURING TRACING** __x__

Perinatal Productions, Narragansett, RI

APPENDIX J • FETAL MONITORING RESOURCES

EFM TRACING-OF-THE-MONTH
007

Patient Information:

18 y.o. G1P0 at term who presented with contractions. At this point in the tracing, she is 6cm/100/-2, LOP, AROM with clear fluid and requesting analgesia.

Tracing Interpretation:

Instrumentation for FHR __direct lead__   UA __external__

Baseline FHR 130-140 bpm   **Contraction Frequency** q 2 min.
STV average   **Contraction Duration** about 60 seconds
Accelerations present   **Contraction Intensity** n/a
Decelerations none   **Resting Tone** n/a

Problem List: **Possible Causes:**   **Intervention:**

None

REASSURING __x__   **NONREASSURING TRACING** _____

Perinatal Productions, Narragansett, RI

EFM TRACING-OF-THE-MONTH
008

Patient Information:

35 y.o. G4P3 at 38 weeks' gestation in early labor. Her cervix is 2cm/80%/-1, LOA, membranes intact. She has been ambulating and has now returned to bed for a monitor strip. She was found to be 5cm and having variable decelerations. An IUPC was placed and amnioinfusion started.

Tracing Interpretation:

Instrumentation for FHR __direct lead__   UA __IUP__

Baseline FHR 140-150 bpm   **Contraction Frequency** q 3 minutes
STV average   **Contraction Duration** 60-80 seconds
Accelerations none   **Contraction Intensity** 60-80 mm/hg
Decelerations variable   **Resting Tone** 20-25 mmHg

Problem List: **Possible Causes:**   **Intervention:**

1. Prior variable decel-   1. Cord compression   1. Continue amnioinfusion
   erations

REASSURING __x__   **NONREASSURING TRACING** _____

Perinatal Productions, Narragansett, RI

APPENDIX J • FETAL MONITORING RESOURCES

EFM TRACING-OF-THE-MONTH
009

Patient Information:

32 y.o. G4P2 who presented with decreased fetal movement at 32 weeks' gestation. At that time, the external fetal monitor revealed the above tracing. She was known to be blood type A positive. Her prior Medical/OB is significant for exposure to Parvovirus.

Tracing Interpretation:

Instrumentation for FHR external   **UA** external

Baseline FHR 130-150 bpm   **Contraction Frequency** none
STV n/a but appears flat   **Contraction Duration** none
Accelerations none   **Contraction Intensity** none
Decelerations none   **Resting Tone** none

Problem List:	Possible Causes:	Intervention:
1. Sinusoidal pattern	1. Fetal anemia 2. Fetal infection or ascites	1. Notify MD 2. Fetal scan

REASSURING _____   **NONREASSURING TRACING** x

Perinatal Productions, Narragansett, RI

EFM TRACING-OF-THE-MONTH
010

Patient Information:

24 y.o G2P0 at 41 weeks' gestation who is in active labor at 8 cm/100%/-1, ROA. Amniotic fluid is clear. Labor has progressed normally, except for a prior episode of hyperstimulation with pitocin. The pitocin is now off.

Tracing Interpretation:

Instrumentation for FHR direct lead   **UA** external toco

Baseline FHR 120-130 bpm   **Contraction Frequency** q 2-4 minutes
STV average   **Contraction Duration** 30-60 sec
Accelerations yes   **Contraction Intensity** n/a
Decelerations none   **Resting Tone** n/a

Problem List:	Possible Causes:	Intervention:
None		

REASSURING x   **NONREASSURING TRACING** _____

Perinatal Productions, Narragansett, RI

APPENDIX J • FETAL MONITORING RESOURCES

EVALUATOR: _____ NAME: _____
DATE: _____

CHECKLIST FOR FETAL MONITORING ANNUAL COMPETENCY EVALUATION

Nursing Practice Competencies	Independent	Needs Supervision	Comments Proposed Action Resolved Date
1. Explains the use of electronic fetal monitor to the patient and her support person(s)			
2. Chooses the appropriate electronic fetal monitoring method based on hospital policy or procedure.			
3. Applies external transducers and adjusts the electronic fetal monitor accordingly.			
4. Describes the limitations of information produced by external transducers.			
5. Prepares the patient, sets up equipment, and completes connections for fetal electrode and intrauterine pressure catheter.			
6. Calibrates the monitor for the use of the intrauterine pressure catheter.			
7. Identifies artifacts and technically inadequate tracings and takes appropriate corrective action.			
8. Obtains and maintains an adequate fetal heart rate and uterine contraction tracing.			
9. Interprets uterine contraction frequency, duration, strength, and baseline resting tone as appropriate based on monitoring method, and determines if abnormal findings are present.			
10. Identifies baseline fetal heart rate, baseline variability, and the presence of periodic changes and determines if findings are reassuring or non-reassuring.			
11. Implements appropriate nursing intervention based on electronic fetal monitor findings.			
12. Identifies the clinical situations based on electronic fetal monitor findings in which immediate physician notification is appropriate.			
13. Communicates the content of electronic fetal monitoring data, its interpretation, and resulting nursing intervention in written and verbal form in an appropriate and timely manner.			
14. Documents appropriate entries on the patient record.			
15. Demonstrates appropriate maintenance of electronic fetal monitoring equipment.			

APPENDIX J • FETAL MONITORING RESOURCES

EVALUATOR: _____ NAME: _____
DATE: _____

CHECKLIST FOR FETAL MONITORING ANNUAL COMPETENCY EVALUATION

AREAS OF RESPONSIBILITY AND EXPECTATION	MEETS STANDARD EXPECTATIONS	NEEDS IMPROVEMENT	REMARKS
PREPARATION OF MONITOR			
1. Is the paper inserted correctly?			
2. Are transducers plugged into monitor?			
ULTRASONIC TRANSDUCER			
1. Has coupling gel been applied to crystals?			
2. Was the FHR calibrated and noted on strip chart?			
3. Is the strap secure and snug?			
4. Is there an adequate recording of FHR?			
TOCOTRANSDUCER			
1. Has it been applied without gel, paste, etc.			
2. Was the pen set adjusted between 15 and 20 mm Hg marks and noted on strip chart?			
3. Was this setting done between contractions?			
4. Is the strap secure and snug?			
5. Is there an adequate recording of uterine activity?			
SPIRAL ELECTRODE			
1. Are the wires attached to their respective posts posts on the leg plate?			
2. Is the spiral electrode attached to the presenting part of the fetus?			
3. Is the inner surface of the leg plate covered with electrode paste or gel?			
4. Is there an adequate recording of FHR?			
INTERNAL CATHETER/STRAIN GAUGE			
1. Is the strain gauge located about half the height of the uterus (approximately at maternal xyphoid)?			
2. Is the catheter filled with sterile water?			
3. Is the black line on the catheter visible at the introitus?			
4. Was the UC calibrated at 50 for 10 seconds and "zeroed" to air?			
5. Was the calibration written on the printout?			
6. Is the stopcock "off" to the syringe?			
7. Is there an adequate recording of uterine activity?			
DOCUMENTATION			
1. Documents maternal - fetal assessments according to policy.			

APPENDIX J • FETAL MONITORING RESOURCES

St. Joseph's Hospital
Breese, Illinois

Name _____

Date _____

ORIENTATION/SKILLS VALIDATION
Women and Infants Center Registered Nurse

TOPIC: **AUSCULTATION OF FETAL HEART TONES**

OBJECTIVE: After completion, the participant will demonstrate how to find and count fetal heart sounds and what to do if you hear a fetal heart rate that is not normal.

LEVEL 1: Orientation period when practitioner is dependent on others to meet practice specifications. *With supervision uses practice standards on providing service. *Action plan required with target date for improvement.

LEVEL 2: Characterized by independence in practice. *Independently uses practice standards in providing service.

LEVEL 3: Practitioner has mastered competencies and can fulfill resource and consultative role. *Assists others in the application of practice standards in providing service.

	SELF EVALUATION		VALIDATOR		
	Have Had Exp. With	Competent to Perform	Level 1	Level 2	Level 3
ASSEMBLE THE EQUIPMENT					
1. The basic types of listening devices are:					
a. A modified stethoscope worn on the head of the listener so that bone conduction from the skull increases hearing ability i.e. DeLee-Hillis fetoscope with headpiece.					
b. A large, heavy bell which increases fetal heart sounds. i.e. Leff stethoscope.					
c. An electronic device that picks up the fetal heart sounds. This is helpful in hard-to-hear fetal heart sounds. It also amplifies the sound so the mother can hear it. Fingers should not touch the bell portion of the fetoscope, because friction sounds can interfere with hearing i.e. Doptone (ultrasound).					
2. Raise the head of the bed so that the woman is in a semi-Fowler's position.					

APPENDIX J • FETAL MONITORING RESOURCES

ORIENTATION/SKILLS VALIDATION
Auscultation of Fetal Heart Tones

		SELF EVALUATION		VALIDATOR		
		Have Had Exp. With	Competent to Perform	Level 1	Level 2	Level 3
3.	Determine fetal position and presentation through Leopold's maneuvers. Determine where the fetal back is. Fetal heart tones are transmitted through the convex portion of the fetus because that is the part in close contact with the uterine wall. In most cephalic and breech presentations, fetal heart sounds are best heard through the fetal back. In a face presentation, the fetal back becomes concave, and the best place to listen for heart sounds is over the more convex chest.					
POSITION THE FETOSCOPE						
1.	Position the fetoscope or doptone on the appropriate quadrant of the mother's abdomen. Use firm pressure. In **ROA**, sounds are best heard in the right lower quadrant. In posterior positions such as **LOP** or **ROP**, sounds are best heard at the mother's side. In the breech position, sounds are best heard above the mother's umbilicus on her left side.					
Guidelines That May Aid You in Hering the Fetal Heart Beat						
2.	Between the 10th and 16th weeks of pregnancy, use a doptone. Begin listening at the upper border of the pubic hair. If you are unable to hear fetal heart tones, slowly move the instrument up toward the mother's umbilicus. The ultrasound instruments is more sensitive than the fetoscope. It will pick up fetal heart tones about the 10th week of gestation. As you search in each location, slowly rotate the instrument in circular motion so the ultrasound waves are directed in a wide circle.					

ORIENTATION/SKILLS VALIDATION
Auscultation of Fetal Heart Tones

		SELF EVALUATION		VALIDATOR		
		Have Had Exp. With	Competent to Perform	Level 1	Level 2	Level 3
3.	Between the 16th and 24th weeks of pregnancy, measure off 2 fingerbreadths above the pubic hairline and listen along the midline of the abdomen.					
4.	After the 24th week of pregnancy, search the abdomen in a methodical manner. Place the fetoscope at position 1 in the illustration. If nothing is heard, move to position 2 in the lower left quadrant. Continue following the numbered positions.					
5.	If you do not detect fetal heart tones at these 8 positions, begin a systematic search of the abdomen. Place the fetoscope at the umbilicus and move it cm by cm outward along a spoke-like pattern. Follow the sequence of numbers in the illustration below.					

APPENDIX J • FETAL MONITORING RESOURCES

ORIENTATION/SKILLS VALIDATION
Auscultation of Fetal Heart Tones

	SELF EVALUATION		VALIDATOR		
	Have Had Exp. With	Competent to Perform	Level 1	Level 2	Level 3
If you hear a soft blowing sound, it may be the blood moving through the uterine arteries, the placenta, or the umbilical cord. Count the mother's pulse rate while listening through the fetoscope to determine whether you are hearing the moderate pulse rate of the mother or the faster fetal heart rate.					

Action Plan & Date

_____
_____
_____

Validator's Signature: _____

269

LEOPOLD'S MANEUVERS

Critical Elements	Met	Not Met
1. First Maneuver:		
a) Stand at side of bed facing the patient.		
b) Lay both hands flat upon abdomen.		
c) Palpate upper abdomen with both hands.		
2. Second Maneuver:		
a) Place palmar surfaces of both hands on either side of abdomen.		
b) Maintain placement of one hand on side of abdomen.		
c) Palpate with the flat surface of the fingers in a circular motion on the opposite side.		
3. Third Maneuver:		
a) Gently grasp lower portion of abdomen just above symphysis pubis between thumb and forefinger.		
b) Observe for moveable body.		
4. Fourth Maneuver:		
a) Stand facing patient's feet.		
b) Use tips of fingers to pressure deep in direction of pelvic inlet.		
c) Identify cephalic prominence.		
5. Document according to policy.		

[   ] PASSED   [   ] NEEDS TO REPEAT

VALIDATED BY: _____ DATE: _____

Adapted from Sioux Valley Hospital, Sioux Falls, South Dakota

PALOS COMMUNITY HOSPITAL
Palos Heights, Illinois
Setting Up/Circulating for Dilatation and Uterine Evacuation
Criterion Checklist

Critical Elements	Met	Not Met
1. Prepares equipment/room/supplies according to physician preference card.		
2. Scrubs, gowns and gloves according to Policy & Procedure.		
3. Sets up operative table without contamination.		
4. Checks all equipment and supplies for completeness and proper functioning.		
5. Positions towel, gown and gloves correctly for surgeon to avoid contamination.		
6. Completes counts according to Policy & Procedure.		
7. Breaks scrub role after completion of all scrub responsibilities.		
8. Identifies patient and verifies operative procedure with patient and consent.		
9. Completes peri-operative assessment on OR Record.		
10. Assesses and documents risks for lithotomy positioning.		
11. Transfers patient to operative table and secures safety straps.		
12. Provides patient privacy.		
13. Assists anesthesiologist during administration of anesthesia and/or surgeon during administration of local anesthesia.		
14. Maintains patient safety and utilizes principles of body alignment during patient positioning.		
15. Preps patient using aseptic technique.		
16. Documents all nursing actions including administration of drugs and solutions intraoperatively.		
17. Handles specimens correctly:		
a. For routine specimens, covers entire specimen with formalin.		
b. For frozen sections, calls pathologist and sends specimens dry without formalin.		
c. Includes LMP on all specimen requisitions.		

Critical Elements	Met	Not Met
18. Assists cleaning of patient.		
19. Maintains patient safety during repositioning to supine position.		
20. Follows safety Policy & Procedure in transfer of patient to and from OR room.		
21. Gives accurate and thorough report to relief RN as appropriate.		
22. Assists in room clean-up.		
23. Completes documentation.		
24. Follows Policy & Procedure regarding patient care and documentation during recovery phase.		
25. Completes appropriate discharge procedure including discharge teaching.		
26. Has read the department information in grief packet and demonstrates knowledge of which materials and information are to be given to patient/family during hospital stay.		

Passed ☐   Needs to repeat ☐

Mock Set-up: _____   Actual: _____

Employee: _____   Preceptor: _____

Manager: _____

Nursing Ed (if involved): _____

APPENDIX K • PERIOPERATIVE EDUCATIONAL PROGRAMS AND COMPETENCE ASSESSMENT TOOLS

PERINATAL SURGICAL COMPETENCY TEST

1. Define the location of the two areas listed and identify the dress code.

   a. semirestricted area _____
   _____

   b. restricted area _____
   _____

2. What part of the surgical gown is considered sterile? _____
   _____

3. Under what circumstances should the door to the actual room where surgery is performed be closed? _____

TRUE OR FALSE

_____ Gloved hands are kept between shoulder-waist level.
_____ Gowned/gloved arm may be folded with hands under axilla.
_____ Only horizontal surfaces of draped tables are sterile.
_____ Scrubbed persons remain close to sterile field at all times.
_____ Unsterile persons do not walk between sterile fields.
_____ Items can only be flipped if they can be delivered without contact with the heat seal edge of the package.
_____ Once a sterile package or container is opened, the edges are considered contaminated.
_____ Pour solutions can be recapped if used for the same patient.
_____ If a package tears while it is being opened, its contents are considered contaminated.
_____ A sterile field can only be left unguarded when covered with a sterile drape/barrier.
_____ Any item with a dry stain is considered contaminated.
_____ Scrubs must be changed if soiled or upon reentry from outdoors.
_____ Scrubs are only worn in restricted areas.

4. Define sterilization _____
   _____

5. Define disinfection _____
   _____

6. List the two methods of sterilization used at this hospital. _____
   _____

7. Why must items be washed prior to sterilization. _____
   _____

APPENDIX K • PERIOPERATIVE EDUCATIONAL PROGRAMS AND COMPETENCE ASSESSMENT TOOLS

8. Items of doubtful sterility should be _____

9. Define shelf life. What can affect an item's shelf life?
   _____
   _____
   _____

10. What color changes occur with the sterilization tapes during steam sterilization?
    _____

11. How should sterile items be stored:
    _____ inches from the floor
    _____ inches from outside wall
    At least _____ inches from ceiling fixtures.

TRUE OR FALSE (if false, why?)

12. _____ Any sterile item dropped to the floor is contaminated.
    _____

13. _____ Shelf life guarantees sterility until the expiration date.
    _____

14. _____ Sterile items should be stored in an area separate from clean items.
    _____

ELECTROCAUTERY: TRUE OR FALSE

15. _____ The terms, monopolar and bipolar refer to the type of grounding pad used.

16. _____ All grounding pads are self adhering and disposable.

17. _____ A grounding pad can be trimmed prior to placement on a small adult.

18. _____ Loops and twists in the cautery cable can deviate the current flow.

19. _____ Cautery current can flow through the drapes to the patient (cause burns).

20. _____ Metal objects touching the patient can be the site of a burn because of the possibility of alternate current paths.

21. _____ Adipose tissue is more susceptible to burns than muscle.

APPENDIX K • PERIOPERATIVE EDUCATIONAL PROGRAMS AND COMPETENCE ASSESSMENT TOOLS

ANSWER:

22. Why is it necessary for the patient to be in final desired placement prior to grounding pad placement?_____

23. Why is diagonal bovie placement dangerous?_____
_____

24. Spinal anesthesia refers to the injection of anesthesia agent into_____
_____

25. Epidural anesthesia refers to the injection of anesthesia into_____
_____

26. _____ an antacid is used as a pre-medication in order to
_____
_____

27. Two advantages of regional anesthesia_____
_____

28. Two advantages of general anesthesia_____
_____

29. Describe a typical induction of general anesthesia/intubation.
_____
_____
_____

30. Describe the Sellick Maneuver. Why is it performed?
_____
_____
_____

31. What is the major complication of spinal or epidural anesthesia?_____
_____

32. What is the purpose of injecting a "test dose" prior to administration of epidural anesthesia?
_____

33. How can you tell if the epidural catheter is in the epidural vein or the intrathecal space?
_____
_____

APPENDIX K • PERIOPERATIVE EDUCATIONAL PROGRAMS AND COMPETENCE ASSESSMENT TOOLS

34. Where is the hyperthermia box located? _____

35. List the contents of the hypothermia box. _____
_____
_____

36. What is the primary drug used to treat malignant hypothermia and from what two locations in the hospital can it be obtained immediately? _____
_____

37. What are the nursing interventions following identification of Malignant Hyperthermia?
_____
_____

38. Instruments are categorized by their: _____

    The 4 categories are _____, _____ _____ and _____.

39. <u>Basic</u> cutting instruments include _____ and _____.

40. Clamping instruments are also referred to as _____.

41. List 4 clamps _____

42. Retractors are designed to _____
_____

43. Name a common self-retaining retractor _____.

44. Grasping instruments are useful for _____
_____

45. Name 3 types of suction tips: _____
_____

46. Most surgical instruments are made of _____.

47. When are instruments counted? _____
_____

48. Why should instruments only be lubricated with a water soluble lubricant?
_____
_____

49. Name 2 types of scissors: a. _____ b. _____

50. When do you utilize these 2 types of scissors? a. _____
    b. _____

OBSTETRIC POSTANESTHESIA NURSING SKILLS CHECKLIST

	SELF-ASSESSED SKILL LEVEL 0=No experience 1=Observed 2=Done with supervision 3=Performs independently	INSTRUCTION 0=None 1=Class 2=Module 3=Demonstration	PERFORMANCE 0=No opportunity to assess 1=Responds appropriately to questions 2=Performs with assistance/supervision 3=Performs independently/proficient 4=Able to teach others	
	CODE	CODE INIT./DATE	CODE INIT./DATE	
I. ADMISSION ASSESSMENT				

A. Performs initial physical assessment: prioritization and demonstration
  1. Respiratory status: airway, breathing, arterial oxygen saturation
  2. Cardiovascular: blood pressure, pulse, ECG
  3. Level of consciousness
  4. Temperature
  5. Surgical site: incision, drains
  6. Fundus, lochia
  7. Nausea and vomiting
  8. Pain
  9. Hydration status
B. Obtains history
  1. Preoperative
  2. Intraoperative
  3. Anesthesia report
C. Assesses psychosocial needs or status
  1. Anxiety
  2. Infant status
  3. Family support				

II. RESPIRATORY SYSTEM				

A. Assesses and/or demonstrates:
  1. Respiratory function
    a. Inspection
    b. Listening/auscultation				

2. Oxygen therapy
   a. Endotracheal tube if applicable
   b. Mask
   c. Nasal cannula
   d. Oral airway
   e. Nasal airway
   f. Bag/mask ventilation
3. Pulse oximetry
   a. Application and use
   b. Interpretation of values
   c. Trouble-shooting

B. Manages airway
   1. Identifies obstruction signs and symptoms
   2. Demonstrates:
      a. Jaw thrust
      b. Chin lift
      c. Head tilt
      d. Head to one side
      e. Lateral decubitus position
   3. Demonstrates operation of suction equipment
   4. Performs stir-up regimen:
      a. Deep breathing
      b. Coughing
      c. Positioning
      d. Mobilization

C. Describes symptoms of and treatments for:
   1. Hypoxia
   2. Mechanical obstruction
   3. Laryngeal edema
   4. Laryngospasm
   5. Bronchospasm
   6. Aspiration

III. CARDIOVASCULAR SYSTEM

A. ECG
   1. Demonstrates correct electrode placement
   2. Sets up cardiac monitor

continues

Continued.

3. Trouble-shoots monitor
4. Recognizes normal sinus rhythm
B. Describes symptoms of and treatments for:
   1. Hypotension
   2. Hypertension
   3. Tachycardia
   4. Bradycardia
   5. Postpartum hemorrhage/hypovolemia
   6. Coagulopathies/emboli
   7. Life-threatening dysrhythmias
   8. Cardiac arrest/defibrillation

IV. CENTRAL NERVOUS SYSTEM

A. Assesses level of consciousness
B. States emergency seizure care
C. Demonstrates assessment of dermatome levels and motor function (see section IX, regional anesthesia)

V. TEMPERATURE REGULATION

A. Describes symptoms of and treatments for:
   1. Hypothermia
   2. Hyperthermia
   3. Shivering
   4. Malignant hyperthermia

VI. FLUIDS AND ELECTROLYTES

A. Describes symptoms of and treatments for:
   1. Fluid overload/pulmonary edema
   2. Hypovolemia
   3. Urinary retention
B. Administers blood products correctly

VII. COMFORT	A. Performs assessment
	B. Administers appropriate medications
	  1. Narcotics
	  2. Patient-controlled analgesia
	  3. Nonsteroidal antiinflammatory drugs
	  4. Epidural analgesics
	C. Provides comfort measures		

VIII. GENERAL ANESTHESIA	A. Assists anesthesia provider with intubation
	B. Assists anesthesia provider with extubation
	C. Describes expected effects/side effects of:
	  1. Induction agents
	  2. Inhaled agents
	  3. Muscle relaxant agents
	  4. Reversal agents
	  5. Adjunct intravenous agents		

IX. REGIONAL ANESTHESIA	A. Demonstrates assessment of dermatome levels and motor function
	B. Describes symptoms of and treatments for:
	  1. High, total, or prolonged blocks
	  2. Hypotension due to anesthesia
	  3. Bradycardia
	  4. Nausea and vomiting
	  5. Urinary retention
	  6. Spinal headache
	  7. Motor/sensory function alteration
	  8. Nerve injury
	  9. Spinal hematoma		

continues

Continued.

X. EMERGENCY MANAGEMENT				

A. Locates/demonstrates use of:
  1. Crash cart
  2. Defibrillator
  3. Anesthesia bags/masks
  4. Emergency trays
  5. Emergency drugs
  6. Suctioning equipment				

XI. DOCUMENTATION				
A. Completes appropriate forms B. Assigns postanesthesia scoring system C. Initiates appropriate patient care plans and protocols, individualizing as needed D. Documents serial assessments E. Completes discharge summary				

O'Brien-Abel, N. et al. (1994). Obstetric post anesthesia nursing: A staff education program. *Journal of Perinatal and Neonatal Nursing, 8(3), 17–32.*

BRIGHAM AND WOMEN'S HOSPITAL
CENTER FOR LABOR & BIRTH
SURGICAL SCRUB COMPETENCY VALIDATION

Critical Elements	Met	Not Met
1. OPENS PACKAGE USING ASEPTIC TECHNIQUE.		
2. PLACES PAPER TOWELS ON EACH SIDE OP PATIENT BEGINNING WITH FARTHEST SIDE FIRST.		
3. SCRUBS X 2 WITH BETADINE SPONGES.		
A. May go over the incision more than once.		
B. Scrubs in a horseshoe fashion, away from incision.		
C. Scrubs the farthest leg first, superior to inferior.		
D. Scrubs inner leg superior to inferior.		
E. Flips the sponge and preps down the mons pubis.		
*CAREFUL TO AVOID INCISION AREA		
4. DRIES WITH PAPER TOWELS X 2.		
A. Peels away towels.		
B. Avoids dragging down abdomen.		
5. PREPS WITH BETADINE STICKS X 2.		
A. Goes over incision *only once*.		
B. Travels superiorly up abdomen to just below breasts.		
C. Preps outside leg first, superior to inferior.		
D. Preps inside leg superior to inferior.		
E. Flips sponge, preps over mons pubis and down.		
*CAREFUL TO AVOID INCISION		
F. Preps all areas missed or "window" with second sponge.		
6. REMOVES SIDE TOWELS.		

NAME: _____

VALIDATED BY: _____

DATE: _____

APPENDIX K • PERIOPERATIVE EDUCATIONAL PROGRAMS AND COMPETENCE ASSESSMENT TOOLS

St. Joseph's Hospital
Breese, Illinois

SKILLS VALIDATION

Name _____

Date _____

TOPIC: **WOMEN AND INFANT CENTER REGISTERED NURSE**
Operating Room

OBJECTIVE: Demonstrate competency when functioning as Circulating Nurse for Cesarean Sections.

LEVEL 1: Orientation period when practitioner is dependent on others to meet practice specifications. *With supervision uses practice standards on providing service. *Action plan required with target date for improvement.

LEVEL 2: Characterized by independence in practice. *Independently uses practice standards in providing service.

LEVEL 3: Practitioner has mastered competencies and can fulfill resource and consultative role. *Assists others in the application of practice standards in providing service.

	Level 1	Level 2	Level 3
Competency to Assess the Physiological Health Status of Patient			
1. Verifies Operative Procedure - Consent form, patient's statement, and surgeon's verification			
2. Notes Condition of Skin - Rashes, bruises, lesions, and previous incisions			
3. Determines Mobility of Body - Range of motion and H & P			
4. Reports Deviation of Diagnostic Studies - Laboratory values and X-ray results			
5. Checks Vital Signs - B.P., Temp, Pulse, and Respirations			
6. Notes Abnormalities, Injuries, and Previous Injuries - Loss of extremity or body part; and congenital anomalies			
7. Identifies Presence of Internal and External Prostheses/Implants			
8. Notes Sensory Impairments - Hearing, visual and tactile deficits			
9. Assesses Cardiovascular Status - Pulse alteration, arrhythmias, edema, and EKG			
10. Assesses respiratory status - Skin color and breath sounds			
11. Assesses renal status - Intake and output; and urinalysis			
12. Notes nutritional status - Nothing by mouth; and weight			
13. Verifies allergies - Medication, food and chemical			

APPENDIX K • PERIOPERATIVE EDUCATIONAL PROGRAMS AND COMPETENCE ASSESSMENT TOOLS

SKILLS VALIDATION
WOMEN AND INFANT CENTER REGISTERED NURSE
Operating Room
Page 2

		Level 1	Level 2	Level 3
14.	Screens for substance abuse - Skin changes, patient's statement, H & P			
15.	Communicates/documents physical health status			
Competency to Assess the Psychosocial Health Status of the Patient/Family				
1.	Elicits perception of surgery			
2.	Elicits expectation of care			
3.	Determines coping mechanisms			
4.	Determines knowledge level			
5.	Determines ability to understand			
6.	Identifies philosophical and religious beliefs			
7.	Identifies cultural practices			
8.	Communicates psychosocial data relevant to planning			
Competency to Create and Maintain a Sterile Field				
1.	Uses principles of aseptic practice in varying situations - Clean Vs. Sterile Field			
2.	Initiates corrective action when breaks in technique occur - Changing gown and gloves; surgical conscience			
3.	Inspects sterile items for contamination before opening - Intake package and sterile indicator			
4.	Maintains sterility while opening sterile items for procedure - Delivery to field and pouring solutions			
5.	Functions within designated dress code - hair covered and wears scrub attire			
6.	Communicates/documents maintenance of sterile field			
Competency to Provide Equipment and Supplies Based on Patient Needs				
1.	Anticipates the need for equipment and supplies - Electrosurgical equipment			
2.	Selects equipment and supplies in an organized and timely manner			
3.	Assures all equipment is functioning before use			
4.	Operates mechanical, electrical, and air-powered equipment according to manufacturer's			

APPENDIX K • PERIOPERATIVE EDUCATIONAL PROGRAMS AND COMPETENCE ASSESSMENT TOOLS

SKILLS VALIDATION
WOMEN AND INFANT CENTER REGISTERED NURSE
Operating Room
Page 3

		Level 1	Level 2	Level 3
5.	Removes malfunctioning equipment from O.R.			
6.	Assures emergency equipment and supplies are available at all times.			
Competency to Perform Sponge, Sharps, and Instrument Counts				
1.	Follows established policies/procedures for counts			
2.	Initiates corrective actions when counts are incorrect			
3.	Communicates/documents results of counts according to policy			
Competency to Physiologically Monitor the Patient During Surgery				
1.	Assists/Monitors Physical Symptoms - Skin color, EKG			
2.	Assists/Monitors Behavioral Changes - Restlessness, and level of consciousness			
3.	Calculates Intake and Output - Fluid intake and blood loss			
4.	Operates Monitor Equipment According to Manufacturer's Instructions - Automatic B.P. Monitor and Temperature Probe			
5.	Initiates Nursing Actions Based on Interpretation of Physiological Changes - Surgeon notification and crash cart			
Competency to Monitor and Control the Environment				
1.	Regulates temperature and humidity as indicated			
2.	Adheres to electrical safety policies/procedures			
3.	Monitors sensory environment			
4.	Maintains traffic patterns			
5.	Adheres to O.R. sanitation policies/procedures			
Sets Up Room Before Procedure				
1.	Checks preference card before case			
2.	Connects suction equipment			
3.	Prepares room for C/Section			
Preparation of Patient				
1.	Selects and stamps correct records for procedure			
2.	Reviews patient's chart before putting on cart			
	a. Checks for signed surgical and blood permits			
	b. Checks for Lab reports			

SKILLS VALIDATION
WOMEN AND INFANT CENTER REGISTERED NURSE
Operating Room
Page 4

			Level 1	Level 2	Level 3
	c.	Checks patient's armband			
	d.	Checks allergies procedure and surgeon(s) with patient when possible			
3.		Patient Transportation			
	a.	Bed - siderails up, IV pole at foot of cart, transport feet first			
	b.	Cover patient's hair with surgical cap			
4.		Positions Patient on O.R. Table			
	a.	Applies BP cuff, monitor electrodes, safety straps			
	b.	Armboards			
5.		Assists Anesthetist with Patient			
6.		Ties Surgeon's and Assistant's gowns			
Intraoperative Procedures					
1.		Preps			
	a.	Shave			
	b.	Skin - Hibiclens			
2.		Documentation of:			
	a.	O.R. Record			
	b.	Charge Record			
	c.	Laboratory Records			
		- Pathology Records			
		- Culture Requisitions			
		- Cytology Requisitions			
3.		Disposition of Specimens			
	a.	Routine Cord Blood			
	b.	Placenta			
4.		Sterile Technique			
	a.	Insertion Foley			
	b.	Be available for counts at correct time			
	c.	Keeps sponges in order during case			
	d.	Documentation of number of sponges			

APPENDIX K • PERIOPERATIVE EDUCATIONAL PROGRAMS AND COMPETENCE ASSESSMENT TOOLS

SKILLS, VALIDATION
WOMEN AND INFANT CENTER REGISTERED NURSE
Operating Room
Page 5

		Level 1	Level 2	Level 3
5.	Knows location and usage of instruments			
6.	Knows location and usage of sutures - Knows importance of suture and needle counts			
7.	Knows correct name and spelling of surgical procedure			
8.	Assists technician with dressing placement			

Comments & Recommendations

_____

_____

_____

_____

Validator's Signature: _____

Action Plan & Date

_____

_____

_____

_____

Supervisor's Signature: _____

St. Joseph's Hospital
Breese, Illinois

SKILLS VALIDATION

Name _____

Date _____

TOPIC: **WOMEN AND INFANT CENTER REGISTERED NURSE**
Post Anesthesia Care Unit

OBJECTIVE: The participant will demonstrate competency in recovering the patient.

LEVEL 1: Orientation period when practitioner is dependent on others to meet practice specifications. *With supervision uses practice standards on providing service. *Action plan required with target date for improvement.

LEVEL 2: Characterized by independence in practice. *Independently uses practice standards in providing service.

LEVEL 3: Practitioner has mastered competencies and can fulfill resource and consultative role. *Assists others in the application of practice standards in providing service.

	Level 1	Level 2	Level 3
Patient Admission			
1. Attaches Blood Pressure Monitor			
2. Obtains initial set of Vital Signs			
3. Completes initial physical assessment			
4. Reviews and implements pertinent Physician's Orders			
5. Calls Pharmacy for any drug orders, i.e. antibiotics, PCA			
Airway Insertion and Removal			
1. Oropharyngeal			
2. Nasal			
Pulse			
1. Radial			
2. Carotid			
3. Femoral			
4. Apical			
5. Brachial			

SKILLS VALIDATION
WOMEN AND INFANT CENTER REGISTERED NURSE
Post Anesthesia Care Unit
Page 2

	Level 1	Level 2	Level 3
Suctioning			
1. Oral-Nasal			
2. Endotracheal			
3. Intermittent			
Oxygen Administration			
1. Nasal Cannula			
2. Face Mask			
3. Rebreathing Mask			
CPR Certification			
Documentation			
1. Vital signs every 10 minutes - Minimum			
2. Respiratory Status			
a. Deep Breathe and Cough			
3. Level of consciousness or degree of post-spinal/epidural anesthesia			
4. Skin condition evaluation			
5. Condition of dressings, tubes, IV sites			
6. Assessment of body functions specific to type of surgical procedure			
7. IV fluid type and volume			
8. Medications and patient response			
9. Procedures/Treatments performed in PACU			
10. Presence of Physician			
11. Understands constant attendance by Recovery Nurse			
12. Condition of Patient at time of discharge			
13. Completes PACU Discharge Criteria			
14. Completes PACU Record			
Transports Patient to Room			
1. Bedrails up, IV pole at foot of cart			

YORK HOSPITAL
MOTHER/CHILD CARE
CROSSTRAINING COMPETENCIES

At the end of the Mother/Child Care program, the professional nurse will be able to:

1. Perform a systematic and thorough postpartum physical assessment based upon knowledge of normal postpartum physiological changes.

2. Provide appropriate care to the postpartum woman without complications.

3. Identify the postpartum woman at risk for postpartum complications.

4. Provide care to nursing and non-nursing mothers.

5. Provide information pertaining to self and newborn care to the postpartum woman and her family based upon individual needs.

6. Perform a systematic and thorough full-term newborn physical assessment based upon knowledge of expected adaptation to extrauterine life.

7. Plan and provide care to normal full-term infants.

8. Identify the full-term infant at risk for complications.

9. Provide appropriate care to the full-term infant with complications.

APPENDIX L • MOTHER-BABY NURSING: COMPETENCE VALIDATION TOOLS AND SKILLS CHECKLISTS

Orientee_____   Mentor_____

COMPETENCY 1.   Perform a systematic and thorough postpartum physical assessment based upon knowledge of normal postpartum physiological changes.

Critical Behavior	Self (*) Assessment	Learning Activities	Method of Evaluation	Performs Independently
1. Understands normal postpartum physiological maternal adaptations.	_____	View video: AWHONN's Cross Training for Obstetrical Nursing Staff: Postpartum Care Study AWHONN's Postpartum Compendium Observes performing a postpartum assessment Practices performing a postpartum assessment	Complete Postpartum Care exam with a score of 90% Mentor reviews charts for appropriate documentation Mentor observes the orientee assessing a postpartum woman	Date/Initials 1. _____
2. Reviews medical record for information pertinent to the nursing plan of care **Rh, rubella status, complications during delivery, and any other pertinent information.**	_____			2. _____
3. Introduces self to patient and explains the purpose of the postpartum physical assessment.	_____			3. _____
4. Provides for patient comfort and privacy by assessing need for pain relief and having patient empty her bladder.	_____			4. _____
5. Obtains necessary vital signs per protocol.	_____			5. _____
6. Inspects the breasts for consistency, tenderness, nipple shape, nipple integrity, and presence of colostrum or milk.	_____			6. _____
7. Palpates uterine fundus noting location consistency and massages if necessary. **Locates the xiphoid process with one hand and places other hand over the symphysis pubis.**	_____			7. _____

(*)   <u>Self Assessment Key</u>
1 - Knowledgeable - able to perform with confidence
2 - Knowledgeable but need practice
3 - Need review and practice

Critical Behavior	Self (*) Assessment	Learning Activities	Method of Evaluation	Performs Independently
COMPETENCY 1. (Continued)				Date/Initials:
8. Observes lochial flow for color, amount, consistency, and odor.	_____			8. _____
9. Obtains information from patient regarding her ability to urinate independently. Notes presence of frequency, urgency, pain or the inability to empty bladder. Assesses bladder status and catheterizes according to protocol if necessary.	_____			9. _____
10. Inspects perineum for presence and intactness of episiotomy and/or lacerations. Notes presence of erythema, ecchymosis, edema, hematoma, pain, and/or drainage in area.	_____			10. _____
11. Inspects incision (cesarean or tubal ligation) for intactness. Note presence of erythema, ecchymosis, edema, and/or drainage in area.	_____			11. _____
12. Inspects intactness of rectal area noting present size, and number of hemorrhoids. Notes occurrence of last bowel movement and presence of constipation.	_____			12. _____
13. Inspects extremities for presence and location of edema, redness, tenderness, and/or varicosities. Performs Homan's sign bilaterally on legs.	_____			13. _____
14. Documents appropriately. a. Progress Notes b. Kardex c. Clinical Pathway d. OB Nursing Care Flow Sheets	_____			14. _____

APPENDIX L • MOTHER-BABY NURSING: COMPETENCE VALIDATION TOOLS AND SKILLS CHECKLISTS

Orientee_____   Mentor_____

COMPETENCY 2: Provide appropriate care to the postpartum woman without complications.

Critical Behavior	Self (*) Assessment	Learning Activities	Method of Evaluation	Performs Independently
1. Receives patient report, reviews physicians' orders and patient chart.	_____	Study AWHONN's Postpartum Compendium	Mentor reviews charts for appropriate documentation	Date/Initials 1. _____
2. Initiates / follows through on plan that supports postpartum assessment and vital signs findings.	_____	Review policies and procedures for postpartum care a. postpartum assessment b. medication administration c. Rhogam d. Rubella e. specimen collection f. discharge of mother and newborn	Mentor observes the orientee providing care to the postpartum woman	2. _____
3. Assesses patient's comfort level and provides for pain relief including administration and/or use of: a. pain medications - oral, IM, PCA b. ice packs c. sitz baths d. pericare measures	_____			3. _____
4. Identifies and meets patient's psychosocial needs by utilizing referral resources within the Postpartum Home Visitation program and available Community agencies.	_____	Review Mother/Baby Referral Resource Manual		4. _____
5. Provides for patient's immunization needs for Rhogam (IM) and Rubella (sc).	_____	Review self learning packet "The Management of pain."		5. _____
6. Collects specimens per protocol as necessary.	_____			6. _____
7. Completes patient discharge per procedure.	_____	Observe peers providing care to a postpartum woman		7. _____
8. Documents appropriately: a. Clinical Pathway b. OB Nursing Care Flow Sheets c. Progress Notes (DAO) d. Kardex e. Referrals	_____	Practice providing care to a postpartum woman		8. _____

(*)   **Self Assessment Key**
1 - **Knowledgeable - able to perform with confidence**
2 - **Knowledgeable but need practice**
3 - **Need review and practice**

APPENDIX L • MOTHER-BABY NURSING: COMPETENCE VALIDATION TOOLS AND SKILLS CHECKLISTS

Orientee_____   Mentor_____

COMPETENCY 3: Identify the postpartum woman at risk for postpartum complications.

Critical Behavior	Self (*) Assessment	Learning Activities	Method of Evaluation	Performs Independently

Postpartum Hemorrhage
1. Assesses for predisposing factors:
   a. previous postpartum hemorrhage
   b. rapid or prolonged labor
   c. uterine over distention due to macrosomia, multiple births, and/or polyhydramnios
   d. use of tocolytic and/or anesthetic agents during labor and/or delivery
   e. operative birth
   f. high parity
   g. intrauterine infections
   h. previous uterine surgery
 	
2. Assesses blood loss according to protocol. Keeps pad count as necessary.
   a. **Scant lochia** - less than 1-inch stain on peripad within 1 hour of assessment
   b. **Light lochia** - less than 4-inch stain on peripad within 1 hour of assessment
   c. **Moderate lochia** - less than 6-inch stain on peripad within 1 hour of assessment
   d. **Heavy lochia** - saturated peripad within 1 hour of assessment
 	
3. Assesses vital signs every 15 minutes when indicated.
 	
4. Accurately records intake and output.
	_____
	
	_____
	
	_____
		View video: AWHONN's Cross Training for Obstetrical Nursing Staff: Pregnancy Induced Hypertension
		
		Review March of Dimes Module: Maternal Assessment-BP
		
		Review March of Dimes Module: Maternal Assessment-urine
		
		Study AWHONN's Postpartum Compendium
			Completes Identification of Postpartum Complication exam with score of 80%
			
			Mentor reviews charts for appropriate documentation
			
			Mentor observes the orientee manage the care of a postpartum woman at risk for a complication
				Date/Initials
				1. _____
				
				2. _____
				
				3. _____
				
				4. _____

(*)   <u>Self Assessment Key</u>
1 - Knowledgeable - able to perform with confidence
2 - Knowledgeable but need practice
3 - Need review and practice

Critical Behavior	Self (*) Assessment	Learning Activities	Method of Evaluation	Performs Independently
COMPETENCY 3. (Continued)				Details/Initials:
5. Plans and take appropriate nursing actions: a. Ensure large-bore needle IV access. b. Obtains appropriate laboratory specimens c. Massages uterus correctly. d. Anticipates need for uterotonic and pain relief medications. e. Administers appropriate IV fluids as necessary. f. Administers prescribed medications as necessary. g. Provide for emotional needs of woman and her family.	_____ _____ _____ _____ _____ _____ _____			5. _____
Endometritis 1. Assess for predisposing risk factors. **a. History of pyelonephritis, cesarean birth, hemorrhage, prolonged labor, prolonged ROM, use of internal monitoring, amnioinfusion, fetal scalp sampling, and/or multiple vaginal examinations.** **b. Anemia, systemic illness, and/or evidence of Socioeconomic and nutritional factors which compromise host defense mechanisms.**	_____ _____			1. _____

2. Assesses for appropriate signs and symptoms.
 a. Appropriate physical and lab findings, which may include:
   1. Fever
   2. Malaise
   3. Lower abdominal pain
   4. Foul-smelling lochia
   5. Urinalysis results
   6. Leukocytosis
   7. Results of all cultures
	_____			2. _____

3. Notifies resource nurse and assists with appropriate nursing actions.	_____			3. _____

Critical Behavior	Self (*) Assessment	Learning Activities	Method of Evaluation	Performs Independently
COMPETENCY 3. (Continued)				Date/Initials:
Urinary Tract Infections				
1. Assess for predisposing risk factors. a. History of birth trauma, anesthesia, frequent vaginal exams, and/or catheterization.	_____			1. _____
2. Assesses for appropriate signs and symptoms. a. Dysuria, frequency, low-grade fever, urgency, and/or lower pelvic pressure, back pain, chills, malaise, hematuria, and nausea and vomiting.	_____			2. _____
3. Obtain urine for analysis, culture and sensitivity.	_____			3. _____
4. Interprets lab results.	_____			4. _____
5. Administer antimicrobials as ordered.	_____			5. _____
6. Assess vital signs every 4 hours.	_____			6. _____
7. Encourages rest, adequate fluid intake, adequate diet, and frequent voiding.	_____			7. _____
8. Teach and/or reinforce appropriate perineal hygiene and hand washing.	_____			8. _____
Thrombophlebitis and Thromboembolism				
1. Assess for predisposing risk factors. a. Normal coagulation changes of pregnancy, cesarean birth, use of forceps, blood vessel and tissue trauma, previous history of thromboembolic disease, varicosities, obesity, age older than 40 years, sepsis, and/or immobility associated with AP bed rest.	_____			1. _____

2. Assess for subjective and objective signs and symptoms.
   a. Positive Homan's sign with circumference of affected leg 2 cms. larger than unaffected leg.
   b. Decreased pulse in affected extremity.
   c. Redness, edema, and/or tenderness in affected lower extremity.
	_____			2. _____

Critical Behavior	Self (*) Assessment	Learning Activities	Method of Evaluation	Performs Independently

COMPETENCY 3. (Continued)
 	
3. Takes appropriate nursing interventions.
   a. Assesses vital signs every 4 hours.
   b. Assesses affected extremity for edema and pain every 4 hours.
   c. Applies antiembolic support stocking.
   d. Applies warm packs to affected extremity.
   e. Elevates affected leg.
   f. Ambulates as ordered.
 	
Pregnancy-induced Hypertension
1. Assesses for predisposing risk factors.
   a. First pregnancy or pregnancy of new genetic makeup.
   b. Multiple gestation
   c. Presence of preexisting diabetes, collagen vascular disease, hypertension, or renal disease.
   d. Hydatidiform mole
   e. Fetal hydrops
   f. Maternal age
   g. African American race
   h. Family history of PIH
   I. Antiphospholipid syndrome
   j. Angiotensinogen gene
   k. Socioeconomic status
   l. Failure to demonstrate hemodilution
   m. Failure to demonstrate a decrease in systemic vascular resistance and second trimester mean arterial pressures.
 	
2. Understands definition of pregnancy-induced hypertension and its classifications.
   a. <u>Definition</u> - onset of hypertension after twenty weeks gestation appearing as a marker of a pregnancy specific vasospastic condition.
   b. <u>Classifications</u>:
     1. <u>Preeclampsia</u> - renal involvement, as evidenced by onset of proteinuria; is mild or severe.
     2. <u>HELLP Syndrome</u> - hepatic involvement evidenced by hemolysis, elevated liver enzymes, and low platelets.
     3. <u>Eclampsia</u> - onset of seizure activity or coma in woman diagnosed with PIH without
	_____
	_____
	_____
	_____
	_____
	_____
	
	_____
	
	_____
				Date/Initials:
				
				3. _____
				
				1. _____
				
				2. _____

APPENDIX L • MOTHER-BABY NURSING: COMPETENCE VALIDATION TOOLS AND SKILLS CHECKLISTS

Critical Behavior	Self (*) Assessment	Learning Activities	Method of Evaluation	Performs Independently
COMPETENCY 3. (Continued)				Date/Initials:
3. Assesses for hypertension, proteinuria, and edema per postpartum protocol for first 48 hours after birth.	_____			3. _____

APPENDIX L • MOTHER-BABY NURSING: COMPETENCE VALIDATION TOOLS AND SKILLS CHECKLISTS

Orientee_____   Mentor_____

COMPETENCY 4:   Provide care to nursing and non-nursing mothers.

Critical Behavior	Self (*) Assessment	Learning Activities	Method of Evaluation	Performs Independently

<u>Nursing Mother:</u>
1. Understands the anatomy and physiology of human lactation.
 	
2. Supports decision of mother to breast-feed.
 	
3. Assists mother with breast-feeding:
   a. properly positions infant at breast;
   b. identifies signs of correct infant latch-on;
   c. describes frequency, duration and establishment of milk supply;
   d. alerts mother to feeding cues of infant;
   e. performs assessment of infant's hydration status.
   f. LATCH scoring
 	
4. Identifies breast-feeding problems and takes appropriate nursing actions
   a. breast refusal (infant sleepy, fussy)
   b. incorrect suck
   c. breaks in nipple integrity
   d. engorgement
 	
5. Teaches mother regarding nipple and breast care, nutrition, and rest.
 	
6. Makes appropriate referrals to lactation consultant, community resources, and support groups.
	_____
	
	_____
	
	_____
	_____
	
	_____
	
	_____
	
	_____
	_____
	
	_____
	_____
	_____
	_____
	
	_____
	
	_____
		Attend Breastfeeding Core Course
		
		Study March of Dimes Module: Breastfeeding
		
		Review policies and procedures for breastfeeding and bottle feeding
		
		Observe peers and lactation consultant providing care to a mother who is breastfeeding
		
		Practice assisting a mother and newborn to feed (breast and/or bottle)
			Complete Breastfeeding exam with a score of 80%
			
			Mentor observes orientee assisting a mother and newborn to breastfeed
			
			Mentor observes orientee assisting a mother and newborn to bottle feed.
			
			Mentor reviews charts for appropriate documentation
				Date/Initials:
				1. _____
				
				2. _____
				
				3a. _____
				3b. _____
				
				3c. _____
				
				3d. _____
				
				3e. _____
				3f. _____
				
				4a. _____
				4b. _____
				4c. _____
				4d. _____
				
				5. _____
				
				6. _____

(*)   <u>Self Assessment Key</u>
1 - Knowledgeable - able to perform with confidence
2 - Knowledgeable but need practice
3 - Need review and practice

Critical Behavior	Self (*) Assessment	Learning Activities	Method of Evaluation	Performs Independently
COMPETENCY 4. (Continued)				Date/Initials:

7. Identifies references to the following:
   a. Contraindications to breast-feeding.
   b. Maternal medications during lactation.
   c. Use of breast-feeding aids appropriately (breast shells, nipple shields, breast pumps, etc.)
   d. Expression and storage of breast milk, including storage guidelines, types/ availability of breast pumps, medela rental stations, etc.
	_____
	_____
	_____
	
	_____
				7a. _____
				7b. _____
				7c. _____
				
				7d. _____

8. Gives appropriate information to mother supplementation and use of pacifier.	_____			8. _____

9. Documents appropriately.
   a. Clinical Pathway
   b. Progress Notes (DAO)
   c. Postpartum Education: Self Assessment Checklist
	_____			9. _____

Non-Nursing Mother:				
1. Supports mother's decision to bottle-feed her newborn.	_____			1. _____

2. Demonstrates/explains formula preparation and storage to mother:
   a. describes differences in formula types:
      1. concentrate
      2. powder
      3. ready to feed
   b. clean method of preparation
   c. discusses appropriate storage methods
   d. describes differences in bottles and nipples
	_____
	
	_____
	_____
	_____
				2a. _____
				
				2b. _____
				2c. _____
				2d. _____

3. Informs mother of typical formula feeding pattern, based upon age of infant, including:
   a. number of feedings
   b. expected volume per feeding
   c. hunger cues of infant
   d. burping or bubbling of infant, including appropriate positioning
   e. stooling and voiding patterns
   f. introduction of supplements, including solids and cow's milk
	_____
	_____
	_____
	_____
	
	_____
	_____
				3a. _____
				3b. _____
				3c. _____
				3d. _____
				
				3e. _____
				3f. _____

APPENDIX L • MOTHER-BABY NURSING: COMPETENCE VALIDATION TOOLS AND SKILLS CHECKLISTS

Critical Behavior	Self (*) Assessment	Learning Activities	Method of Evaluation	Performs Independently
COMPETENCY 4. (Continued)				Date/Initials:
4. Discusses safety issues regarding bottle feeding with parents, including:				
a. use of bulb syringe	_____			4a. _____
b. discouragement of propping infant with bottle	_____			4b. _____
c. feeding at room temperature and discouraging use of microwave for warming formula	_____			4c. _____
d. examining expiration date on formula care	_____			4d. _____
e. discarding unused formula within 48 hours	_____			4e. _____
f. discarding unused formula in bottle immediately after use.	_____			4f. _____
5. Discusses lactation suppression with mother, including:				
a. Use of tight-fitting bra 24 hours/day until breast are soft;	_____			5a. _____
b. use of ice to breast and analgesics for relief of discomfort;	_____			5b. _____
c. avoidance of nipple/breast stimulation	_____			5c. _____

6. Documents appropriately.
   a. Progress Notes (DAO)
   b. Postpartum Education: Self Assessment Checklist
   c. Newborn Flow Sheet
   d. Newborn Clinical Pathway
	_____			6. _____

APPENDIX L • MOTHER-BABY NURSING: COMPETENCE VALIDATION TOOLS AND SKILLS CHECKLISTS

Orientee_____   Mentor_____

COMPETENCY 5: Provide information pertaining to self and newborn care to the postpartum woman and her family based upon individual needs.

Critical Behavior	Self (*) Assessment	Learning Activities	Method of Evaluation	Performs Independently
1. Incorporates assessed Barriers to Learning in implementation of the patient's educational plan	_____	Views video: Review Self Learning Packet: "Nurses as Patient Educators."	Completes "Nurses as Patient Educators" exam with a score of 80%	Date/Initials 1._____
2. Utilizes "Guidelines for Care" to individualize patient teaching in regard to maternal self-care.		Review "Guidelines for Care"	Mentor observes the orientee individualizing educational needs of the mother and family based on assessed level of knowledge and barriers to learning	
a. Postpartum danger signs	_____			2a._____
b. Breast care for either nursing or non-nursing mothers	_____			2b._____
c. Uterine massage	_____	Review policies and procedures about postpartum education		2c._____
d. Vaginal bleeding	_____			2d._____
e. Post Cesarean and/or Tubal Ligation Care	_____			2e._____
f. Episiotomy Care	_____	Observe peers providing education to a mother and family	Mentor reviews charts for appropriate documentation	2f._____
g. Return of bowel function	_____			2g._____
h. Nutrition for nursing or non-nursing mothers	_____			2h._____
I. Rest and exercise	_____			2i._____
j. Postpartum psychological adjustment	_____	Practice providing education to a mother and family		2j._____
k. Contraception	_____			2k._____
l. Resumption of intercourse	_____			2l._____
m. Follow-up care	_____			2m._____
n. Home support/family relationships	_____			2n._____
o. Sibling rivalry, if appropriate	_____			2o._____
3. Utilizes "Guidelines for Care" to individualize patient teaching in regard to infant care				
a. Rooming-in & Hospital safety	_____			3a._____
b. Guidelines for calling pediatrician	_____			3b._____
c. Car seat safety	_____			3c._____
d. Infant safety issues	_____			3d._____
e. Positioning and holding	_____			3e._____
f. Bathing and skin care	_____			3f._____
g. Nail care	_____			3g._____
h. Cord care and diapering	_____			3h._____

(*)   **Self Assessment Key**
1 - Knowledgeable - able to perform with confidence
2 - Knowledgeable but need practice
3 - Need review and practice

Critical Behavior	Self (*) Assessment	Learning Activities	Method of Evaluation	Performs Independently
COMPETENCY 5: (Continued)				Date/Initials:
3. (Continued)				
i. Clothing infant	_____			3i. _____
j. Voiding and stooling patterns	_____			3j. _____
k. Care of the circumcised/ uncircumcised male infant	_____			3k. _____
l. Taking axillary and rectal temperatures	_____			3l. _____
m. Jaundice	_____			3m. _____
n. Colic and irritability	_____			3n. _____
o. Normal characteristics of the newborn	_____			3o. _____
p. Infant development, stimulation, and attachment	_____			3p. _____
q. Newborn reflexes	_____			3q. _____
r. Feeding issues	_____			3r. _____

4. Documents appropriately.
   a. Clinical Pathway
   b. Progress Notes (DAO)
   c. Kardex
   d. Postpartum Education: Self Assessment Checklist
	_____			4. _____

APPENDIX L • MOTHER-BABY NURSING: COMPETENCE VALIDATION TOOLS AND SKILLS CHECKLISTS

Orientee_____   Mentor_____

COMPETENCY 6: Perform a systematic and thorough full-term newborn physical assessment based upon knowledge of expected adaptation to extrauterine life.

Critical Behavior	Self (*) Assessment	Learning Activities	Method of Evaluation	Performs Independently

1. Understands the physiological changes which take place during the newborn transitional period.
 	
2. Observe newborn in quiet, alert state, noting breathing pattern, overall skin color, posture, and muscle tone.
 	
3. Weigh and measure newborn.
 	
4. Assess vital signs per protocol:
  a. Axillary temperature (36.5 & 37.2 C).
    1. < 36.5 initiates warmer placement
    2. > 37.2
  b. Heart rate and condition affecting HR (100 to 140 BPM)
    1. Sleeping
    2. Crying
    3. Stimulation
    4. Placement of stethoscope
    5. Regularity
    6. Murmurs
  c. Respirations (40 to 60 BPM)
    1. Conditions affecting respirations:
      a. sleeping
      b. crying
    2. Regularity
    3. Placement of stethoscope
    4. Lung sounds - clear, moist, rales, equality
	_____
	
	_____
	
	_____
	
	_____
	
	_____
	
	_____
		View video: AWHONN's Cross Training for Obstetrical Nursing Staff: Newborn care
		
		Study March of Dimes Module: Thermoregulation
		
		Review policies and procedures for newborn assessment
		
		Review AWHONN's Postpartum Compendium
		
		Observes peers assessing a newborn
		
		Practices assessing a newborn
			Completes Newborn Care exam with a score of 80%
			
			Mentor observes the orientee assessing a newborn
			
			Mentor reviews charts for appropriate documentation
				Date/Initials
				
				1._____
				
				2._____
				
				3._____
				
				4a._____
				
				4b._____
				
				4c._____

(*)   <u>Self Assessment Key</u>
1 - Knowledgeable - able to perform with confidence
2 - Knowledgeable but need practice
3 - Need review and practice

APPENDIX L • MOTHER-BABY NURSING: COMPETENCE VALIDATION TOOLS AND SKILLS CHECKLISTS

Critical Behavior	Self(*) Assessment	Learning Activities	Method of Evaluation	Performs Independently
COMPETENCY 6. (Continued)				Date/Initials:
5. Observes skin color for presence of duskiness, cyanosis, jaundice, bruising, or edema.	_____			5. _____
6. Inspects skin for warmth, turgor, presence of peeling rashes or lesion.	_____			6. _____
7. Inspects head for presence of molding, caput, cephalohematom, and fullness of fontanelles.	_____			7. _____
8. Inspects cord condition for intactness, dryness, signs of infection, presence of clamp (removal).	_____			8. _____
9. Inspects healing of circumcision when appropriate.	_____			9. _____
10. Assesses movement symmetry of limbs, face.	_____			10. _____

11. Assesses elimination pattern
   a. Stools - color, consistency and number
   b. Urine - color, amount and number
	_____
	_____
				11a. _____
				11b. _____

12. Assesses muscle tone and elicits reflexes.	_____			12. _____

13. Documents appropriately
   a. Newborn Clinical Pathway
   b. Progress Notes (DAO)
   c. Newborn Flow Sheet
	_____			13. _____

APPENDIX L • MOTHER-BABY NURSING: COMPETENCE VALIDATION TOOLS AND SKILLS CHECKLISTS

Orientee _____   Mentor_____

COMPETENCY 7:   Plan and provide care to normal full-term infants.

Critical Behavior	Self (*) Assessment	Learning Activities	Method of Evaluation	Performs Independently

1. Initiates/follows through on plan that supports newborn physical assessment findings.
 	
2. Provides care for umbilical cord stump:
  a. applies triple dye q day
  b. removes cord clamp after 24 hours of age, if dry
  c. teaches parents how to cleanse with alcohol after discharge
  d. keeps diaper away from drying cord
  e. teaches parents signs and symptoms of infection
 	
3. Correctly prepares and cares for newborn with circumcision:
  a. places newborn NPO 2 hours prior to procedure
  b. maintains infant safety during procedure
  c. assesses circumcision site for bleeding 1 hour after procedure
  d. teaches parents to care for circumcision
    1. Gomco care
    2. Plastibell care
  e. responds to bleeding per policy/ procedure
	_____
	
	_____
	_____
	
	_____
	
	_____
	_____
	
	_____
	
	_____
	
	_____
	
	_____
	
	_____
		Reviews policies and procedures for newborn care:
		a. Cord care
		b. Circumcision care
		c. Capillary blood sampling
		d. Breastfeeding
		e. Formula feeding
		f. Medication administration
			Mentor observes the orientee providing care to the newborn
			
			Mentor reviews charts for appropriate documentation
				Date/Initials
				1._____
				
				2a._____
				2b._____
				
				2c._____
				
				2d._____
				2e._____
				
				3a._____
				
				3b._____
				
				3c._____
				
				3d._____
				
				3e._____

(*)   <u>Self Assessment Key</u>
1 - Knowledgeable - able to perform with confidence
2 - Knowledgeable but need practice
3 - Need review and practice

APPENDIX L • MOTHER-BABY NURSING: COMPETENCE VALIDATION TOOLS AND SKILLS CHECKLISTS

Critical Behavior	Self (*) Assessment	Learning Activities	Method of Evaluation	Performs Independently
COMPETENCY 7: (Continued)				Date/Initials:
4. Correctly prepares and administers Hepatitis B Vaccine:				
a. checks for physician's order	_____			4a. _____
b. obtains signed informed consent from parents after practitioner explanation	_____			4b. _____
c. Draws up medication	_____			4c. _____
d. Administers medication correctly (lateral thigh)	_____			4d. _____
e. Explains use of vaccine	_____			4e. _____
5. Correctly performs capillary blood sampling for MDT and supplemental screening				
a. Understands need for testing and teaches parents same	_____			5a. _____
b. selects and prepares collection site	_____			5b. _____
c. collects specimen per policy/procedure	_____			5c. _____
6. Provides for care by mother through rooming-in.	_____			6. _____
7. Provides for appropriate feeding by parents or nurse.	_____			7. _____

8. Documents appropriately.
    a. Newborn Clinical Pathway
    b. Progress Notes
    c. Newborn Flow Sheet
	_____			8. _____

APPENDIX L • MOTHER-BABY NURSING: COMPETENCE VALIDATION TOOLS AND SKILLS CHECKLISTS

Orientee_____   Mentor_____

COMPETENCY 8:   Identify the full-term infant at risk for complications.

COMPETENCY 9:   Provide appropriate care to the full-term infant with complications.

Critical Behavior	Self (*) Assessment	Learning Activities	Method of Evaluation	Performs Independently
Respiratory 1. Recognizes the signs & symptoms of newborn respiratory distress. 2. Provides adequate oxygenation and ventilation as necessary. 3. Maintains neutral thermal environment for infant. 4. Provides adequate nutrition. Hypoglycemia 1. Recognizes the signs & symptoms of hypoglycemia. 2. Performs glucose screening as necessary according to protocol. 3. Provides supplemental glucose or additional bottle/breast feeds as necessary. Hyperbilirubinemia 1. Assesses for jaundice according to protocol. 2. Interprets lab results appropriately. Neonatal Sepsis 1. Recognizes signs & symptoms of infections in newborns. Hypothermia 1. Recognizes signs & symptoms of newborn hypothermia 2. Provides warmth for infant according to protocol.	_____ _____ _____ _____ _____ _____ _____ _____ _____ _____ _____ _____	Study March of Dimes Module: Respiratory Dysfunction Study March of Dimes Module: Hypoglycemia Study March of Dimes Module: Assessment of Risk in the Newborn: Birth Injury Review AWHONN's Postpartum Compendium	Completes March of Dimes Modules with a score of 80% Mentor observing the orientee providing care to the infant at visit	Date/Initials 1._____ 2._____ 3._____ 4._____ 1._____ 2._____ 3._____ 1._____ 2._____ 1._____ 1._____ 2._____

(*)   Self Assessment Key
1 - Knowledgeable - able to perform with confidence
2 - Knowledgeable but need practice
3 - Need review and practice

YORK HOSPITAL

York, Pennsylvania

POSTPARTUM EMOTIONAL ADJUSTMENT

1. During a home visit, you provide anticipatory guidance to the mother concerning postpartum emotional adjustment. Which of the following will you recommend?

    a. Have friends or a family member take the baby overnight so you can sleep
    b. Have quick easy foods available such as yogurt, sandwiches, fruit so that you will eat even if you do not feel like eating
    c. When friends or family offer their help, accept their assistance so you can rest and recuperate
    d. All of the above
    e. b. & c. only

2. What is the cause of postpartum depression?

    a. The hormonal changes that occur after the birth of a baby
    b. The mother's mother had postpartum depression after she gave birth
    c. The life style changes that occur with the birth of a new baby
    d. All of the above

3. During a telephone assessment the mother reveals to you that she is having difficulty sleeping. What is your best response?

    a. "You should lie down whenever the baby sleeps"
    b. "Tell me more about your difficulty sleeping"
    c. "I am sure you are. Most new mothers have their sleep disturbed by a crying baby"
    d. Isn't your husband getting up with the baby at night"

4. Choose the statement(s) that will alert you that this mother may have postpartum depression?

    a. "I am having difficulty sleeping and I cry all the time"
    b. "I don't want anyone else to care for my baby girl. I am afraid something will happen to her"
    c. "When I lay down to sleep I hope that I don't wake up"
    d. All of the above

5. You have read the postpartum referral form and have determined that this patient is at risk for postpartum emotional adjustment. What would make you think this?

   a. The patient is an 18 year old with a history of sexual abuse
   b. The patient's mother has a history of manic-depression
   c. The patient had postpartum depression after her last pregnancy
   d. b. & c.
   e. All of the above

6. You have **assessed** that the patient is at risk for postpartum depression but currently has no symptoms. What is your immediate nursing plan?

   a. Reassess the patient for symptoms during your follow-up phone call in one week
   b. Educate the patient about postpartum emotional adjustment and her risk
   c. Provide her with information about available referrals in the community related to postpartum emotional adjustment
   d. b. & c.
   e. All of the above

7. You follow-up with a phone call within one week of the home visit and feel that the patient needs professional help. What has the patient told you?

   a. "I just can't do this anymore"
   b. "I don't want to hurt the baby, I just don't want to hold her"
   c. "I can't stop crying. My husband is frustrated and doesn't know what to do about it"
   d. b. & c.
   e. All of the above

8. When you suspect a mother has postpartum depression, who should be your first referral?

   a. Her family doctor or Obstetrician
   b. A counselor
   c. The New Mother's Group
   d. Crisis Intervention
   e. A Social Worker

9. You are visiting a new mother and she greets you at the door crying. Your initial thoughts are?

   a. This mother must have postpartum depression. I haven't even come in and she is crying
   b. This mother is probably experiencing the baby blues, she will probably be fine as soon as I answer her questions
   c. This mother must have the baby blues, but I had better ask a few questions and check her history to be sure
   d. This mother must need help. I better call the doctor before I leave here.

10. You are on the phone with a mother who is frantic. She is crying and says she is afraid she will hurt her baby. What will you do?

    a. Hang up and call her doctor
    b. Keep her on the phone while someone else calls Crisis Intervention
    c. Talk soothingly to her and try to find out more details
    d. b. & c.
    e. All of the above

ANSWERS:

1. e

2. d

3 b

4. e

5. e

6. e

7. e

8. a

9. c

10. d

APPENDIX M • PROMOTING AND ASSISTING WITH BREASTFEEDING COMPETENCE ASSESSMENT TOOLS

BREASTFEEDING COMPETENCY CHECKLIST

	DATE MET	LACTATION CONSULTANT OR PRECEPTOR SIGNATURE
I. Locates breastfeeding packet and gives it upon admission to all labor patients who plan on nursing		
II. Instructs and/or assists mother with correct latch on and feels confident giving rationale		
III. Instructs mother in length of each feeding at each breast and rationale		
IV. Instructs mother regarding frequency of feedings and feels confident giving rationale		
V. Instructs mother regarding four different infant positions and rationale		
VI. Instructs mother how to determine adequacy of infant feedings		
VII. States what time and where the breastfeeding class is daily		
VIII. Verbalizes indication for breast shells and rationale		
IX. Demonstrates assembly/cleaning of breast shells and rationale for using each type		
X. Instructs the mother how to prevent/minimize engorgement and steps to take if it occurs		
XI. Verbalizes indication for use of manual/electric breast pumps and rationale		
XII. Instructs mother in the use of hand, single electric, and double electric pumps		
XIII. Demonstrates set-up and cleaning of manual, single, and double electric breast pump		
XIV. Instructs mother how to hand express her breast milk and rationale		
XV. Charges for breast pump supplies given to inpatient postpartum mothers		
XVI. Knows how to label, and where to store colleced breast milk until mother and/or baby are discharged		
XVII. Documents problem statement, interventions, and evaluation for all of the following: pumping, sore nipples, flat nipples, engorgement		
XVIII. Instructs mother how to call the Lactation Consultants, once discharged		

Palos Community Hospital, Palos Heights, Illinois

APPENDIX M • PROMOTING AND ASSISTING WITH BREASTFEEDING COMPETENCE ASSESSMENT TOOLS

SIOUX VALLEY HOSPITAL
Sious Falls, South Dakota
LATCH SCORE

The LATCH Scoring Table

	0	1	2
L Latch	Too sleepy or reluctant. No latch achieved	Repeated attempts. Hold nipple in mouth. Stimulate to suck	Grasps breast. Tongue down. Lips flanged. Rhythmic sucking
A Audible swallowing	None	A few with stimulation	Spontaneous and intermittent < 24 hours old. Spontaneous and frequent < 24 hours old
T Type of nipple	Inverted	Flat	Everted (after stimulation)
C Comfort (Breast/Nipple)	Engorged. Cracked, bleeding, largeblisters, or bruises. Severe discomfort	Filling. Reddened/small blisters or bruises. Mild/moderate discomfort	Soft. Tender
H Hold (Positioning)	Full assist (staff holds infant at breast)	Minimal assist (i.e., elevate head of bed; place pillows for support.) Teach one side; mother does other. Staff holds and then mother takes over	No assist from staff. Mother able to position/hold infant

From Jensen, D., Wallace, S., Kelsey, P. (1994). LATCH: A breastfeeding charting system and documentation tool. <u>Journal of Obstetric, Gynecologic, and Neonatal Nursing</u>, <u>23</u>(1), 27-32.

Complete the LATCH Score case studies.

Case #1 · Baby sleepy will not latch on · No swallowing heard · Mom has everted nipples · Breasts/nipples are soft/tender · Nursing staff holds and positions baby during entire nursing LATCH SCORE: _____	**Case #2** · Baby holds breast/nipple in mouth, both lips are flanged, tongue is under areola, baby's gum line covers mother's lactiferous sinus. Nursing staff must repeatedly stimulate baby to suck. · No swallowing heard · Mother's nipples are everted · Breast/nipples are soft/tender · Mom is able to hold and position baby by herself. LATCH SCORE: _____
Case #3 · Repeated attempts with no latch on · No swallows heard · Mother's nipples are flat · Breast/nipples soft/tender · Mother needs full assistance with breastfeeding from staff LATCH SCORE: _____	**Case #4** · Baby grasps nipple and breast tissue, lips flanged, baby's cheeks are full, no dimpling of cheeks, rhythmic sucking noted · Swallowing head resembling forceful expiration of air · Mom's nipples/breast are soft/tender · Mother's nipples are everted · Mom positions and holds baby without help LATCH SCORE: _____

APPENDIX M • PROMOTING AND ASSISTING WITH BREASTFEEDING COMPETENCE ASSESSMENT TOOLS

BREASTFEEDING
PROMOTING A BABY FRIENDLY ENVIRONMENT
POST-TEST

INSTRUCTIONS: Please complete test at the end of class session and turn into instructor.

MULTIPLE CHOICE: Please circle correct answer
1. Breast milk is superior to commerical formulas because breast milk is:
   a. Easier to measure and is always the same no matter what the infant's demands are.
   b. Capable of providing antibodies which help protect the infant from infection.
   c. Available in several different forms and is always accessible to the hospitalized infant.

DEFINE
2. Define the components of the LATCH score:
   L:_____
   A:_____
   T:_____
   C:_____
   H:_____

TRUE OF FALSE
3. Which of the following would indicate that the baby is correctly latched on to the breast?
   _____Baby's cheeks are sucked in and baby has continuous head movement.
   _____The baby is making clicking and sucking noises at the breast, and the lips are sucked in.
   _____The baby's lips are flanged out and sucking sounds are heard.
   _____Equal amounts, top and bottom, of the breast areola are sucked into the baby's mouth.
   _____The baby's nose and chin are to the breast, you see circular movements of the baby's jaw and wiggling of the baby's ears.

MULTIPLE CHOICE: Please circle correct answer
4. Which form of breast milk expression is recommended for a mother whose infant is hospitalized?
   a. Bicycle horn style hand pumps
   b. Pistan or cylinder style
   c. Hospital grade electric pump
   d. Manual expression
   e. Whatever works best for the mother

5. A six day old baby Hernandez just spend 20 minutes breast feeding and still is acting fussy & hungry. Which of the following statements from his mother would make you suspect that he is having problems latching onto the breast? (4 correct answers)
   a. "He acts hungry no matter how long I breastfeed him."
   b. "He falls asleep after just a few sucks."
   c. "He detaches from the breast, seems content and relaxed, then falls asleep after eating."
   d. "He roots, fidgets, fusses and cries both during and after the feeding."
   e. "It hurts to have him feed because my nipples are sore and are cracking."

APPENDIX M • PROMOTING AND ASSISTING WITH BREASTFEEDING COMPETENCE ASSESSMENT TOOLS

6. According to the protocol for breastfeeding the suspected sepsis infant, under which condition would the infant need supplementation with formula or expressed breast milk after breastfeeding?
   a. The baby is awake and acting hunger 1 ½ - 2 hours after feeding.
   b. Mother says she doesn't have any milk yet.
   c. Baby has lost more than 10% of his or her birth weight.
   d. The IV fluids are being weaned by glucose.

7. A two day old breastfeeding baby is awake and sucking on her fist 1 hour and 50 minutes after her previous feeding. Her mother is in her room in post partum. The best nursing action for this mother/baby couple at this time would be to:
   a. Give the baby a pacifier and hold off the feeding until 3 hours have elapsed from the last feeding to keep the baby on schedule.
   b. Call the mother in her room, inform her that the baby is ready to eat and ask her to come and breastfeed the baby.
   c. Give the baby 15-20 cc in a bottle to keep her quiet until feeding time.
   d. Call the post partum floor and tell the nurse taking care of the mother to tell the mother that it is time for the baby to eat.

8. According to the Specialty Care Nurseries Policy entitled, "Breast Milk: Collection, Storage andUse" polyethylene bags or bottle liners should not be used for milk storage because...
   a. They are expensive and not readily available.
   b. The antibody titers are lowered by storage in the bags.
   c. It is more difficult to properly label the bags.

TRUE OR FALSE

9. _____ Expressed milk should be refrigerated immediately upon completion of expression unless it will be used within 1 hour of expressing.

10. _____ Bacteriological screening of a mother's own milk is necessary before feeding it to her baby.

MULTIPLE CHOICE

11. Which of the following are true when breast milk is thawed in the microwave? (2 possible answers)
    a. There is no effect on the IgA levels
    b. Activity of lysozyme is decreased
    c. Growth of E. Coli is inhibited
    d. Amount of Vitamin C is reduced

APPENDIX M • PROMOTING AND ASSISTING WITH BREASTFEEDING COMPETENCE ASSESSMENT TOOLS

12. When a mother is using the cradle hold to breast feed her baby, she should:
    a. Hold the baby's head with one hand and the baby's body will be to her side, under her arm.
    b. Make sure the baby's tummy is to mom's and his ear, shoulder and hip form a straight line.
    c. Hold her breast areola between her index and middle fingers so the baby can latch on more effectively.

13. For expressed breast milk that was frozen and now is thawed, how long is it good to be used if kept in the refrigerator?
    a. 8 hours
    b. 24 hours
    c. 48 hours

APPENDIX N • THE NEWBORN: HEALTHY FULL-TERM NURSERY, SPECIAL CARE NURSERY, AND NEONATAL INTENSIVE CARE UNIT COMPETENCE VALIDATION TOOLS AND SKILLS CHECKLISTS

APGAR SCORES

At one minute of life, baby girl Smith has a heart rate of 140, weak cry, extremities well flexed, moves away from the bulb syringe and is pale in color. At five minutes of age, she is crying, but pale.

	Heart Rate	Respiration	Muscle Tone	Reflex Irritability	Skin Color	Totals
1 min						
5 min						
10 min						

At one minute of life, baby boy Johnson has a heart rate of 152, crying vigorously intermittently, extremities well flexed, moves away from bulb syringe, and has acrocyanosis. At five minutes of age, he is completely pink.

	Heart Rate	Respiration	Muscle Tone	Reflex Irritability	Skin Color	Totals
1 min						
5 min						
10 min						

At one minute of life, baby boy Jones has a heart rate of 90; no spontaneous respirations, some flexion of his extremities, no response to bulb syringe, skin color is blue.

	Heart Rate	Respiration	Muscle Tone	Reflex Irritability	Skin Color	Totals
1 min						
5 min						
10 min						

At five minutes of life, heart rate is 110, breath sounds are present bilaterally with weak cry, some flexion of extremities, grimaces in response to the bulb syringe, and has acrocyanosis.

	Heart Rate	Respiration	Muscle Tone	Reflex Irritability	Skin Color	Totals
1 min						
5 min						
10 min						

At one minute of life, baby girl Brown has a heart rate of 140, she is crying vigorously, moving around, her extremities are well flexed, coughs, her color is blue. At five minutes of life, her color has changed to pale.

	Heart Rate	Respiration	Muscle Tone	Reflex Irritability	Skin Color	Totals
1 min						
5 min						
10 min						

At one minute of life, baby girl Green has a heart rate of 100, no cry, some flexion, grimaces in response to bulb syringe, skin color is pale. At five minutes of life, her heart rate is 132, she has a weak cry, is sneezing and has acrocyanosis.

	Heart Rate	Respiration	Muscle Tone	Reflex Irritability	Skin Color	Totals
1 min						
5 min						
10 min						

Reference

Letko, M. (1996). Understanding the Apgar score. Journal of Obstetric, Gynecologic, and Neonatal Nursing, 25(4), p. 299-303.

Source: Patricia A. Creehan RNC, MS (1997)

APPENDIX N • THE NEWBORN: HEALTHY FULL-TERM NURSERY, SPECIAL CARE NURSERY, AND NEONATAL INTENSIVE CARE UNIT COMPETENCE VALIDATION TOOLS AND SKILLS CHECKLISTS

HealthEast Perinatal Services
Minneapolis, Minnesota

Special Care Nursery
Skill Validation Tools

APPENDIX N • THE NEWBORN: HEALTHY FULL-TERM NURSERY, SPECIAL CARE NURSERY, AND NEONATAL INTENSIVE CARE UNIT COMPETENCE VALIDATION TOOLS AND SKILLS CHECKLISTS

SPECIAL CARE NURSERY
RN/RNLP COMPETENCY CHECKLIST

EMPLOYEE_____

DATE CHECKLIST STARTED_____

DATE CHECKLIST COMPLETED_____

Dates are placed in the boxes as skills are completed

	Observed Skill Performed by Preceptor	Skill Performed With Supervision	Skill Performed Independently	Preceptor's Signature
I. Demonstrate ability to: A. Care for a newborn 1. During uncomplicated delivery				
2. During Cesarean/high risk delivery				
B. Perform Apgar score				
C. Measure blood pressure with Dynamap				
D. Perform Gestational Age Assessment				
E. Perform newborn physical assessment				
F. Silverman Score				
G. Venipuncture 1. Initiate an IV				
2. Care for an infant with a peripheral IV				
3. Care for a PVAD				
H. Oxygen Therapy 1. Set up and maintain oxygen				
2. Wean off oxygen				
I. Use wall suction for infant whois: 1. intubated				
2. non-intubated				
J. Assist with umbilical catherization				
K. Discontinue umbilical catheter				
L. Gastric lavage				
M. Gavage feed				
N. Chest physiotherapy				
O. Specimen collection 1. Hemacult				
2. Umbilical line				

APPENDIX N • THE NEWBORN: HEALTHY FULL-TERM NURSERY, SPECIAL CARE NURSERY, AND NEONATAL INTENSIVE CARE UNIT COMPETENCE VALIDATION TOOLS AND SKILLS CHECKLISTS

	Observed Skill Performed by Preceptor	Skill Performed With Supervision	Skill Performed Independently	Preceptor's Signature
P. Medication Administration 1. IV				
2. IM				
Q. Assist with pneumogram				
R. Process a readmission from the Perinatal Center				
S. Discharge an infant to home				
T. Assist with: 1. Spinal tap				
2. Intubation				
U. Chest tubes 1. Assist with insertion				
2. Care for infant with chest tubes				
V. Operate equipment safely: 1. Stabilet				
2. ICU Bed				
3. Cardiac/Respiratory Monitor				
4. O₂ Analyzer				
5. Crash Cart				
6. Bed Scale				
7. Transilluminator				
8. Neomate Pump				
9. Infant transporter				
10. Pulse oximeter				

		DATE REVIEWED
II.	Review policies in the Newborn Manual related to the skills identified in this checklist	
III.	Review in Nursery Policy and Procedures Manual: A. Infant abduction	
	B. Criteria for admission to Special Care Nursery	
	C. Routine newborn assessment	
	D. Blood/blood component transfusion in children	
	E. Infants requiring Pediatric/Neonatology consultation	
	F. Titration of IV and oral fluids in SCN	
	G. Suctioning the Newborn	

APPENDIX N • THE NEWBORN: HEALTHY FULL-TERM NURSERY, SPECIAL CARE NURSERY, AND NEONATAL INTENSIVE CARE UNIT COMPETENCE VALIDATION TOOLS AND SKILLS CHECKLISTS

	H.	Neonatal Resuscitation	
	I.	Procedure for Infant Transfer	
	J.	Visiting in Special Care Nursery	
	K.	Oxygen Therapy and/or mechanical ventilation of newborns	
	L.	Immediate care of extremely premature live born infant	
	M.	Department of Pediatric Rules and Regulations	
	N.	Department of Obstetrics Rules and Regulations	
IV.		Viewed the following video tapes A. Gestational Age and Growth Evaluation	
	B.	Newborn Physical Assessment	
			DATE REVIEWED
	C.	Neonatal Stabilet	
	D.	Mec-Gard	
	E.	Infant Nasal CPAP Systems	
	F.	Infant Abduction	
	G.	The Compromised Neonate 1. Assessment and Basic Care	
		2. Support in Acute Respiratory Compromise	
		3. Implications of Early Neonatal Infection	
	H.	Biliblanket Phototherapy System	
	I.	Starting a Peripheral Intravenous Line on an Infant	
	J.	Space Labs - PC Express	
	K.	Check-Up for Life: Neonatal Screening	

APPENDIX N • THE NEWBORN: HEALTHY FULL-TERM NURSERY, SPECIAL CARE NURSERY, AND NEONATAL INTENSIVE CARE UNIT COMPETENCE VALIDATION TOOLS AND SKILLS CHECKLISTS

HEALTHEAST: PERINATAL SERVICES
SPECIAL CARE NURSERY RN COMPETENCY CHECKLIST

Name _____   Skill Level (circle) C D E

SKILLS	SELF-ASSESSMENT			EXPECTATION/ACTION PLAN					COMMENTS/RESOURCES
C = Required for Core Competent Staff in Special Care Nursery. D = Advanced Care Skills in Special Care Nursery. E = Level III Nursery Skills (ONLY AT SJNE)	CAN FUNCTION INDEPENDENTLY	NEED REVIEW	HAVE NOT DONE	CLASS OR LEARNING MODULE	DISCUSSED OR REVIEWED POLICY	ASSISTED OR OBSERVED	RETURN DEMONSTRATION	PERFORMED INDEPENDENTLY	RESOURCES @ = HEPS POLICY BOOK # = HENSA POLICY BOOK S = LEARNING MODULE-SCN SOC = STANDARD OF CARE V = VALIDATION TOOL OM = OPERATION MANUAL *Items may take longer than 6 months to complete.
I. EQUIPMENT LOCATION, USE & CLEANING OF:	/////	/////	/////	/////	/////	/////	/////	/////	
1. Air-Oxygen Mixer (Blender)					D		D	E	OM
2. Oxyhooa					C		C	C	OM, @O-1
3. Ventilator Sechrist (St. John's Only)					C		D	E	OM, @V-2
4. Biliblanket					C		C	C	OM
5. Phototherapy Radiometer					C		C	C	
6. Phototherapy Unit (Bililights)					C		D	D	
7. CR (Cardio-Respiratory Monitor) Lead application, When to use, & Alarm limits					C		C		
a. 78832A/78833A (Midway Only)					C		C	C	OM
b. 505/506					C		C	C	OM
c. 556					C		C V	C	OM
8. Doppler for Flow Detector in Infants (Midway Only)					C		C	C	
9. Incubator Humidifier-Dewette (St. John's Only)					C		C	C	OM
10. Reflux Wedge					C		C V		OM @C-13
II. NEUROLOGICAL	/////	/////	/////	/////	/////	/////	/////	/////	
1. Minimal Stress				S-1	C		C	C	SOC Minimal Stress
2. Ultrasound (Ordering and Assisting)					C	C		C	Clinipac

APPENDIX N • THE NEWBORN: HEALTHY FULL-TERM NURSERY, SPECIAL CARE NURSERY, AND NEONATAL INTENSIVE CARE UNIT COMPETENCE VALIDATION TOOLS AND SKILLS CHECKLISTS

SKILLS	SELF-ASSESSMENT			EXPECTATION/ACTION PLAN					COMMENTS/RESOURCES
	CAN FUNCTION INDEPENDENTLY	NEED REVIEW	HAVE NOT DONE	CLASS OR LEARNING MODULE	DISCUSSED OR REVIEWED POLICY	ASSISTED OR OBSERVED	RETURN DEMONSTRATION	PERFORMED INDEPENDENTLY	
3. CT Scan (Ordering and Assisting)					C	C		C	Clinipac
4. Lumbar Puncture (Ordering, Set-Up and Assisting)				S-2	C	C	C V		@L-2
5. BSER (Basal Stem Evoked Response)					C				@B-8
III. RESPIRATORY	//////	//////	//////	//////	//////	//////	//////	//////	SOC Resp. Distress
1. Oxygen Administration	//////	//////	//////	//////		//////	//////	//////	@O-1 & O-2
a. Blow By				NRP	C		C	C	
b. Mask				NRP	C		C	C	
c. Headbox					C		C	C	
d. Cannula					C		C	C	@O-2
e. Endotracheal Tube (Assisting with Intubation & Securing)				NRP S-3	C		C	C	@I-6
f. Nasal CPAP				S-3	C		E	E*	@C-7
g. Mechanical Ventilation—Stable Infant				S-3	C		E	E*	@V-2, SOC Resp. Vent.
h. Mechanical Ventilation—Initial Set Up				S-3	E		E	E*	
2. Respiratory Treatments	//////	//////	//////	//////	//////	//////	//////	//////	
a. Nebulizations (Ordering & Expected Outcomes)					C				Clinipac
b. CPT/Vibrations (Ordering & Expected Outcomes)					C				
c. Oxy-Pneumogram					C		C	C	@O-4

APPENDIX N • THE NEWBORN: HEALTHY FULL-TERM NURSERY, SPECIAL CARE NURSERY, AND NEONATAL INTENSIVE CARE UNIT COMPETENCE VALIDATION TOOLS AND SKILLS CHECKLISTS

SKILLS	SELF-ASSESSMENT			EXPECTATION/ACTION PLAN					COMMENTS/RESOURCES
	CAN FUNCTION INDEPENDENTLY	NEED REVIEW	HAVE NOT DONE	CLASS OR LEARNING MODULE	DISCUSSED OR REVIEWED POLICY	ASSISTED OR OBSERVED	RETURN DEMONSTRATION	PERFORMED INDEPENDENTLY	
d. Suctioning	/////	/////	/////	/////		/////	/////	/////	@S-2
1) Nasal Pharyngeal (NP)				M-16	See Mother–Baby Checklist	V			
2) Endotracheal Tube (ETT)				S-4	C		D V	D*	
e. Chest Tubes	/////	/////	/////	S-5	/////	/////	/////	/////	@C-6
1) Needle Aspiration (Assisting)					C		C V	C*	
2) Assisting with Placement					C		D V	D*	
3) Ongoing Care of Chest Tubes (St. John's Only)					D		E V	E*	
f. X-Ray				S-6	C		C	C	
g. ABG Interpretation				S-7	C		D	D	@A-7
3. Apnea and Bradycardia Observation				S-8	C		C	C	@A-11
IV. CARDIOVASCULAR	/////	/////	/////	/////	/////	/////	/////	/////	
1. Venous Access	/////	/////	/////	/////	/////	/////	/////	/////	
a. Peripheral Venipuncture				S-9	C		C V	C	
b. Heparin Locks					C		C	C	@H-5
c. Lab Draws					C		C V	C	
d. UVC (Umbilical Vein Catheter) Line				S-10	C		D V	D*	@U-1
2. Arterial Access	/////	/////	/////	/////		/////	/////	/////	@A-7
a. UAC (Umbilical Artery)				S-10	C		D V	D*	@U-1
b. Percutaneous Lines					D		D St. John's Only	D*	@P-9

APPENDIX N • THE NEWBORN: HEALTHY FULL-TERM NURSERY, SPECIAL CARE NURSERY, AND NEONATAL INTENSIVE CARE UNIT COMPETENCE VALIDATION TOOLS AND SKILLS CHECKLISTS

SKILLS	SELF-ASSESSMENT			EXPECTATION/ACTION PLAN					COMMENTS/RESOURCES
	CAN FUNCTION INDEPENDENTLY	NEED REVIEW	HAVE NOT DONE	CLASS OR LEARNING MODULE	DISCUSSED OR REVIEWED POLICY	ASSISTED OR OBSERVED	RETURN DEMONSTRATION	PERFORMED INDEPENDENTLY	
c. PA Stick for ABG's				S-19	C				@A-7 & @C-5
d. Direct B/P Monitoring					C			D*	@B-4
3. Fluid & Electrolytes	/////	/////	/////	/////	/////	/////	/////	/////	
a. Maintenance Fluid				S-11	C		C	C	
b. TPN & FAT Emulsion Therapy					C		C	C*	@H-6, F-2
c. I & O					C		C	C	
d. Volume Expanders				NRP	C		C	C	
4. Blood Administration	/////	/////	/////	/////		/////	/////	/////	@B-6
a. PRBC's (Packed Red Blood Cells)					D		D	D*	
b. Recording Blood Out					C		C	C	
c. Exchange Transfusion					C				@E-11
d. Emergency Blood Transfusion					C				@B-6a
5. Cardiac Diagnostics	See Mother–Baby Nurse Skills Checklist								
V. GASTROINTESTINAL	/////	/////	/////	/////	/////	/////	/////	/////	
1. Lavage				S-12	C		C V	C	@L-1
2. Gavage Feeding				S-12	C		C V	C	@G-2, G-3
3. Preterm Breast-Feeding				S-13	C		C	C	
4. Preterm Bottle Feeding					C		C	C	
5. Clinitest Stool					C		C	C	@C-16

APPENDIX N • THE NEWBORN: HEALTHY FULL-TERM NURSERY, SPECIAL CARE NURSERY, AND NEONATAL INTENSIVE CARE UNIT COMPETENCE VALIDATION TOOLS AND SKILLS CHECKLISTS

SKILLS	SELF-ASSESSMENT			EXPECTATION/ACTION PLAN					COMMENTS/RESOURCES
	CAN FUNCTION INDEPENDENTLY	NEED REVIEW	HAVE NOT DONE	CLASS OR LEARNING MODULE	DISCUSSED OR REVIEWED POLICY	ASSISTED OR OBSERVED	RETURN DEMONSTRATION	PERFORMED INDEPENDENTLY	
6. NG/OG Drainage	/////	/////	/////	/////		/////	/////	/////	@G-2 & G-4
a. Straight					C		C	C	
b. With Suction					C		D	D*	
7. Guaiac Stool					C		C	C	
8. Nutritional Needs				S-14	C				@C-4
VI. GENITOURINARY	/////	/////	/////	/////	/////	/////	/////	/////	
1. Diaper Weights					C		C	C	
2. Catheterization					C				@C-17
3. Suprapubic Tap (Assist)					C		C	C	@S-6
VII. INTEGUMENTARY	/////	/////	/////	/////	/////	/////	/////	/////	SOC
1. Sheepskin					C		C	C	
2. Tegaderm					C		C	C	
3. Repositioning				S-1	C		C	C	
4. Tape					C				
VIII. THERMOREGULATION	/////	/////	/////	/////	/////	/////	/////	/////	
1. Isolette (Use & Weaning)					C		C	C	@I-7 & I-8
2. Infant Care Center					C		C	C	

APPENDIX N • THE NEWBORN: HEALTHY FULL-TERM NURSERY, SPECIAL CARE NURSERY, AND NEONATAL INTENSIVE CARE UNIT COMPETENCE VALIDATION TOOLS AND SKILLS CHECKLISTS

SKILLS	SELF-ASSESSMENT			EXPECTATION/ACTION PLAN					COMMENTS/RESOURCES
	CAN FUNCTION INDEPENDENTLY	NEED REVIEW	HAVE NOT DONE	CLASS OR LEARNING MODULE	DISCUSSED OR REVIEWED POLICY	ASSISTED OR OBSERVED	RETURN DEMONSTRATION	PERFORMED INDEPENDENTLY	
IX. MEDICATIONS	/////	/////	/////	/////	/////	/////	/////	/////	
1. Intravenous	/////	/////	/////	/////		/////	/////	/////	@I-3, I-10, & M-4
a. Medication Infusion Pump				S-15	C		C	C	
b. Micro AVI Pump					C		C	C	
c. IV Medication Push				NRP	C		C	C	@B-5, I-10
2. PO					C		C	C	
3. IM					C		C	C	
4. ETT				NRP	C				
5. Rectal					C		C	C	
6. Medication References					C				
X. SEPSIS	/////	/////	/////	/////	/////	/////	/////	/////	
1. Infections in the Newborn				S-16	C				
2. Isolation-Care of the Infant					C		C		@I-5
XI. MISCELLANEOUS	/////	/////	/////	/////	/////	/////	/////	/////	
1. Pre/Post Op Care (SJNE ONLY)					C		D	D*	
2. SCN Parent Teaching Flowsheet					C		C	C	
3. NICU Initial Admission Assessment					C		C	C	
4. NICU Shift Assessment					C		C	C	

APPENDIX N • THE NEWBORN: HEALTHY FULL-TERM NURSERY, SPECIAL CARE NURSERY, AND NEONATAL INTENSIVE CARE UNIT COMPETENCE VALIDATION TOOLS AND SKILLS CHECKLISTS

SKILLS	SELF-ASSESSMENT			EXPECTATION/ACTION PLAN					COMMENTS/RESOURCES
	CAN FUNCTION INDEPENDENTLY	NEED REVIEW	HAVE NOT DONE	CLASS OR LEARNING MODULE	DISCUSSED OR REVIEWED POLICY	ASSISTED OR OBSERVED	RETURN DEMONSTRATION	PERFORMED INDEPENDENTLY	
5. Lab Values and Resources				S-17	C				Phlebotomy Manual
6. Transports	//////	//////	//////	//////		//////	//////	//////	@T-3 & T-7
a. Preparation					C		C	C	
b. Professional Building (St. John's Only)					C				
c. Ambulance					C		D	D*	
7. Ready Unit Preparation/Equipment Check					C		C	C	
8. Developmental Care (Optimal Stress)				S-1	C				
9. SIDS (Sudden Infant Death Syndrome) Previous Loss				S-18	C				
10. Attendance at High Risk Births					C		DS	DS	
11. Receiving Transfer from Another Facility					C				@A-6a
12. Teaching Parents CPR					C				@C-14
13. Visitation in Nursery					C				@T-2

Skills Competency Reviewed: Date/Year _____

Employee _____

Preceptor/Educator _____

Clinical Manager _____

APPENDIX N • THE NEWBORN: HEALTHY FULL-TERM NURSERY, SPECIAL CARE NURSERY, AND NEONATAL INTENSIVE CARE UNIT COMPETENCE VALIDATION TOOLS AND SKILLS CHECKLISTS

INITIAL AND SIGNATURE BOXES FOR PRECEPTORS OR OTHER STAFF WHO ASSIST WITH ORIENTATION OR TRAINING.

Initials	Signature	*Symbol/Date

VALIDATION TOOLS REQUIRED	DATE DONE
SPINAL TAP	
ETT SUCTIONING	
CHEST TUBES	
MECHANICAL VENTILATION	
X-RAY	
INFANT IV START	
BLOOD DRAW FROM UMB. LINE	
INSERTION OF GASTRIC TUBE & GAVAGE FEEDING	
LAVAGE OF GASTRIC CONTENTS	
IV MEDICATION INFUSION	
REFLUX PRECAUTIONS	
PHOTOTHERAPY	
CR MONITOR 556	
Oxygen Headbox	

* OPTIONAL-If you are reviewing a number of items with a new orientee you can establish your own UNIQUE symbol or letter to correlate with the date you are providing the information.

APPENDIX N • THE NEWBORN: HEALTHY FULL-TERM NURSERY, SPECIAL CARE NURSERY, AND NEONATAL INTENSIVE CARE UNIT COMPETENCE VALIDATION TOOLS AND SKILLS CHECKLISTS

SKILL VALIDATION TOOL

BLOOD DRAW FROM UMBILICAL ARTERIAL LINE

NAME:_____ SITE:_____

OBJECTIVES: Nurse will draw blood samples from umbilical line while maintaining sterility and preventing air in the line per HealthEast Perinatal policy and procedures.

SKILL STEPS	SUCCESSFULLY MET? YES	*Optional Date/Initials
1. Assemble supplies.	___	___
2. Clear line:		
a. correct use of stopcock.	___	___
b. pre-draw blood.	___	___
3. Obtain blood samples.	___	___
4. Replace pre-draw blood.	___	___
5. Flush line.	___	___
6. Correct Documentation.	___	___

COMMENTS:_____

_____

_____

*Validator should date and initial steps completed if not a full return demonstration.

SETTING: ____ CLINICAL AREA   ____ SIMULATED OR SKILLS DAY

VALIDATOR_____

DATE OF COMPLETION:_____

APPENDIX N • THE NEWBORN: HEALTHY FULL-TERM NURSERY, SPECIAL CARE NURSERY, AND NEONATAL INTENSIVE CARE UNIT COMPETENCE VALIDATION TOOLS AND SKILLS CHECKLISTS

SKILL VALIDATION TOOL

INSERTION OF GASTRIC TUBE AND GAVAGE FEEDING

NAME: _____ SITE: _____

OBJECTIVES: Nurse will use proper technique for insertion of gastric tube and gavage feeding according to HEPS policies G-2 and G-3.

SKILL STEPS	SUCCESSFULLY MET? YES	*Optional Date/Initials
1. Assemble Equipment.	____	____
2. Positions Infant on back with HOB elevated.	____	____
3. Measures infant for placement properly.	____	____
4. Inserts gastric tube per policy.	____	____
5. Checks aspirate.	____	____
6. Gavage feeding given by gravity.	____	____
7. Proper removal of gastric tube.	____	____
8. Documents procedure, feeding amount and tolerance.	____	____

COMMENTS: _____
_____
_____

*Validator should date and initial steps completed if not a full return demonstration.

VALIDATOR _____

DATE OF COMPLETION: _____

APPENDIX N • THE NEWBORN: HEALTHY FULL-TERM NURSERY, SPECIAL CARE NURSERY, AND NEONATAL INTENSIVE CARE UNIT COMPETENCE VALIDATION TOOLS AND SKILLS CHECKLISTS

SKILL VALIDATION FORM

FOR: LAVAGE OF GASTRIC CONTENTS

NAME: _____ SITE: _____

OBJECTIVES: Nurse will use proper technique for insertion of gastric tube and lavage of gastric contents according to HEPS policies G-2 and L-1.

SKILL STEPS	SUCCESSFULLY MET? YES	*Optional Date/Initials
1. Assemble Equipment.	____	____
2. Positions Infant on back with HOB elevated.	____	____
3. Measures infant for placement properly.	____	____
4. Inserts gastric tube per policy.	____	____
5. Checks aspirate.	____	____
6. Perform Lavage per HE Policy.	____	____
7. Proper removal of gastric tube.	____	____
8. Documents procedure, results and tolerance.	____	____

COMMENTS: _____
_____
_____

*Validator should date and initial steps completed if not a full return demonstration.

VALIDATOR _____

DATE OF COMPLETION: _____

APPENDIX N • THE NEWBORN: HEALTHY FULL-TERM NURSERY, SPECIAL CARE NURSERY, AND NEONATAL INTENSIVE CARE UNIT COMPETENCE VALIDATION TOOLS AND SKILLS CHECKLISTS

INFANT IV START VALIDATION TOOL

NURSE_____ SITE_____

OBJECTIVE: Nurse will demonstrate the ability to perform an IV start on infant per HealthEast procedural standards.

	Successfully Met? YES	*Optional Date/Initials

STEPS:

1. Collect and prepare appropriate supplies & equipment. ___ ___

2. Explain procedure to patient and family. ___ ___

3. Identify four potential sites. ___ ___

4. Select the appropriate needle/catheter for infant and use. ___ ___

5. Discuss or Demonstrate methods of identifying arteries from veins. ___ ___

6. Demonstrate correct procedure for preparing site. ___ ___

7. Perform successful venepuncture on infant. ___ ___

8. Demonstrate proper taping & restraining technique. ___ ___

9. Complete documentation and label IV tubing and site. ___ ___

*Validator should date and initial steps completed if not a full return demonstration.

Three return demonstrations are required. (Small placental veins may be substituted for one return demonstration.)

VALIDATOR/DATE   COMMENTS (Actual IV, Lab Draw, or placenta)

#1_____   _____
OBSERVED BY/DATE

#2_____   _____
OBSERVED BY/DATE

#3_____   _____
OBSERVED BY/DATE

#4_____   _____
OBSERVED BY/DATE

SKILL VALIDATION TOOL

OXYGEN HEADBOX: SET UP & INITIATING

NAME:_____ SITE:_____

OBJECTIVES: Nurse will use correct technique in setting up headbox oxygen

SKILL STEPS	SUCCESSFULLY MET? YES	*Optional Date/Initials
1. Assemble appropriate equipment.	____	____
2. Connects equipment correctly.	____	____
3. Turns blender on to desire FiO2 with flowmeter at 10-12 L.	____	____
4. Correct size headbox (with baffle pad depending on type used).	____	____
5. Continues to augment supplemental Oxygen via mask or tube, if initiated, until desire concentration of Oxygen obtained.	____	____
6. Turns on humidifier, adjusts to correct temperature control.	____	____
7. Calibrates the O2 analyzer to R/A, sets analyzer alarms, and places in correct headbox port.	____	____
8. Correctly applies pulse oximeter, knows appropriate saturation limits.	____	____
9. Adjusts the correct knobs when changing the FiO2 need.	____	____
10. Documents all appropriate readings and vital signs on the NICU flow sheet at correct intervals.	____	____
11. Demonstrates cleaning, maintenance of equipment.	____	____
12. Demonstrates charging mechanism for Oxygen administration.	____	____

COMMENTS:_____
_____

*Validator should date and initial steps completed if not a full return demonstration.

VALIDATOR_____

DATE OF COMPLETION:_____

APPENDIX N • THE NEWBORN: HEALTHY FULL-TERM NURSERY, SPECIAL CARE NURSERY, AND NEONATAL INTENSIVE CARE UNIT COMPETENCE VALIDATION TOOLS AND SKILLS CHECKLISTS

SKILL VALIDATION TOOL

INFANT CHEST TUBE (ASSISTING WITH PLACEMENT, MANAGEMENT, & DRESSING CHANGES)

NAME: _____ SITE: _____

OBJECTIVES: Nurse will demonstrate appropriate setup of Thoraklex, assist with chest tube placement, and dressing change.

SKILL STEPS	SUCCESSFULLY MET? YES	*Optional Date/Initials

A. Setting up Thoraklex
   1. Connect pt tube to chest catheter.   ____   ____

   2. Place unit below chest level.   ____   ____

   3. Connect wall suction to suction adapter ____   ____
      on Thoraklex.

   4. Two suction   (a) wall 80-120 cm H20   ____   ____
      settings   (b) Thoraklex 0-20 cm H20 ____ ____

   5. Fill air leak indicator with 15 cc   ____   ____
      sterile water (if concerned about
      possible air leak)

   6. Check negative pressure indicator on   ____   ____
      Thoraklex. Should read "yes".
      *"yes" may flash with respirations if
       using only gravity drainage.

   7. Band or securely tape all connections. ____   ____

B. Assisting with Chest tube placement per   ____   ____
   HEPS C-6.

C. Dressing change for Chest tube per HEPS C-6. ____ ____

COMMENTS:_____

_____

_____

*Validator should date and initial steps completed if not a full return demonstration.

VALIDATOR_____

DATE OF COMPLETION:_____

APPENDIX N • THE NEWBORN: HEALTHY FULL-TERM NURSERY, SPECIAL CARE NURSERY, AND NEONATAL INTENSIVE CARE UNIT COMPETENCE VALIDATION TOOLS AND SKILLS CHECKLISTS

SKILL VALIDATION TOOL

SUCTIONING OF INFANT WITH ENDOTRACHEAL TUBE

NAME: _____ SITE: _____

OBJECTIVES: Nurse will use suctioning appropriately to maintain adequate oxygenation for the infant with an ET tube.

SKILL STEPS	SUCCESSFULLY MET? YES	*Optional Date/Initials
1. Assess need: coarse breath sounds, coughing, agitation, inability to adequately oxygenate, suction every 4 hours all 2.5 ETT size, and lavage only prn.	____	____
2. Hyperoxygenates (10% above baseline) for 3-4 breaths before, during and 3-4 breaths after if needed.	____	____
3. Using sterile technique inserts catheter into ET tube.	____	____
4. Applies intermittent suction, does not exceed 10 seconds.	____	____
5. Clears suction catheter with sterile water.	____	____
6. Assesses effectiveness and determines if procedure needs to be repeated.	____	____
7. Documents how patient tolerates the procedure and the type of secretions obtained.	____	____

COMMENTS: _____
_____
_____

*Validator should date and initial steps completed if not a full return demonstration.

VALIDATOR _____

DATE OF COMPLETION: _____

APPENDIX N • THE NEWBORN: HEALTHY FULL-TERM NURSERY, SPECIAL CARE NURSERY, AND NEONATAL INTENSIVE CARE UNIT COMPETENCE VALIDATION TOOLS AND SKILLS CHECKLISTS

SKILL VALIDATION TOOL

NASOPHARYNGEAL SUCTIONING WITH WALL AND/OR BULB SUCTION-INFANT

NAME: _____   SITE: _____

OBJECTIVES: Nurse will use bulb, wall suction with and without Delee mucus trap appropriately to clear secretions.

SKILL STEPS	SUCCESSFULLY MET? YES	*Optional Date/Initials
A. Bulb syringe:		
1. Assesses need	____	____
2. Properly inserts and suctions	____	____
B. Wall Suction:		
1. Uses appropriate wall suction pressure.	____	____
a. Uses appropriate sized catheter.	____	____
b. Sets up Delee correctly.	____	____
2. Uses universal precautions.	____	____
3. Suctions adequately and appropriately per procedure.	____	____
4. Documents how infant tolerates the procedure and the type of secretions obtained.	____	____

COMMENTS: _____
_____
_____

*Validator should date and initial steps completed if not a full return demonstration.

VALIDATOR: _____

DATE OF COMPLETION: _____

Phototherapy

	Correct	Incorrect
1. Properly prepares isolette	( )	( )
A) Prewarmed to 34° c (Air)	( )	( )
B) Bed made to prevent soilage of linen	( )	( )
C) Temperature skin probe set at 36.5° c	( )	( )
D) Air temperature probe removed	( )	( )
E) Inner wall of isolette removed	( )	( )
2. Obtains appropriate lights as ordered	( )	( )
A) Bank lights	( )	( )
B) Spot light	( )	( )
C) Blanket or pad light	( )	( )
3. Properly prepares infant	( )	( )
A) Protects eyes with approved opaque covering	( )	( )
B) Provides maximum skin exposure	( )	( )
C) Covers diaper area to control waste soilage on bed while maintaining maximum skin exposure	( )	( )
D) Skin temp probe on with appropriate cover	( )	( )
4. Provides adequate hydration	( )	( )
5. Adjusts isolette temp as necessary, once lights on	( )	( )
6. Properly documents treatment, light irradiance, protective eye covering, patient tolerance, bilirubin levels	( )	( )
7. Draws blood samples and does feedings with phototherapy lights off.	( )	( )
8. Provides teaching material about jaundice to parents.	( )	( )
9. Charges for equipment	( )	( )

RN Signature _____ Date: _____

Evaluator _____ Date: _____

APPENDIX N • THE NEWBORN: HEALTHY FULL-TERM NURSERY, SPECIAL CARE NURSERY, AND NEONATAL INTENSIVE CARE UNIT COMPETENCE VALIDATION TOOLS AND SKILLS CHECKLISTS

SKILL VALIDATION TOOL

FOR: Mechanical Ventilation for an Infant

NAME: _____ **SITE:** _____

OBJECTIVES:

1. The nurse will be able to demonstrate the ability to care for an infant on mechanical ventilation in accordance with HEPS V-2.

SKILL STEPS FOR DS STAFF	SUCCESSFULLY MET?	
	YES	*Optional Date/Initials
Intubation:		
1. Identifies necessary equipment & its correct usage in intubation.	_____	_____
*Ambu bag, mask, & manometer.	_____	_____
*Laryngoscope, blade size 1 & 0.	_____	_____
*ET Tube and stylet.	_____	_____
*Adhesive tape, liquid adhesive, & skin protector.	_____	_____
*Stethoscope.	_____	_____
2. Demonstrates proper positioning of infant during intubation.	_____	_____
3. Properly assists with intubation.	_____	_____
Intubated Infant on Mechanical Ventilation:		
1. Lists potential problems during mechanical ventilation of a neonate.	_____	_____
2. Auscultates correct placement of ETT: Listening for presence and equality of bilateral breath sounds.	_____	_____
3. Properly tapes ET tube securely.	_____	_____
4. Auscultates breath sounds bilaterally and states findings with vital signs and position changes.	_____	_____
5. Measures ETT from lip to hub to ensure consistently correct placement.	_____	_____
6. Suctions as correctly.	_____	_____
7. Check ventilator setting with MD orders at start of each shift and record setting hourly.	_____	_____
8. Has Intubation box and Ambu bag with manometer and mask at bedside.	_____	_____
Ventilator Modes:		
1. Describe IMV.	_____	_____
2. Describe CPAP.	_____	_____
Ventilator Components:		
Define and locate the following on the ventilator.		
1. FI02.	_____	_____
2. Rate.	_____	_____
3. PMAX.	_____	_____
4. PEEP.	_____	_____
5. I:E Ratio.	_____	_____
6. Temperature sensor.	_____	_____
7. Alarm controls.	_____	_____
Documentation:		
1. Properly documents settings on flowsheet.	_____	_____

APPENDIX N • THE NEWBORN: HEALTHY FULL-TERM NURSERY, SPECIAL CARE NURSERY, AND NEONATAL INTENSIVE CARE UNIT COMPETENCE VALIDATION TOOLS AND SKILLS CHECKLISTS

SKILL STEPS FOR DS STAFF	SUCCESSFULLY MET? YES	*Optional Date/Initials
Troubleshooting: Demonstrates the ability to troubleshoot ventilators and intervene appropriately for the problems listed below.		
1. High Pressure.		
ET tube obstructed by secretions.	_____	_____
High resistance from water in the tubes.	_____	_____
Decrease in compliance (Pneumothorax).	_____	_____
Patient fighting ventilator (Anxiety).	_____	_____
Obstruction in ventilator (Kinked tube).	_____	_____
2. Low Pressure.		
Leak.	_____	_____
Disconnection.	_____	_____
3. Uses ambu bag if unable to solve problem quickly.	_____	_____
CPAP: Describes how to set up, initiate, & manage.		
1. Assemble nasal prongs and adaptor to ventilator tubing.	_____	_____
2. Place prongs on infant and secure.	_____	_____
3. Listen for breath sounds.	_____	_____
4. Insert orogastric tube and leave open to air to allow decompression of stomach.	_____	_____
5. Assess nares for skin breakdown Q 2 hrs and PRN.	_____	_____
6. Wean from CPAP slowly per MD orders.	_____	_____
7. Assess need for restarting CPAP and getting MD order.	_____	_____
Ambu Bag: Correctly uses to ventilate an intubated infant.		
1. Start Oxygen flow in ambu bag at 2L/Min.	_____	_____
2. Uses Pressure Manometer.	_____	_____
3. Attaches Ambu Bag to ET tube.	_____	_____
4. Coordinates manual & spontaneous resp.	_____	_____
5. Administers breaths at vent. set rate.	_____	_____
6. Auscultates effectiveness of bagging.	_____	_____
7. Assesses appropriate return to IMV.	_____	_____

SKILL STEPS FOR ES STAFF	SUCCESSFULLY MET? YES	*Optional Date/Initials
Mechanical Ventilation-Unstable Neonate:		
1. Verbalize indications, administration, and considerations for Pressor use.	_____	_____
2. Demonstrates ability to handle a crisis (role of nurse leader in the care of an unstable preterm infant).	_____	_____
3. Provide care for 3 unstable infants (as defined by NNP) under supervision.	_____	_____
4. Admit an infant when ventilator is initiated.	_____	_____

COMMENTS _____

*Validator should date & initial steps completed if not a full return demonstration.

VALIDATOR: _____ DATE OF COMPLETION: _____

YORK HOSPITAL
POSTPARTUM HOME VISITATION
CORE COMPETENCIES

At the end of this Postpartum Home Visitation program, the professional nurse will be able to:

1. Describe the operation of the Postpartum Home Visitation program.

2. Demonstrate a systematic and thorough evaluation of maternal adaptation during the puerperium.

3. Demonstrate a systematic and thorough newborn physical assessment based upon knowledge of normal adaptation to extrauterine life.

4. Provide care and support to the mother in her chosen method of infant feeding.

5. Evaluate knowledge and provide information to the postpartum woman pertaining to self and newborn care based upon her individual needs and those of her family.

6. Demonstrate a systematic and thorough evaluation of the family's adaptation based upon family systems theory.

7. Demonstrate therapeutic interpersonal skills while providing care to the postpartum follow-up patient.

8. Manage identified patient care needs requiring intervention or referral per protocol.

9. Demonstrate collection and care of lab specimen(s) obtained in the home.

APPENDIX O • MOTHER-BABY HOMECARE COMPETENCE ASSESSMENT TOOLS

Orientee _____   Mentor _____

COMPETENCY 1. Describe the operation of the Postpartum Home Visitation program.

Critical Behavior	Self (*) Assessment	Learning Activities	Method of Evaluation	Performs Independently
1. Locates policies, procedures and protocols. a. Breastfeeding b. Capillary blood samples c. Home Visit d. Scale e. Telephone Call Assessment f. When to call the doctor g. Car repair	_____	Attend Postpartum Home Visitation course View video: AWHONN's Cross-Training for Obstetrical Nursing Staff: Home Follow-up of Early Postpartum Discharge	Completes Postpartum Home Care Exam with a score of 90%. Mentor observes the orientee performing policies and procedures of the Home Visit Program.	Date/Initials 1. _____
2. Employs safety precautions during home visits.	_____	Study Self-Learning Packet on Postpartum Home care.		2. _____
3, Performs handwashing prior to each assessment.	_____			3. _____
4. Communicates with the management of variances on pathway with Care Manager	_____	Reviews Home Visitation policies, procedures, and protocols.		4. _____
5. Follows through with home visit schedule. a. Enter appropriate cost center b. Protocols for sick calls, etc.	_____			5. _____

(*)   <u>Self-Assessment Key</u>
1 - **Knowledgeable - able to perform with confidence**
2 - **Knowledgeable, but needs practice**
3 - **Needs review and practice**

APPENDIX O • MOTHER-BABY HOMECARE COMPETENCE ASSESSMENT TOOLS

Orientee _____   Mentor _____

COMPETENCY 2. Demonstrate a systematic and thorough evaluation of maternal adaptation during the puerperium.

Critical Behavior	Self (*) Assessment	Learning Activities	Method of Evaluation	Performs Independently
				Date/Initials:
1. Understands normal postpartum physiological and psychologic maternal adaptations.	_____	View video: AWHONN's Cross Training for Obstetrical Nursing Staff: Postpartum Care	Completes Basic Postpartum Care exam with a score of 90%.	1. _____
2. Reviews postpartum referral form for information that takes into account perinatel events and risks to direct assessment.	_____	Study Self-Learning Packet for Postpartum Emotional Adjustment	Mentor reviews charts for appropriate documentation.	2. _____
3. Provides for patient comfort and privacy prior to assessment by having patient empty her bladder and determining appropriate location to perform physical assessment.	_____	View Video: "Beyond the Blues"; "Fragile Beginnings"	Mentor observes the orientee assessing a postpartum mother.	3. _____
4. Obtains vital signs with blood pressure	_____	Observes peers performing a postpartum assessment.		4. _____
5. Inspects the breasts for consistency, tenderness, nipple integrity, and presence of colostrum or milk.	_____	Practices performing a postpartum assessment and documenting on Hollister Forms and Pathway.		5. _____
6. Palpates uterine fundus noting location, and consistency.	_____			6. _____
7. Observes lochial flow for color, amount, consistency, and odor.	_____			7. _____
8. Obtains information from patient regarding her ability to urinate independently. Notes presence of frequency, urgency, pain, or the inability to empty bladder.	_____			8. _____

APPENDIX O • MOTHER-BABY HOMECARE COMPETENCE ASSESSMENT TOOLS

Critical Behavior	Self (*) Assessment	Learning Activities	Method of Evaluation	Performs Independently
COMPETENCY 2. (Continued)				Date/Initials:
9. Inspects perineum for presence and intactness of episiotomy and/or lacerations. Notes presence of erythema, ecchymosis, edema, hematoma, pain, and/or drainage in area.	_____			9. _____
10. Inspects incision (cesarean or tubal ligation) for intactness. Note presence of erythema, ecchymosis, edema, and/or drainage in area.	_____			10. _____
11. Inspects intactness of rectal area noting present size, and number of hemorrhoids. Notes occurrence of last bowel movement and presence of constipation.	_____			11. _____
12. Inspects extremities for presence and location of edema, redness, tenderness, and/or varicosities. Performs Homan's sign bilaterally on legs.	_____			12. _____
13. Assesses for pain level of discomfort, location, measures that alleviate.	_____			13. _____
14. Assesses the psychosocial adjustment to early motherhood, such as self-confidence, attachment issues, parenting issues, level of social support, blues and/or depression, specific concerns.	_____			14. _____
15. Assesses sexual change and adjustments such as issues of sexual relationship with partner, and plans for future pregnancies, contraceptive use.	_____			15. _____

16. Documents appropriately.
   a. Hollister Forms - Maternal Care Plan
   b. Postpartum Clinical Pathway Follow-up
	_____			16. _____

(*)   **Self-Assessment Key**
1-Knowledgeable - able to perform with confidence
2-Knowledgeable, but needs practice
3-Needs review and practice

APPENDIX O • MOTHER-BABY HOMECARE COMPETENCE ASSESSMENT TOOLS

Orientee _____   Mentor _____

COMPETENCY 3. Demonstrate a systematic and thorough newborn physical assessment based upon knowledge of normal adaptation to extrauterine life.

Critical Behavior	Self (*) Assessment	Learning Activities	Method of Evaluation	Performs Independently
1. Reviews perinatal history to identify potential risks.	_____	View video: AWHONN's Cross-Training for Obstetrical Nursing Staff: Newborn Care	Completes Basic Newborn Care exam with a score of 90%.	Date/Initials 1. _____
2. Observe newborn in quiet, alert state, noting breathing pattern, overall skin color, posture, and muscle tone.	_____	Observes peers performing a newborn assessment in the home.	Mentor reviews charts for appropriate documentation.	2. _____
3. Weigh newborn according to protocol.	_____	Practice performing a newborn assessment using the Hollister: Infant Care Plan and Newborn Home Care Pathway.	Mentor observes the orientee assessing a newborn in the home.	3. _____
4. Assess vital signs per protocol:				4. _____
a. Axillary temperature (36.5 and 37.2 C).	_____			

b. Heart rate and condition affecting HR (100 to 140 BPM)
     1. Sleeping
     2. Crying
     3. Stimulation
     4. Placement of stethoscope
     5. Regularity
     6. Murmurs
	_____			

c. Respirations (40 to 60 RPM)
     1. Conditions affecting respirations:
       a. Sleeping
       b. Crying
     2. Regularity
     3. Placement of stethoscope
     4. Lung sounds - clear, moist, rales, equality
	_____			

5. Observes skin color for presence of duskiness, cyanosis, jaundice, bruising or edema.	_____			5. _____

APPENDIX O • MOTHER-BABY HOMECARE COMPETENCE ASSESSMENT TOOLS

Critical Behavior	Self (*) Assessment	Learning Activities	Method of Evaluation	Performs Independently
COMPETENCY 3. (Continued)				Date/Initials:
6. Inspects skin for warmth, turgor, presence of peeling rashes or lesion	_____			6. _____
7. Inspects head for presence of molding, caput, cephalohematom, and fullness of fontanelles.	_____			7. _____
8. Inspects cord condition for intactness, dryness, signs of infection, presence of clamp (removal).	_____			8. _____
9. Palpates liver for enlargement esp. in the presence of jaundice.	_____			9. _____
10. Inspects healing of circumcision when appropriate.	_____			10. _____
11. Assesses movement symmetry of limbs, face.	_____			11. _____
12. Assesses elimination pattern a. Stools - color, consistency and number	_____			12. _____
b. Urine - color, amount and number	_____			
13. Assesses muscle tone and elicits reflexes.	_____			13. _____

14. Documents appropriately
   a. Hollister Form - Infant Care
   b. Newborn Follow-Up Clinical Pathway
	_____			14. _____

(*)   Self-Assessment Key
1 - **Knowledgeable - able to perform with confidence**
2 - **Knowledgeable but need practice**
3 - **Need review and practice**

APPENDIX O • MOTHER-BABY HOMECARE COMPETENCE ASSESSMENT TOOLS

Orientee _____   Mentor _____

COMPETENCY 4. Provide care and support to the mother in her chosen method of infant feeding.

Critical Behavior	Self (*) Assessment	Learning Activities	Method of Evaluation	Performs Independently
1. Understands the anatomy and physiology of human lactation.	_____	Attends Postpartum Home Visit Course	Mentor observes the orientee assisting mother to feed her newborn in the home (breast or bottle).	Date/Initials: 1. _____
2. Assists mother with breast-feeding: a. properly positions infant at breast;	_____	Review March of Dimes Module: Breastfeeding the Health Newborn: A Nursing Perspective		2a. _____
b. identifies signs of correct infant latch-on;	_____			2b. _____
c. describes frequency, duration and establishment of milk supply;	_____	Attend Breastfeeding Course for Home Visit and Office Nurses.	Mentor reviews charts for appropriate documentation.	2c. _____
d. alerts mother to feeding cues of infant;	_____	Attend Breastfeeding Advanced Course.	Mentor observes the orientee individualizing newborn feeding plan of care based on feeding assessment.	2d. _____
e. performs assessment of infant's hydration status.	_____	Observes peers and/or lactation consultant assisting a mother feed her newborn (breast or bottle) in the home.		2e. _____
f. LATCH scoring	_____			2f. _____
3. Identifies breast-feeding problems and initiates breastfeeding protocols.		Practices assisting mother to feed newborn in the home.		
a. Breast refusal (infant sleepy, fussy)	_____			3a. _____
b. incorrect suck	_____			3b. _____
c. breaks in nipple integrity	_____			3c. _____
d. engorgement	_____			3d. _____
e. newborn hydration status	_____			3e. _____
f. newborn weight	_____			3f. _____
g. diminished lactation	_____			3g. _____
4. Reinforces teaching to mother regarding nipple and breast care, nutrition, rest, and infant growth spurts.	_____			4. _____
5. Makes appropriate referrals to lactation consultant, pediatrician, community resources, and support groups	_____			5. _____

APPENDIX O • MOTHER-BABY HOMECARE COMPETENCE ASSESSMENT TOOLS

Critical Behavior	Self (*) Assessment	Learning Activities	Method of Evaluation	Performs Independently

COMPETENCY 4. (Continued)
6. Demonstrates appropriate use of lactation aids.
   a. Breast shells
   b. Nipple shields
   c. Breast pumps (including type/availability and medela rental stations)
   d. Expression and storage of breast milk including storage guidelines).
	_____			Date/Initials:
				6. _____

7. Utilizes references for the following:
   a. Contraindications to breast-feeding
   b. Maternal medications during lactation
				7. _____

8. Gives appropriate information to mother about supplementation and use of pacifier.	_____			8. _____

9. Documents appropriately.
 	
   a. Hollister Form - Infant Care
   b. Newborn Home Visits Pathway
	_____			9. _____

Non-Nursing Mother:
 	
1. Demonstrates/explains formula preparation and storage to mother:
 	
   a. describes differences in formula types:
      1. Concentrate
      2. Powder
      3. Ready to feed
 	
   b. clean method of preparation
 	
   c. discusses appropriate storage methods
 	
   d. describes differences in bottles and nipples
	
	_____
	
	_____
	
	_____
	
	_____
				Non-Nursing Mother:
				
				1. _____

APPENDIX O • MOTHER-BABY HOMECARE COMPETENCE ASSESSMENT TOOLS

Critical Behavior	Self (*) Assessment	Learning Activities	Method of Evaluation	Performs Independently

COMPETENCY 4. (Continued)
 	
2. Reinforces mother's knowledge of typical formula feeding pattern, based upon age of infant, including:
 	
   a. number of feedings
   b. expected volume per feeding
   c. hunger cues of infant
   d. burping or bubbling of infant, including appropriate positioning
   e. stooling and voiding patterns
   f. introduction of supplements, including solids and cow's milk
	
	_____
	_____
	
	_____
	_____
	
	_____
	
	_____
				Date/Initials:
				
				2. _____

(*)   **Self-Assessment Key**
1 - Knowledgeable - able to perform with confidence
2 - Knowledgeable but need practice
3 - Need review and practice

APPENDIX O • MOTHER-BABY HOMECARE COMPETENCE ASSESSMENT TOOLS

Orientee _____   Mentor _____

COMPETENCY 5. Evaluate knowledge and provide information to the postpartum woman pertaining to self and newborn care based upon her individual needs and those of her family.

Critical Behavior	Self (*) Assessment	Learning Activities	Method of Evaluation	Performs Independently
1. Assess mother's level of knowledge of self and newborn care.	_____	View video Review Self-Learning Packet "Nurses as Patient Educators" Review "Guidelines for Care" Reviews policies and procedures about postpartum education Observe peers providing education to a mother & family Practice providing education to a mother and family	Mentor observes the orientee individualizing educational needs of the mother and family based on assessed level of knowledge and barriers to learning Mentor reviews charts for appropriate documentation	**Date/Initials** 1. _____
2. Assess Barriers to Learning prior to reinforcement of the knowledge gained from patient's in-hospital educational plan.	_____			2. _____
3. Utilizes "Guidelines for Care" to reinforce patient teaching in regard to maternal self-care.				3. _____
a. Postpartum danger signs	_____			
b. Breast care for either nurses or non-nursing mothers	_____			
c. Uterine massage	_____			
d. Vaginal bleeding	_____			
e. Post Cesarean and/or Tubal Ligation Care	_____			
f. Episiotomy care	_____			
g. Return of bowel function	_____			
h. Nutrition for nursing or non-nursing mothers	_____			
i. Rest and exercise	_____			
j. Postpartum psychological adjustments	_____			
k. Contraception	_____			
l. Resumption of intercourse	_____			
m. Follow-up care	_____			
n. Home support/family relationships	_____			
o. Sibling rivalry, if appropriate	_____			

APPENDIX O • MOTHER-BABY HOMECARE COMPETENCE ASSESSMENT TOOLS

Critical Behavior	Self (*) Assessment	Learning Activities	Method of Evaluation	Performs Independently
COMPETENCY 5. (Continued)				Date/Initials:
4. Utilizes "Guidelines for Care" to individualize patient teaching in regard to newborn care.				4. _____
a. Rooming-in & Hospital safety	_____			
b. Guidelines for calling pediatrician	_____			
c. Car seat safety	_____			
d. Infant safety issues	_____			
e. Positioning and holding	_____			
f. Bathing and skin care	_____			
g. Nail care	_____			
h. Cord care and diapering	_____			
i. Clothing infant	_____			
j. Voiding and stooling patterns	_____			
k. Care of the circumcised/uncircumcised male infant	_____			
l. Taking axillary and rectal temperatures	_____			
m. Jaundice	_____			
n. Colic and irritability	_____			
o. Normal characteristics of the newborn	_____			
p. Infant development, stimulation, and attachment	_____			
q. Newborn reflexes	_____			
r. Feeding issues	_____			
5. Provides wellness information that promotes the health and well being of the mother, newborn, and family.				
a. Follow-up appointment	_____			5a. _____
b. Immunization	_____			5b. _____
c. VBAC	_____			5c. _____
d. Postpartum emotional adjustment	_____			5d. _____
e. Stress management	_____			5e. _____
f. Occupation	_____			5f. _____

(*)   **Self-Assessment Key**
1 - Knowledgeable - able to perform with confidence
2 - Knowledgeable but need practice
3 - Need review and practice

APPENDIX O • MOTHER-BABY HOMECARE COMPETENCE ASSESSMENT TOOLS

Orientee _____   Mentor _____

COMPETENCY 6. Demonstrate a systematic and thorough evaluation of the family's adaptation based upon family systems theory.

Critical Behavior	Self (*) Assessment	Learning Activities	Method of Evaluation	Performs Independently
1. Assesses adjustment of mother and family members/support person		Attend the Postpartum Home Visit course	Mentor reviews charts for appropriate documentation.	Date/Initials: 1. _____
a. Adaptation to role changes b. Integration of newborn into family unit	_____ _____	Review March of Dimes Module: Parent/Infant Relationships	Mentor observes the orientee assessing the family system of the mother and baby.	
2. Obtains information about the sibling(s) adjustment and demonstration of age appropriate regression	_____			2. _____
3. Provides strategies for meeting sibling(s) needs.	_____			3. _____
4. Provides anticipatory guidance to mother in seeking supportive care for herself and her newborn from extended family members and friends.	_____			4. _____
5. Assesses for environmental safety and financial resources.	_____			5. _____
6. Documents appropriately.	_____			6. _____
a. Hollister form - Family Care Plan b. Follow-up clinical Pathways				

(*)   Self-Assessment Key
1 - Knowledgeable - able to perform with confidence
2 - Knowledgeable but need practice
3 - Need review and practice

APPENDIX O • MOTHER-BABY HOMECARE COMPETENCE ASSESSMENT TOOLS

Orientee _____ Mentor _____

COMPETENCY 7. Demonstrate therapeutic interpersonal skills while providing care to the postpartum follow-up patient.

Critical Behavior	Self (*) Assessment	Learning Activities	Method of Evaluation	Performs Independently
				Date/Initials:
1. Develop interactive rapport with mother and/or family.	_____	Study self-learning packet on General Telephone Skills	Completes the General Telephone Skills exam with a score of 90%.	1. _____
2. Able to recognize and overcome cultural barriers.	_____	Observe peers interacting with mothers and families in the home and on the telephone.	Mentor observes the orientee performing a home visit.	2. _____
3. Demonstrates effective interviewing skills.	_____			3. _____
4. Demonstrates effective listening skills.	_____	Practice using effective communication techniques being aware of open-ended and leading questions.	Mentor observes the orientee performing a telephone assessment.	4. _____
5. Obtains sensitive information.	_____			5. _____

(*) **Self-Assessment Key**
1 - Knowledgeable - able to perform with confidence
2 - Knowledgeable but need practice
3 - Need review and practice

APPENDIX O • MOTHER-BABY HOMECARE COMPETENCE ASSESSMENT TOOLS

Orientee _____   Mentor _____

COMPETENCY 8. Manage identified patient care needs requiring intervention or referral per protocol.

Critical Behavior	Self (*) Assessment	Learning Activities	Method of Evaluation	Performs Independently
				Date/Initials:
1. Identifies variances from the norm in the mother, newborn, and family assessments.	_____	Attends Postpartum Home Visitation Course	Mentor observes the orientee employing critical thinking skills in the development of a plan of care for mother, newborn, and family.	1. _____
2. Prescribes appropriate intervention for variances to postpartum and newborn follow-up clinical pathways.	_____	Review policies, procedures and guidelines for referral	Mentor observes the orientee follow-through on an appropriate plan of care for mother, newborn and family.	2. _____
3. Notifies physician of variances based on guidelines.	_____	Review "Education Guidelines"		3. _____
4. Provides education to mother and family about variances from norm.	_____	Observe peers utilizing critical thinking skills to develop plan of care for mother, newborn, and family.		4. _____

5. Refers mother and family to appropriate community resources.
  a. VNA
  b. City/state health
  c. ACCESS
  d. Children & Youth
  e. Postpartum Emotional Adjustment
  f. Perinatal coaching
  g. Mom's and mentors
  h. Others
	_____	Interact with community agencies about the services they provide to mother, newborn, and family
		
		Practice employing critical thinking skills in the planning of follow-up care for a mother, newborn, and family.
			Mentor reviews charts for appropriate documentation.	5. _____

6. Works collaboratively with care manager, physicians, other health care providers, and community agencies.	_____			6. _____

APPENDIX O • MOTHER-BABY HOMECARE COMPETENCE ASSESSMENT TOOLS

Orientee _____   Mentor _____

COMPETENCY 9. Demonstrate collection and care of lab specimen(s) obtained in the home.

Critical Behavior	Self (*) Assessment	Learning Activities	Method of Evaluation	Performs Independently
1. Performs capillary blood sampling per protocol: a. MDT b. Microbili c. Neogen d. Chemstick 2. Transports blood samples per protocol: a. MDT b. Neogen c. Microbili	 _____ _____ _____ _____ _____ _____ _____	Review policy and procedure on Capillary Blood Sampling View video: Newborn Screening: The First Steps Observe peers collect and transport blood samples. Practice collecting and transporting blood samples.	Mentor observes the orientee collect and transport blood samples. Mentor reviews charts for appropriate documentation.	Date/Initials: 1a. _____ 1b. _____ 1c. _____ 1d. _____ 2a. _____ 2b. _____ 2c. _____

(*)   Self-Assessment Key
1 - Knowledgeable - able to perform with confidence
2 - Knowledgeable but need practice
3 - Need review and practice

APPENDIX P • TOOL FOR EVALUATION OF ORIENTEE BY PRECEPTOR

SIOUX VALLEY HOSPITAL
Sioux Falls, South Dakota

Name: _____   Date: _____
         Orientee

PRECEPTOR WEEKLY EVALUATION OF ORIENTEE

Week 1 2 3 4 5 6 7 8 9 10 11 12   Key: 1--Needs improvement; not performing at level expected
                                           2--Making progress; progressing but not yet competent
                                           3--Meets expectation; meets minimum competency standards
                                           4--Exceeds expectations; exceeds minimum competency standards

Rate on a scale of 1-4 (circle one)	Needs Improvement	Making Progress	Meets Expectations	Exceeds Expectations
Technical/Clerical				
1. Documentation	1	2	3	4
2. Assessment	1	2	3	4
3. Admit and Transfer	1	2	3	4
4. IV Medications	1	2	3	4
5. Nutritional Support	1	2	3	4
Interpersonal Relations				
6. Works well with others	1	2	3	4
7. Communicates successfully with families	1	2	3	4
8. Communicates successfully with patients	1	2	3	4
9. Communicates successfully with doctors	1	2	3	4
10. Teaching	1	2	3	4
Critical Thinking				
11. Knows own limits; seeks help when needed	1	2	3	4
12. Setting priorities	1	2	3	4
13. Recognizes changes in patient condition and implements intervention as needed	1	2	3	
14. Able to delegate effectively	1	2	3	4

APPENDIX P • TOOL FOR EVALUATION OF ORIENTEE BY PRECEPTOR

Rate on a scale of 1-4 (circle one)	Needs Improvement	Making Progress	Meets Expectations	Exceeds Expectations
Competency Outcomes				
15. Organization	1	2	3	4
16. Ability to work independently	1	2	3	4
17. Self-confidence	1	2	3	4
18. Knowledge of resources	1	2	3	4
Employee Role				
19. Confidentiality	1	2	3	4
Unit Specific Skills				
20. Basic Breast Feeding	1	2	3	4
21. Blood Administration	1	2	3	4
22. Foley Insertion/Intermittent Self-Cath	1	2	3	4
23. PCA Pump	1	2	3	4
24. Circumcision	1	2	3	4
25. One touch/Hematocrits	1	2	3	4

1. Preceptee's accomplishments/strengths demonstrated this week:

2. Goals/learning needs for next week (must have a goal for any area rated 1, suggest goal for any area rated 2 listed above):

3. Plan to meet goals:

_____ _____
Preceptor's signature   Orientee's signature

March of Dimes
Continuing Education for Nurses

Assessment of Risks in the Term Newborn (1997)
Susan Bakewell-Sachs, Ph.D., CRNP, RN, CS
Valerie D. Shaw, MS, RN, CPN
Amy L. Tashman, MSN, RNC
5.0 CH

Diabetes in Pregnancy (2nd ed.) (1998) (Due out by March 1st)
Jo M. Kendrick, RNC, MSN, CDE

**Easing the Transition from Hospital to Home:
Postpartum Discharge Planning and Homecare Service**
Kathleen Rice Simpson, MSN, RNC
5.1 CH (.4 CEUs for CNMs)

Ethical Decision Making for Perinatal Nurses
Kathleen Lagana, PhD, RN, PCNS
Karen Duderstadt, MS, RN, PNP, PCNS
6.0 CH (.5 CEUs for CNMs)

Genetics for the Perinatal Nurse
Janet Williams, PhD, RN, CPNP, CGC
4.0 CH (.3 CEUs for CNMs)

Hemodynamic Monitoring of the Critically Ill Obstetric Patient
Mildred Harvey, MSN, RNC
7.0 CH

The Mature Gravida: Pregnancy at Age 35 and Older
Virginia A. Passero, PhD, RNC
4.8 CH (.4 CEUs for CNMs)

**Nursing Management of Multiple Birth Families:
Preconception through Postpartum**
Joan Drukker Dauphinee, MS, RN
Nancy Bowers, RN
7.0 CH (ACNM Pending)

Obstetrical Emergencies for the Perinatal Nurse
Denise White, MSN, RNC
Judith H. Poole, MN, RNC, FACCE
4.8 CH

APPENDIX Q • THE MARCH OF DIMES NURSING MODULES PROGRAM: CONTINUING EDUCATION FOR PERINATAL NURSES

Perinatal Impact of Substance Abuse
Susan M. Weiner, MSN, RNC
6.0 CH

Preconceptional Health Promotion
Merry-K. Moos, MPH, FNP, RN
7.0 CH

Pregnancy: Psychosocial Perspectives
Leah Ramer, PhD, RN
18.3 CH (1.5 CEUs for CNMs)

Preterm Labor: Prevention and Nursing Management
Margaret Comerford Freda, EdD, RN, CHES, FAAN
Ellen Tate Patterson, DSN, RN
6.6 CH

Window of Opportunity: Interviewing by the Perinatal Nurse
Mary Lou Moore, PhD, RNC, FACCE, FAAN
Susan Rumsey Givens, MPH, RNC, ACCE
5.2 CH

Hypertensive Disorders of Pregnancy
Judith H. Poole, PhD(c), MN, RNC, FACCE
3.4 CH

Adolescent Pregnancy (Revised)
Deborah Raines, PhD, RN

Antepartal Assessment/Lab Values
Mary Lee Barron, RN-CS, MSN, FNP

Antepartal Complications and Home Visitation
Suzanne Colemen, MS, RNC
Debianne Peterman, MN, RNC

Art and Science of Labor Support
Sylvia Wood, MSN, RN, CNM

Assessment of Risk in the Health Newborn
Valerie D. Shaw, MS, RN, CPN
Amy L. Tashman, MSN, RNC

Assessment of Risk in the Preterm/Low-birthweight Infant
Carol Trotter, RNC, MPH, NNP, PhD(c)
Lyn Varga, RNC, MSN, NNP

Assessment of Risks in the Term Newborn
Susan Bakewell-Sachs, Ph.D., CRNP, RN, CS
Valerie D. Shaw, MS, RN, CPN
Amy L. Tashman, MSN, RNC

Diabetes in Pregnancy (2nd ed.)
Jo M. Kendrick, RNC, MSN, CDE

Discharge of the High Risk Neonate
Susan Blackburn, PhD, RN, FAAN
Susan Bakewell-Sacks, PHD, CRNP, RN, CS

HIV and STDs
Maureen Shannon, MS, CNM, FNP
Barbara Peterson Sinclair, MSN, RN

High Risk Pregnancy: Chronic Medical Conditions
Patricia M. Sauer, RNC, MSN

All of the publications are available through:

March of Dimes Perinatal Data Center
P.O. Box 1657
Wilkes-Barre, PA 18703-1657
1-800-367-6630
FAX 717-825-1987

LABOR AND DELIVERY CONCEPTS

The March of Dimes Learning Modules Integration with the 1997 Joint Commission on Accreditation of Healthcare Organizations (JCAHO) Standards.

Human Resources Planning

HR. 3 The leaders ensure that the competence of all staff members is assessed, maintained, demonstrated, and improved continually.

HR.3.1 The hospital encourages and supports self-development and learning for all staff.

HR.4 An orientation process provides initial job training and information and assesses the staff's ability to fulfill specified responsibilities.

HR.4.1 The hospital orients and educates staff about their responsibilities related to patient care.

HR.4.2 Ongoing inservice and other education and training maintain staff and improve staff competence.

HR.4.3 The hospital regularly collects aggregate data on competence patterns and trends to identify and respond to the staff's learning needs.

(All modules meet this criteria)

Patient Assessment

PE.1 Each patient's physical, psychological, and social status are assessed.
    Abuse during pregnancy
    Antepartal screening of the pregnant woman
    Adolescent pregnancy
    Assessment of the newborn at risk
    The mature gravida: Pregnancy at age 35 and older
    Obstetrical emergencies for the perinatal nurse
    Preterm labor: Prevention and nursing management
    Window of opportunity: Interviewing by the perinatal nurse
    Multiple gestation
    Culturally sensitive caregiving
    Hypertension during pregnancy

PE.1.2 **Nutritional status is assessed when warranted by the patient's needs or condition.**
    Preconceptional health promotion
    Diabetes in pregnancy
    Breastfeeding the healthy newborn
    Hypoglycemia in the newborn

PE.1.5 The need for discharge planning assessment is determined.
Easing the transition from hospital to home: Postpartum discharge planning and homecare services

PE.1.8 Possible victims of abuse are identified using criteria developed by the hospital.
Abuse during pregnancy

Additional Requirements for Specific Patient Populations

PE.5 The assessment process for an infant, child, or adolescent is individualized (age specific).
Adolescent pregnancy
Assessment of the newborn at risk
The mature gravida: Pregnancy at age 35 and older

PE. 7 The assessment and reassessment of patients receiving treatment for alcoholism or other drug dependencies includes specific historical and cultural information.
Perinatal impact of substance abuse
Culturally sensitive caregiving

PE.8 Patients who are possible victims of alleged or suspected abuse or neglect have special needs relative to the assessment process.
Abuse during pregnancy

APPENDIX R • UNLICENSED ASSISTIVE PERSONNEL: POSITION DESCRIPTIONS, COMPETENCE VALIDATION TOOLS, AND SKILLS CHECKLISTS

St. Elizabeth Health Center
Organizational Education

Women's & Children's Care Center
Health Care Associate
Orientation Skills Checklist

NAME: _____   DATE OF HIRE: _____

SPECIALTY: _____   PRECEPTOR: _____

PURPOSE: The Orientation Skills Checklist is utilized for:

1. Self evaluation of competencies prior to orientation. This assessment is the basis for planning individualized clinical orientation.

2. Periodic evaluation of the orientee's progress during orientation.

3. Documentation of the orientee's progress during orientation.

DIRECTIONS:
1. The orientee reviews the Orientation Skills Checklist prior to the beginning of clinical orientation and performs a self-evaluation. This is reviewed by the preceptor.

2. The orientee and the preceptor evaluate the orientee's performance at the end of the clinical orientation.

CRITERIA FOR CLINICAL EVALUATION: Place a check-mark in the appropriate columns to identify the orientee's level of performance at the beginning and end of orientation. Utilize the following performance criteria.

- A. **DEPENDENT:**
  - unable to demonstrate behavior
  - lacks confidence, coordination and efficiency
  - needs continuous verbal, physical and supportive cues

- B. **ASSISTED:**
  - skillful in parts of behavior
  - improved confidence, coordination and efficiency
  - needs to improve organizational skills
  - requires occasional verbal, physical and supportive cues

- C. **INDEPENDENT:**
  - proficient, coordinated and confident
  - organized
  - does not require cues

- D. **REVIEWED INFORMATION**
  - orientee may not have had opportunity during orientation to perform identified skills
  - information and resources related to skill were identified and reviewed with orientee

APPENDIX R • UNLICENSED ASSISTIVE PERSONNEL: POSITION DESCRIPTIONS, COMPETENCE VALIDATION TOOLS, AND SKILLS CHECKLISTS

Skills Checklist for Health Care Associate	Self Eval Date _____			End Point Date _____			Can Identify Resources Available	N/A Does Not Apply to Job
	DEPENDENT	ASSISTED	INDEPENDENT	DEPENDENT	ASSISTED	INDEPENDENT		
COMMUNICATION SKILLS Demonstrates good interpersonal skills with patient/families/staff								
Respects patient confidentiality								
Observes the proper chain of command for problem solving and communications								
Documents and reports pertinent patient care information appropriately								
Answers patient call lights appropriately and in a timely manner								
Demonstrates ability to properly operate tube system								
Demonstrates ability to operate computer								
Demonstrates ability to operate/answer the phone								
Demonstrates ability to properly operate fax machine								
Utilizes reference materials and policy/procedure manuals appropriately								
SAFETY Demonstrates knowledge of universal precautions								
Demonstrates knowledge of personal protection equipment								
Demonstrates knowledge of electrical safety								
Demonstrates knowledge of isolation procedures								

Demonstrates knowledge of emergency #911 for:
     Resuscitation team - Code Blue/Code Pink
     Assist Team								

Identifies location of fire extinguishers								
Utilizes siderails and electric beds appropriately								
Demonstrates knowledge of seizure precautions								

APPENDIX R • UNLICENSED ASSISTIVE PERSONNEL: POSITION DESCRIPTIONS, COMPETENCE VALIDATION TOOLS, AND SKILLS CHECKLISTS

Skills Checklist for Health Care Associate	Self Eval Date			End Point Date			Can Identify Resources Available	N/A Does Not Apply to Job
	DEPENDENT	ASSISTED	INDEPENDENT	DEPENDENT	ASSISTED	INDEPENDENT		
Verbalizes knowledge of evacuation procedure								
EQUIPMENT/PROCEDURES Demonstrates care of a patient with an IV/IVAC								
Demonstrates care of a patient with a PCA pump								
Performs dressing changes								
BASIC RESPIRATORY CARE Incentive spirometer								
Emergency O_2 Kit								
Pulse Oximetry								
Oxygen therapy								
Suctioning								
COLLECTION OF SPECIMENS Routine urine								
Clean catch urine								
Catheterized urine								
24-hour urine								
Stool								
Blood (Phlebotomy)								
NUTRITION Checks trays/menus								
Assists in passing trays								
Passes water								

APPENDIX R • UNLICENSED ASSISTIVE PERSONNEL: POSITION DESCRIPTIONS, COMPETENCE VALIDATION TOOLS, AND SKILLS CHECKLISTS

Skills Checklist for Health Care Associate	Self Eval Date _____			End Point Date _____			Can Identify Resources Available	N/A Does Not Apply to Job
	DEPENDENT	ASSISTED	INDEPENDENT	DEPENDENT	ASSISTED	INDEPENDENT		
ENVIRONMENT								
Assists in stocking of supplies								
Assists in daily cleaning								
Performs simple maintenance								
Maintains a safe environment								
BASIC PATIENT CARE								
Makes beds:								
Occupied								
Unoccupied								
Bassinets								
Isolettes								
Warming tables								
Drainage								
Bed pan								
Emesis basin								
Foley bag								
Isolation								
Handwashing								
Universal precautions								
Gowning/glove/mask								
Supportive Measures								
Ted hose								
Flexitone binder								
Transfer techniques								
Bed to cart								
Bed to wheelchair								
Bed to chair								
Assist with ambulation								

APPENDIX R • UNLICENSED ASSISTIVE PERSONNEL: POSITION DESCRIPTIONS, COMPETENCE VALIDATION TOOLS, AND SKILLS CHECKLISTS

Skills Checklist for Health Care Associate	Self Eval Date			End Point Date			Can Identify Resources Available	N/A Does Not Apply to Job
	DEPENDENT	ASSISTED	INDEPENDENT	DEPENDENT	ASSISTED	INDEPENDENT		
MATERNAL CARE Admit to room								
Height & Weight								
Bath/shower								
Pericare								
Sitzbath								
PM Care								
Ice Bags								
Vital Signs Temperature								
Pulse								
Respirations								
BP								
Enema Administration Fleets								
Tap water/soap suds								
Urine dipstick								
Catheterization Prepartum patient								
Postpartum patient								
Removal of Foley								
Care of a preoperative patient								
Care of postoperative patient								

APPENDIX R • UNLICENSED ASSISTIVE PERSONNEL: POSITION DESCRIPTIONS, COMPETENCE VALIDATION TOOLS, AND SKILLS CHECKLISTS

Skills Checklist for Health Care Associate	Self Eval Date			End Point Date			Can Identify Resources Available	N/A Does Not Apply to Job
	DEPENDENT	ASSISTED	INDEPENDENT	DEPENDENT	ASSISTED	INDEPENDENT		
Newborn/Pediatric Care Initial bath								
Daily bath								
Height								
Weight								
Cord care								
Circumcision care								
Diaper Changing								
Weighing Diapers								
Initial feeding								
Daily feeding								
Transporting infants								
Suction with bulb syringe								
Picture taking								
Urine collection bag								
Car seats								
Infants seats								

APPENDIX R • UNLICENSED ASSISTIVE PERSONNEL: POSITION DESCRIPTIONS, COMPETENCE VALIDATION TOOLS, AND SKILLS CHECKLISTS

Skills Checklist for Health Care Associate	Self Eval Date _____			End Point Date _____			Can Identify Resources Available	N/A Does Not Apply to Job
	DEPENDENT	ASSISTED	INDEPENDENT	DEPENDENT	ASSISTED	INDEPENDENT		
Vital signs Rectal temperature								
Axillary temperature								
Tympanic temperature								
Respirations								
Apical pulse								
BP								
Urines								
Dipstick								
Specific gravity								
Heelsticks								
Cares for infant with feeding tube								
PLAN OF CARE Assists with development of patient care plan by identifying patient problems/needs								
Performs data collection								
Organizes and implements patient care for an assigned group of patients								
Assists with discharge planning as directed by the health care professional								
Reinforces patient teaching								
Discharges patients								
Transfers patients								

Skills Checklist for Health Care Associate	Self Eval Date _____			End Point Date _____			Can Identify Resources Available	N/A Does Not Apply to Job
	DEPENDENT	ASSISTED	INDEPENDENT	DEPENDENT	ASSISTED	INDEPENDENT		
DOCUMENTATION Verbalizes knowledge of charting by standards								
Documents according to hospital policy								
Documents using approved hospital abbreviations								
Demonstrates accurate order transcription skills								
AGE SPECIFIC INFORMATION Verbalizes knowledge of basic developmental and physical needs for the following patient populations: Newborns								
Pediatric								
Maternity								

APPENDIX R • UNLICENSED ASSISTIVE PERSONNEL: POSITION DESCRIPTIONS, COMPETENCE VALIDATION TOOLS, AND SKILLS CHECKLISTS

Skills Checklist for Licensed Health Care Associate	Self Eval Date			End Point Date			Can Identify Resources Available	N/A Does Not Apply to Job
	DEPENDENT	ASSISTED	INDEPENDENT	DEPENDENT	ASSISTED	INDEPENDENT		
LICENSED HCA **MEDICATION ADMINISTRATION PROCEDURES** Administers medications utilizing the "5 Rights"								
Operates the ADM machine								
Administers to Adults: Oral medications								
Topical								
IM								
Subcutaneous								
Administers to Infants/Pediatric Patients: Oral medications								
Topical								
IM								
Subcutaneous								
Administers respiratory medications: MDI								
Orders medications appropriately								
Transcribes medication orders								
Performs narcotic checks								
Documents medications accurately								
Administers 1-2-3 enema								

Health Care Associate
Orientation Skills Checklist

I have completed the Health Care Associate Orientation Skills Checklist:

_____   _____
Orientee Signature   Date

I have reviewed the Health Care Associate Skills Checklist.

_____   _____
Care Center Preceptor Signature   Date

_____   _____
Physical Therapy Preceptor Signature   Date

_____   _____
Environmental Services Preceptor Signature   Date

_____   _____
Educator   Date

_____   _____
Care Center Leader   Date

pm/checklist/wchca.lst/ljc
3/4/96

APPENDIX R • UNLICENSED ASSISTIVE PERSONNEL: POSITION DESCRIPTIONS, COMPETENCE VALIDATION TOOLS, AND SKILLS CHECKLISTS

ST. ELIZABETH HEALTH CENTER, A MEMBER OF HM HEALTH SERVICES

Name:	Center/Department - Clinical Services Women's/Children's
Position: Health Care Associate	

POSITION SUMMARY

The Health Care Associate works with his/her team partner(s), the Health Care Professional and the Hospitality Associate, to provide direct patient care. As a member of the Patient Care Team, the Associate is cross-trained to perform a wide range of essential patient services.

The Associate performs a variety of basic age-specific duties to assist in the care of patients under the direction of a Registered Nurse (RN). All clinical care will be done under the direction of the RN who has determined appropriate tasks for delegation. The Health Care Associate makes observations as directed by the RN and reports deviations to the RN.

POSITION QUALIFICATIONS

Required:

- High School Diploma/GED

Desired:

- State-tested Nurse Assistant or completion of a hospital-based Nurse Assistant orientation program
- Experience in providing direct patient care
- Computer literacy.
- Previous experience in Care Center specialty area.

Ongoing:

- Maintains Care Center specific certifications (see reverse).
- Attends hospital's mandatory education programs.
- Maintains required health screens.

AGE-APPROPRIATENESS

[1]	Neonate	Birth to 1 month
[1]	Infant	1 month to 1 year
[1]	Early Childhood	1 year to 5 years
[1]	Late Childhood	6 years to 12 years
[1]	Adolescence	13 years to 17 years
[1]	Young Adult	18 years to 25 years
[1]	Adult	26 years to 54 years
[ ]	Senior Adult	55 years to 64 years
[ ]	Geriatric	65 years and above
[2]	All Age Groups	Birth and above

APPENDIX R • UNLICENSED ASSISTIVE PERSONNEL: POSITION DESCRIPTIONS, COMPETENCE VALIDATION TOOLS, AND SKILLS CHECKLISTS

ST. ELIZABETH HEALTH CENTER, A MEMBER OF HM HEALTH SERVICES

Name:	Center/Department - Clinical Services

Position: Health Care Associate

Performance Management Philosophy:

In accordance with the continuing mission to be a healing, reconciling presence, and a just structure through the delivery of health services in our community, each individual will provide service in an atmosphere sensitive to physical, emotional, social, and spiritual needs with respect to the beliefs and values of co-workers, patients, and their families. Individuals will function in the spirit of teamwork with others to provide quality, efficient customer service. As members of this organization, individuals will be empowered and encouraged to use their skills and creativity to achieve common organizational and team goals.

VALUE-BASED BEHAVIORS

INTERDEPENDENCE:

Actively supports and participates within a team.

Holds self and team members responsible for accomplishing team goals.

Takes responsibility for seeking and communicating necessary information in an accurate and timely manner.

Seeks, offers, and accepts constructive feedback.

Participates in the decision-making process and supports the outcome.

STEWARDSHIP:

Makes the best use of time and talents to enhance the quality of service.

Uses supplies, equipment and services cost-effectively to insure our ability to serve the needs of the present and the future.

Willingly shares resources to avoid unnecessary duplication.

Supports efforts to respond to needs in the local community.

Consistently upholds the values of the organization.

RESPECT:

Expresses appreciation and gratitude to others.

Approaches others in a spirit of hospitality.

Respects the individuality and dignity of each person.

Respects the privacy and confidentiality of each person.

Remains calm in stressful circumstances, contributing to a peaceful and just outcome.

APPENDIX R • UNLICENSED ASSISTIVE PERSONNEL: POSITION DESCRIPTIONS, COMPETENCE VALIDATION TOOLS, AND SKILLS CHECKLISTS

ST. ELIZABETH HEALTH CENTER, A MEMBER OF HM HEALTH SERVICES

Name:	Center/Department - Clinical Services
Position: Health Care Associate	

COMPASSION:

Responds to the physical, emotional, social, and spiritual needs of others.

Gives caring service to all, understanding and valuing differences in others.

Demonstrates willingness to provide services, anticipating the needs of others.

Responds to requests in an appropriate time frame.

Listens to others with sensitivity, balancing the needs of the individual with those others and the organization

EXCELLENCE:

Directs all activities toward meeting the needs and exceeding the expectations of all served.

Offers suggestions and implements ways to improve the quality of service.

Supports the challenge of change that leads to the improvement of service.

Performs job responsibilities in a professional manner.

Demonstrates a strong commitment to self-development.

APPENDIX R • UNLICENSED ASSISTIVE PERSONNEL: POSITION DESCRIPTIONS, COMPETENCE VALIDATION TOOLS, AND SKILLS CHECKLISTS

ST. ELIZABETH HEALTH CENTER, A MEMBER OF HM HEALTH SERVICES

Name:	Center/Department - Clinical Services

Position: Health Care Associate

ESSENTIAL RESPONSIBILITIES:

All clinical care will be done under the direction of the RN who has determined appropriate tasks for delegation. The Health Care Associate makes observations as directed by the RN and reports deviations to the RN.

- Performs designated respiratory therapy (excluding medications).

- Performs general patient care including, but not limited to: bathing, mouth care, changing linens, dressing patient, back rubs, elimination, hygiene, and other needs as expressed.

- Performs venipuncture for blood collection.

- Collects specimens (i.e. urine, sputum) and ensures timely transport of specimens to the lab.

- Performs electrocardiogram (ECG).

- Observes patient's responses and reports any adverse reaction or other pertinent information to Registered Nurse and Physician.

- Performs wound care as directed by the Health Care Professional RN.

- Performs urinary catheterizations and enemas. Whenever possible, a male Health Care Associate will perform these procedures for male patients and a female Health Care Associate will perform these procedures for female patients.

- Obtains and records vital signs, height, and weight.

- Lifts, ambulates, and transports patients. Seeks assistance as needed.

- Performs designated bedside lab tests.

- Positions patient and performs range of motion. Assists physical therapist as needed.

- Delivers menus. Prepares patient for meals, distributes food trays, feeds patient, and removes trays. Distributes drinking water.

- Accurately charts patient information following the guidelines for charting by standards.

- Transcribes and implements physician orders.

- Performs computer order/entry functions as required by care center.

- Anticipates patient's needs and responds in a timely manner to patient and other caregiver requests.

- Provides friendly assistance to patient's family members and visitors.

- Answers phones courteously, and quickly addresses the caller's needs.

- Initiates emergency procedures when necessary.

APPENDIX R • UNLICENSED ASSISTIVE PERSONNEL: POSITION DESCRIPTIONS, COMPETENCE VALIDATION TOOLS, AND SKILLS CHECKLISTS

**ST. ELIZABETH HEALTH CENTER, A MEMBER OF
HM HEALTH SERVICES**

Name:	Center/Department - Clinical Services
Position: Health Care Associate	

- Observes universal precautions and aseptic techniques.

APPENDIX R • UNLICENSED ASSISTIVE PERSONNEL: POSITION DESCRIPTIONS, COMPETENCE VALIDATION TOOLS, AND SKILLS CHECKLISTS

ST. ELIZABETH HEALTH CENTER, A MEMBER OF HM HEALTH SERVICES

Name:	Center/Department - Clinical Services
Position: Health Care Associate	

- Performs other designated procedures.

OTHER RESPONSIBILITIES:

- Assists in daily cleaning of patient rooms and care center. Helps prepare room(s) for incoming patients.

- Performs simple maintenance (light bulbs, batteries).

- Inventories unit and determines supply needs. Conveys needs to appropriate personnel.

- Assists with patient education and discharge planning.

- Assesses maintenance needs. Initiates maintenance requisition to repair equipment, furniture, and building fixtures.

- Acts as a liaison and support person for family members.

- Participates in orientations of students and new employees.

- Attends required staff meetings and inservices.

APPENDIX R • UNLICENSED ASSISTIVE PERSONNEL: POSITION DESCRIPTIONS, COMPETENCE VALIDATION TOOLS, AND SKILLS CHECKLISTS

ST. ELIZABETH HEALTH CENTER, A MEMBER OF HM HEALTH SERVICES

Name:	Center/Department -Clinical Services Women's and Children's
Position: Health Care Associate - Licensed	

POSITION SUMMARY

The licensed Health Care Associate works with his/her team partner(s), the Health Care Professional and the Hospitality Associate, to provide direct patient care. As a member of the Patient Care Team, the licensed Associate is cross-trained to perform a wide range of essential patient services including designated medication administration.

The licensed Associate performs a variety of basic age-specific duties to assist in the care of patients under the direction of a Registered Nurse (RN). All clinical care will be done under the direction of the RN who has determined appropriate tasks for delegation. The licensed Health Care Associate makes observations as directed by the RN and reports deviations to the RN.

POSITION QUALIFICATIONS

Required:

- High School Diploma/GED
- License to administer designated medications (Licensed Practical Nurse, Respiratory Technician)

Desired:

- State-tested Nurse Assistant or successful completion of a hospital-based Nurse Assistant course.
- Experience in providing direct patient care
- Computer literacy.
- Previous experience working in Care Center specialty area.

Ongoing:

- Maintains Care Center specific certifications (see reverse).
- Attends hospital's mandatory education programs.
- Maintains current license.
- Maintains required health screens.

AGE-APPROPRIATENESS

[1]	Neonate	Birth to 1 month
[1]	Infant	1 month to 1 year
[1]	Early Childhood	1 year to 5 years
[1]	Late Childhood	6 years to 12 years
[1]	Adolescence	13 years to 17 years
[1]	Young Adult	18 years to 25 years
[1]	Adult	26 years to 54 years
[ ]	Senior Adult	55 years to 64 years
[ ]	Geriatric	65 years and above
[2]	All Age Groups	Birth and above

APPENDIX R • UNLICENSED ASSISTIVE PERSONNEL: POSITION DESCRIPTIONS, COMPETENCE VALIDATION TOOLS, AND SKILLS CHECKLISTS

ST. ELIZABETH HEALTH CENTER, A MEMBER OF HM HEALTH SERVICES

Name:	Center/Department -Clinical Services

Position: Health Care Associate - Licensed

Performance Management Philosophy:

In accordance with the continuing mission to be a healing, reconciling presence, and a just structure through the delivery of health services in our community, each individual will provide service in an atmosphere sensitive to physical, emotional, social, and spiritual needs with respect to the beliefs and values of co-workers, patients, and their families. Individuals will function in the spirit of teamwork with others to provide quality, efficient customer service. As members of this organization, individuals will be empowered and encouraged to use their skills and creativity to achieve common organizational and team goals.

VALUE-BASED BEHAVIORS

INTERDEPENDENCE:

Actively supports and participates within a team.

Holds self and team members responsible for accomplishing team goals.

Takes responsibility for seeking and communicating necessary information in an accurate and timely manner.

Seeks, offers, and accepts constructive feedback.

Participates in the decision-making process and supports the outcome.

STEWARDSHIP:

Makes the best use of time and talents to enhance the quality of service.

Uses supplies, equipment and services cost-effectively to insure our ability to serve the needs of the present and the future.

Willingly shares resources to avoid unnecessary duplication.

Supports efforts to respond to needs in the local community.

Consistently upholds the values of the organization.

RESPECT:

Expresses appreciation and gratitude to others.

Approaches others in a spirit of hospitality.

Respects the individuality and dignity of each person.

Respects the privacy and confidentiality of each person.

Remains calm in stressful circumstances, contributing to a peaceful and just outcome.

APPENDIX R • UNLICENSED ASSISTIVE PERSONNEL: POSITION DESCRIPTIONS, COMPETENCE VALIDATION TOOLS, AND SKILLS CHECKLISTS

ST. ELIZABETH HEALTH CENTER, A MEMBER OF HM HEALTH SERVICES

Name:	Center/Department -Clinical Services
Position: Health Care Associate - Licensed	

COMPASSION:

Responds to the physical, emotional, social, and spiritual needs of others.

Gives caring service to all, understanding and valuing differences in others.

Demonstrates willingness to provide services, anticipating the needs of others.

Responds to requests in an appropriate time frame.

Listens to others with sensitivity, balancing the needs of the individual with those others and the organization

EXCELLENCE:

Directs all activities toward meeting the needs and exceeding the expectations of all served.

Offers suggestions and implements ways to improve the quality of service.

Supports the challenge of change that leads to the improvement of service.

Performs job responsibilities in a professional manner.

Demonstrates a strong commitment to self-development.

APPENDIX R • UNLICENSED ASSISTIVE PERSONNEL: POSITION DESCRIPTIONS, COMPETENCE VALIDATION TOOLS, AND SKILLS CHECKLISTS

ST. ELIZABETH HEALTH CENTER, A MEMBER OF HM HEALTH SERVICES

Name:	Center/Department -Clinical Services
Position: Health Care Associate - Licensed	

ESSENTIAL RESPONSIBILITIES:

All clinical care will be done under the direction of the RN who has determined appropriate tasks for delegation. The licensed Health Care Associate makes observations as directed by the RN and reports deviations to the RN.

- Performs designated respiratory therapy according to license, training, and demonstrated competency.

- Performs general patient care including, but not limited to: bathing, mouth care, changing linens, dressing patient, back rubs, elimination, hygiene, and other needs as expressed.

- Performs venipuncture for blood collection.

- Performs arterial blood gas puncture as governed by licensure, training, and demonstrated competency.

- Collects specimens (i.e. urine, sputum) and ensures timely transport of specimens to the lab.

- Performs electrocardiogram (ECG).

- Observes patient's responses and reports any adverse reaction or other pertinent information to Registered Nurse and Physician.

- Performs wound care as directed by the Health Care Professional RN.

- Performs urinary catheterizations and enemas. Whenever possible, a male Health Care Associate will perform these procedures for male patients and a female Health Care Associate will perform these procedures for female patients.

- Obtains and records vital signs, height, and weight.

- Lifts, ambulates, and transports patients. Seeks assistance as needed.

- Performs designated bedside lab tests.

- Positions patient and performs range of motion. Assists physical therapist as needed.

- Delivers menus. Prepares patient for meals, distributes food trays, feeds patient, and removes trays. Distributes drinking water.

- Accurately charts patient information following the guidelines for charting by standards.

- Transcribes and implements physician orders

- Performs computer order/entry functions as required by care center.

- Anticipates patient's needs and responds in a timely manner to patient and other caregiver requests.

- Provides friendly assistance to patient's family members and visitors.

- Answers phones courteously, and quickly addresses the caller's needs.

- Initiates emergency procedures when necessary.

APPENDIX R • UNLICENSED ASSISTIVE PERSONNEL: POSITION DESCRIPTIONS, COMPETENCE VALIDATION TOOLS, AND SKILLS CHECKLISTS

**ST. ELIZABETH HEALTH CENTER, A MEMBER OF
HM HEALTH SERVICES**

Name:	Center/Department -Clinical Services
Position: Health Care Associate - Licensed	

- Observes universal precautions and isolation procedures. Maintains aseptic technique.

ST. ELIZABETH HEALTH CENTER, A MEMBER OF
HM HEALTH SERVICES

Name:	Center/Department -Clinical Services

Position: Health Care Associate - Licensed

- Performs other designated procedures.

OTHER RESPONSIBILITIES:

- Administers medications and performs IV therapy as governed by licensure, training, and demonstrated competency.

- Assists in daily cleaning of patient rooms and care center. Helps prepare room(s) for incoming patients.

- Performs simple maintenance (light bulbs, batteries).

- Inventories unit and determines supply needs. Conveys needs to appropriate personnel.

- Assists with patient education and discharge planning.

- Assesses maintenance needs. Initiates maintenance requisition to repair equipment, furniture, and building fixtures.

- Acts as a liaison and support person for family members.

- Participates in orientations of students and new employees.

- Attends required staff meetings and inservices.

APPENDIX R • UNLICENSED ASSISTIVE PERSONNEL: POSITION DESCRIPTIONS, COMPETENCE VALIDATION TOOLS, AND SKILLS CHECKLISTS

MATERNITY SERVICES ORIENTATION
UNIT SECRETARY SKILLS CHECKLIST

Skills	Never Done	Needs Review	Performs Independently	Preceptor Initials Date
1. Typing/Computer Skills				
2. Transcribing M.D. orders (entering orders in computer)				
3. Phone Skills (Proper etiquette, transferring, answer in timely manner, etc.)				
4. Paging system				
5. Call lights/emergency				
6. Fax machine				
7. Addressograph				
8. Printer				
9. Shredder				
10. Greeting visitors and patients				
11. Providing visitors and patients with information				
12. Log Book				
13. Charges				
14. Distribute Mail				
15. Gathering information for birth certificates				
16. Data gathering and report preparation				
17. Assemble chart and label chart for LDR, MB Cesarean Section, 23 hour observation, infant, Outpatient				
18. Discharge patients in computer				
19. Transferring patients in computer				
20. Scheduling inductions, NST's, Cesarean Sections				
21. Responsible that par level chart supplies are maintained				
22. Filing prenatal, lab reports, ultrasound, x-ray reports				
23. Know how to call baby to admitting, pediatrics				
24. Maintaining patient boards (admissions, discharges, transfers				
25. Primary phone answerer				
26. Preparation for Mother (Baby, discharge)				

Lake Forest Hospital, Lake Forest, Illinois

APPENDIX R • UNLICENSED ASSISTIVE PERSONNEL: POSITION DESCRIPTIONS, COMPETENCE VALIDATION TOOLS, AND SKILLS CHECKLISTS

Skills	Never Done	Needs Review	Performs Independ-ently	Preceptor Initials Date
Strengths:				
Need for Improvement:				
Comments:				

_____   _____
Orientee Signature   *Preceptor Signature*

APPENDIX R • UNLICENSED ASSISTIVE PERSONNEL: POSITION DESCRIPTIONS, COMPETENCE VALIDATION TOOLS, AND SKILLS CHECKLISTS

MATERNITY SERVICES ORIENTATION SUPPORT TECH SKILLS CHECKLIST

Skills	Never Done	Needs Review	Performs Independently	Preceptor Initials Date
1. Orientation to the unit:				
a. mother/baby				
b. labor/delivery/recovery				
c. nursery				
d. Sue's office				
e. locker room				
f. utility rooms				
2. Listen to report				
3. Scrub				
4. Pass water				
5. Pass trays				
6. Collect trays				
7. Collect menus				
8. Set-up circumcision trays				
9. Clean circumcision trays				
10. Clean cribs				
11. Stock cribs				
12. Take cribs to LDR when needed				
13. Set-up rooms for new-patients				
14. Restock rooms, check glove and needle boxes				
15. Transporting patients				
16. Discharging patients				
17. Clean kitchen				
18. Clean and supply sitz baths				
19. Empty linen				
20. Put away clean linen				
21. Assist with making beds				
22. Assist housekeeper-strip linen from discharge rooms				
23. Run errands i.e.: pharmacy, lab, materials management				
24. Assist secretaries				
a. Xeroxing				
b. Stamp or label charts				
c. Filing				
d. Fill in PKU slips				
e. Fill in birth certificate information from pre-admit forms				
f. Enter charges in the computer				
g. Enter nurse station revisions in the computer				
h. Shredding				
i. Answer phones and call lights				
j. Assembling charts				

APPENDIX R • UNLICENSED ASSISTIVE PERSONNEL: POSITION DESCRIPTIONS, COMPETENCE VALIDATION TOOLS, AND SKILLS CHECKLISTS

Skills	Never Done	Needs Review	Performs Independently	Preceptor Initials Date
Support Tech - LDR:				
1. Set-up labor room for admissions				
2. Set-up delivery table				
3. Post delivery cleaning: instruments, washroom, & restock				
4. Assist with transporting of patient				
5. Pass food trays				
6. Run errands				
7. Assemble charts				
8. Answer phones				
9. Answer call lights				
10. Empty linen				
11. Clean metal carts with cavicide				
12. Make baby hats				
13. Make generic charts for moms and babies				
Strengths:				
Need for Improvement:				
Comments:				

APPENDIX R • UNLICENSED ASSISTIVE PERSONNEL: POSITION DESCRIPTIONS, COMPETENCE VALIDATION TOOLS, AND SKILLS CHECKLISTS

MATERNITY SERVICES ORIENTATION
PATIENT CARE TECH SKILLS CHECKLIST

Skills	Never Done	Needs Review	Performs Independently	Preceptor Initials Date
1. Orientation to the unit:				
a. mother/baby				
b. labor/delivery/recovery				
c. nursery				
d. Sue's office				
e. locker room				
f. utility rooms				
2. Vital signs mother and infant: temperature, pulse, respirations and blood pressure (mother only)				
3. Orient patient to room and routine				
4. Check supplies infants crib and restock with enough supplies for your shift				
5. Report vital signs to the nurse and record them on the chart				
6. Assist patients to the bathroom or shower or with bedbath				
7. Assist patient with pericare				
8. Report to nurse pt. status				
9. Assist with passing trays				
10. Assist with circumcision				
a. Set-up				
b. Obtain 4 x 4's and petrolatum for dressing				
11. Return infant to mother and check I.D. band				
12. Demonstrate cic care				
13. Demonstrate cord care				
14. Assist mom with infant feeding				
15. Check on baby pictures				
16. Assist moms to the sitz bath				
17. Clean and restock sitz bath				
18. Make ice packs				
19. Assemble and stamp or label charts				
20. Infant bath PRN				
21. Update infants clinical record				
22. Make beds				
23. Empty foley catheters				
24. Collect and record Intake and Output				
25. Universal precautions				
26. Assist Secretaries				
a. Xeroxing				
b. Stamp or label charts				
c. Filing				
d. Fill in PKU slips				
e. Fill in birth certificate information from pre-admit forms				
f. Enter charges in the computer				

APPENDIX R • UNLICENSED ASSISTIVE PERSONNEL: POSITION DESCRIPTIONS, COMPETENCE VALIDATION TOOLS, AND SKILLS CHECKLISTS

Skills	Never Done	Needs Review	Performs Independ-ently	Preceptor Initials Date
g. Enter nurse station revisions in the computer				
h. Shredding				
i. Answer phones and call lights				
j. Assemble charts				
k. Assist support techs				
Additionally, the following skills are needed in LDR:				
1. Orient patient and S.O. to room				
2. Instruct pt. in changing clothes				
3. Instruct pt. to give urine sample and check sample with Chem. Strip				
4. Obtain vital signs				
5. Set-up room for an epidural				
6. Assist R.N. in delivery room				
7. Notification of delivery				
a. admitting, time, sex, type of delivery, and pediatrician				
b. pediatrician				
c. mother/baby				
8. Assist R.N. in preparing for C-section				
9. Transport patient				
Strengths:				
Need for Improvement:				
Comments:				

_____   _____
Orientee Signature   Preceptor Signature

APPENDIX R • UNLICENSED ASSISTIVE PERSONNEL: POSITION DESCRIPTIONS, COMPETENCE VALIDATION TOOLS, AND SKILLS CHECKLISTS

Patient Care Associate Clinical Evaluation of Performance

Candidate's Name _____ Clinical Dates _____

Clinical Instructor's Name _____

The purpose of this document is to give the Patient Care Associate feedback on their performance in the clinical practicum of the PCA course. It is not meant to be used in lieu of, or as, a formal performance evaluation. Candidate's will be rated by the clinical instructor in all areas. Comments will be made as necessary. The candidate will have an opportunity to review all the information before the document is forwarded to the manager for filing.

CORPORATE VALUES

Corporate values are the principles and commitments which shape the identity of a corporation and permeate its activities. The values of the Sisters of Mercy Health System are:

Dignity	Accept all as created in God's image
Justice	Honor each person's rights for common good
Stewardship	Use talents and resources wisely
Service	Respond with compassion to others' needs
Excellence	Strive to attain high standards of performance

*** The following expectations must be present consistently in interactions which include staff-patient, staff-visitor, staff-staff, staff-physician, etc.

Explanation of Rating Scale -- **YES** = Performs Above Expected Level   **yes** = Performs at the Expected Level
Inconsistently Performs = Performs Inconsistently at Expected Level   **NO** = Does Not Meet Expectations

Performance Expectation	YES	yes	Inconsistently Performs	NO	*Comments*
1. Acknowledges and maintains the right to privacy and confidentiality.					
2. Gives appropriate feedback in a constructive and sensitive manner to the person involved.					
3. Assumes responsibility for problem solving: does not assign fault.					
4. Demonstrates the ability to maintain a poised, calm and composed manner.					
5. Acknowledges individuals in a prompt and courteous manner.					
6. Responds to identified/expressed need in a prompt and courteous manner.					
7. Offers additional assistance before concluding each interaction.					
8. Communications are courteous, utilizing appropriate statements.					
9. Focuses attention and communication on the individual being served.					
10. Demonstrates congruency between verbal and nonverbal communication.					
11. Keeps hospital and work areas neat and clean.					
12. Respects medical center and guest's property.					
13. Presents neat and clean appearance, in accordance with medical center policy.					
14. Adheres to medical center and department specific safety regulations.					

St. John's Mercy Medical Center, St. Louis Missouri

APPENDIX R • UNLICENSED ASSISTIVE PERSONNEL: POSITION DESCRIPTIONS, COMPETENCE VALIDATION TOOLS, AND SKILLS CHECKLISTS

CLINICAL COMPETENCIES

Performance Expectation	YES	yes	Inconsistently Performs	NO	Comments
1. Administers daily hygiene measures, including but not limited too: bathing, mouth and skin care, etc. Changes linens.					
2. Performs routine daily activities. Assists with ambulation. Assists with passing trays, snacks, ice water and feeding patients. Performs passive and active ROM. Turns and positions patients, observes skin condition.					
3. Gathers and records patient data, including vital signs, calorie counts, appetite, intake and output, stools, simple dressing changes, weights, specimens and all assigned patient care activities.					
4. Performs unit specific computer functions, i.e. ADL, ordering equipment and supplies, entering lab specimens.					
5. Demonstrates proficiency in clinical skills related to unit. Provides catheter care. Administers enemas.					
6. Observes changes or unusual occurrences in patient condition and reports them immediately to the appropriate professional.					
7. Provides patients and their families with explanation of care and psychological support under the direction of the nurse.					
8. Demonstrates knowledge of and practices sound infection control techniques.					
9. Assesses safety needs and provides for a safe environment for patients and co-workers. Applies and monitors patient safety devices appropriately, i.e. wrist restraints, jackets.					
10. Participates in admission, discharge and transfer of patients and their belongings. Orients patient to the environment. Completes necessary documentation.					
11. Accepts delegation of tasks.					
12. Prioritizes appropriately and utilizes good judgement in use of time.					
13. Organizes and completes tasks in a timely manner.					
14. Acquires adequate supplies to perform daily care.					
15. Demonstrates flexibility regarding workload, assignments and change. Accepts and completes special assignments as directed.					

Instructor's Signature_____Date Reviewed_____

Candidate's Signature_____Date Reviewed_____

Initiated by: D. Biggs, RN 6/96   Reviewed:

APPENDIX R • UNLICENSED ASSISTIVE PERSONNEL: POSITION DESCRIPTIONS, COMPETENCE VALIDATION TOOLS, AND SKILLS CHECKLISTS

SKILLS CHECKLIST FOR NEONATE METABOLISM SCREEN

Candidate's Name _____ Preceptor _____
Classroom Training Date _____ Competency Varified _____

The candidate is required to:
1. Read and understand the PKU procedure (sign acknowledgement list).
2. View the video of proper capillary phlebotomy techniques (sign acknowledgement list).

COMPETENCY RATING SCALE
1. No experience or opportunity to perform.
2. Requires 50-100% supervision/direction to perform skill/task/procedure.
3. Requires less than 50% supervision/direction to perform skill/task/procedure.
4. Requires no supervision to perform.

To varify competency of the NMS procedure, the candidate must complete a minimum of 5-10 supervised procedures with documentation of progress or identification of areas where improvement is needed by an individual designated as proficient in the procedure.

Procedure Number	1	2	3	4	5	6	7	8	9	10	11	12	13	14	15	16	17	18	19	20
Initial Demonstration Dt.																				
Skill/Task to Be Performed																				
1. Familar with proper collection times																				
2. Orders test correctly																				
3. Completes all info on DOH form																				
4. Is familiar with Repeat Screening form																				
5. Inventories and orders supplies																				

APPENDIX R • UNLICENSED ASSISTIVE PERSONNEL: POSITION DESCRIPTIONS, COMPETENCE VALIDATION TOOLS, AND SKILLS CHECKLISTS

Procedure Number	1	2	3	4	5	6	7	8	9	10	11	12	13	14	15	16	17	18	19	20
6. Gathers supplies for skin puncture																				
7. Wash hands in Nursery																				
8. Wears gloves																				
9. Identifies patient																				
10. Chooses proper site for skin puncture																				
11. Warms skin puncture site																				
12. Cleans site with alcohol pad																				
13. Perform skin puncture correctly																				
14. Wipe away first drop of blood																				
15. Collect specimen properly																				
16. After collection, hold gauze over site until bleeding stops																				
17. Apply bandaid (FTN) or gauze wrap (SCN)																				
18. Remove ALL collection equipment from crib & dispose of properly																				
19. Place one CHC label on back of DOH req and one in chart																				
20. Before collecting sample from another baby, wash hands and change gloves																				

Procedure Number	1	2	3	4	5	6	7	8	9	10	11	12	13	14	15	16	17	18	19	20
21. Verify that specimen was collected																				
22. Send specimen to lab																				
Comments/ Action Items																				

SKILLS CHECKLIST FOR VENIPUNCTURE

Candidate's Name _____ Preceptor _____

Classroom Training Date _____ Competency Verified _____

The candidate is required to read the proper patient identification and specimen labeling procedures (sign acknowledgment list).

COMPETENCY RATING SCALE

1. No experience or opportunity to perform.
2. Requires 50-100% supervision/direction to perform skill/task/procedure.
3. Requires less than 50% supervision/direction to perform skill/task/procedure.
4. Requires no supervision to perform.

To verify competency of the venipuncture blood collection procedure, the candidate must complete 25-35 supervised procedures with documentation of progress or identification of areas where improvement is needed by an individual designated as proficient in the procedure. Competency is at the discretion of the preceptor; however, the candidate must have a rating of (4) in all categories consistently for a minimum number of procedures.

Procedure Number	1	2	3	4	5	6	7	8	9	10	11	12	13	14	15	16	17	18	19	20
Initial Demonstration Dt.																				
Skill/Task to Be Performed																				
1. Inventories and orders supplies																				
2. Wash hands. Wear gloves.																				
3. Approach patient.																				
4. Identify patient.																				

APPENDIX R • UNLICENSED ASSISTIVE PERSONNEL: POSITION DESCRIPTIONS, COMPETENCE VALIDATION TOOLS, AND SKILLS CHECKLISTS

Procedure Number	1	2	3	4	5	6	7	8	9	10	11	12	13	14	15	16	17	18	19	20
20. Pushes the evacuated tube onto the back of the needle, keeping the holder absolutely still.																				
21. Draws evacuated tubes in appropriate order.																				
22. Instructs pt. to open hand, and appropriately removes tourniquet.																				
23. Pulls evacuated tube off needle.																				
24. Places a piece of gauze over the puncture site.																				
25. Withdraws the needle. Applies pressure to site, or instructs pt to do this.																				
26. Removes needle from the tube holder and places uncapped needle in sharps disposal unit.																				
27. Invert tubes gently several times to mix blood with additive.																				
28. Labels tubes appropriately. Verify specimen collection.																				
29. Discards materials contaminated with blood into the biohazard bag.																				
30. Appropriately discards other waste materials.																				
31. Inspects puncture site; applies bandage, if needed.																				
32. Removes all equipment from bedside.																				

LABOR AND DELIVERY CONCEPTS

CONCEPT 1: ADMISSION OF THE LABORING PATIENT

- State the criteria for admission to the Birth Center.
- Discuss the risk factors which preclude use of the Birth Center.
- State the admission and screening procedure for the Birth Center.

Admission Data Collection

- Identify important information or pertinent facts found in the maternal history/prenatal record, which must be considered when planning care for the laboring patient.
- Discuss the concept of a "birth plan" and why it is an important part of admission data collection/assessment.

Admission Assessment/Procedures

- List the key assessments/procedures involved in admission of a laboring patient.
- State the purpose and the procedure/technique involved for the following:
  - obtaining maternal vital signs
  - obtaining FHR by fetascope/doptone/EFM
  - performing Leopold's maneuvers
  - palpating contractions
  - assessing status of membranes by Nitrazine test
  - assessing presence of "show"
  - assessing maternal edema/reflexes
  - obtaining an admission Hct
  - obtaining a urine dipstick/SSA.

Distinguish normal from abnormal findings in these assessment procedures. Discuss possible reasons for variations and appropriate nursing interventions.

- Explain the procedure for performing/assisting with a vaginal exam and the indications/contraindications for performing this exam.
- Discuss the procedure for assisting with a sterile speculum exam, including the indications for this exam.
- Review the appropriate procedure for initiating IV access.
- Discuss what orientation/information is necessary to prepare the patient and family for admission to the Birth Center.
- Discuss nursing documentation related to admission of a laboring patient.

CONCEPT 2: THE PROCESS OF LABOR

- Define the following:
  - gynecoid, android, anthropoid and platypelloid pelvis types
  - pelvic inlet, midpelvis and pelvic outlet
  - cervical effacement and dilatation
  - fetal lie, presentation, position, presenting part, station and engagement
- State the 5 p's or factors which determine the progress of labor.
- Explain the normal maternal adaptations to labor—cardiovascular, respiratory, gastrointestinal, renal, musculoskeletal, neurologic, endocrine and emotional/behavioral. Discuss what findings you will observe during labor as a result of these adaptations.
- Discuss the normal fetal adaptations to labor and what findings you will observe during labor as a result of these adaptations.
- Define the normal mechanisms of labor: engagement, descent, flexion, internal rotation, extension, restitution/external rotation, and expulsion.
- Briefly define the four stages of labor and the normal duration of each stage for nulliparas and multiparas.

CONCEPT 3: FIRST STAGE OF LABOR

Latent Phase

- Define latent phase—describe the normal contraction pattern, rate of effacement/dilatation, rate of fetal descent, appearance of "show," and maternal behavior/sources of discomfort seen in this phase.
- State the policy for assessing and recording maternal vital signs, FHR and contractions during this phase.
- Distinguish normal from abnormal findings in maternal vital signs. Explain possible reasons for variations and appropriate nursing interventions.
- Discuss reassuring vs non-reassuring FHR patterns seen during this phase. State the appropriate procedure to be followed in the case of non-reassuring data.
- Discuss patient needs and nursing interventions related to diet/hydration, activity, elimination, hygiene and comfort/support during this phase.
- Discuss the role of family/support person(s) in meeting patient needs during this phase.
- Describe the signs of true vs false labor.
- Discuss the discharge instructions that are given to undelivered patients, as well as the paperwork necessary for discharging a patient undelivered.

Active/Transition Phase

- Define active phase—further define transition as part of this phase. Describe the normal contraction pattern, rate of dilatation, rate of fetal descent, appearance of "show," and maternal behavior/sources of discomfort/pain seen during this phase.

- State the policy for assessing and recording maternal vital signs, FHR and contraction pattern during this phase. Explain the rationale for increased monitoring.

- Distinguish normal from abnormal findings in maternal vital signs. Discuss possible reasons for alterations and appropriate nursing interventions.

- Discuss reassuring vs non-reassuring FHR patterns seen during this phase. State the appropriate procedure to be followed in the case of non-reassuring data.

- Explain the procedure for applying the electronic fetal monitor for external monitoring/obtaining a strip for evaluation and communicating with the physician regarding follow-up actions and care.

- Explain use of the Friedman graph (SMH 333) in monitoring the progress of labor. Distinguish normal from abnormal progress in cervical dilatation and normal from abnormal patterns of uterine activity. Discuss possible reasons for abnormal progress and appropriate nursing interventions.

- State the indications for performing a vaginal exam during this stage.

- Discuss the nursing interventions required after SROM.

- Outline patient needs and nursing interventions related to hydration, activity, elimination and comfort/support during this phase—especially focus on psychoprophylaxis and alternative comfort measures, e.g., use of whirlpool.

- List the analgesia/anesthesia options available to labor patients on the Birth Center and indications/contraindications for their use.

- Discuss the role and needs of the family during this phase.

- List the nursing priorities, in order of priority, during this stage.

- Discuss patient education related to this stage.

- Discuss nursing documentation required during this stage.

CONCEPT 4: SECOND STAGE OF LABOR/DELIVERY OF NEONATE

- Define the second stage of labor—describe the normal contraction pattern, rate of fetal descent, appearance of "show," maternal behavior/sources of pain and perineal changes seen during this stage.

- State the policy for assessing and recording maternal vital signs, FHR and contraction pattern during this phase. Explain the rationale for increased monitoring.

- Distinguish normal from abnormal findings in maternal vital signs. Discuss possible reasons for variations and appropriate nursing interventions.

- Discuss reassuring vs non-reassuring FHR patterns seen during this stage. State the appropriate procedure to be followed in the case of non-reassuring data.

- Distinguish normal from abnormal patterns of fetal descent and/or uterine activity. Discuss possible reasons for abnormal patterns and appropriate nursing interventions.

- Discuss effective breathing/pushing techniques and the method of instructing patient and support person(s) in these techniques. Identify when restraint in pushing is necessary and nursing interventions to facilitate this.

- List and describe the maternal positions which will facilitate fetal descent during this stage.

- Discuss the proper technique for applying suprapubic and fundal pressure to facilitate fetal descent and when these interventions should be employed.

- Outline patient needs and nursing interventions related to pain relief/support during this stage.

- Discuss the role and needs of the family during this stage.

- List the equipment and supplies which must be assembled for a delivery.

- List and describe the various birthing positions available to the patient—relate these positions to use of the birthing bed.

- State the causes of perineal/vaginal lacerations/tears.

- Outline the advantages vs disadvantages of episiotomies.

- Discuss nursing interventions to maintain perineal integrity and avoid episiotomy.

- Define the following: median episiotomy, mediolateral episiotomy, extensions, lacerations (1st to 4th degree), periuretheral lacerations, sulcus tears (unilateral or bilateral).

- Discuss the proper procedure for assisting with a forceps or vacuum delivery.

- List the nursing priorities, in order of priority, during this stage.

- Discuss patient education related to this stage.

- Discuss nursing documentation required during this stage.

CONCEPT 5: THIRD STAGE OF LABOR/DELIVERY OF PLACENTA

- Define the third stage of labor.

- List the key points involved in the immediate, postdelivery assessment of the newborn.

- Discuss the Apgar score as a method of assessment and state the policy for obtaining and recording an Apgar score.

- State the policy for assessing and recording an initial set of newborn vital signs and performing an initial screening assessment of the newborn.

- Distinguish normal from abnormal findings in Apgar score and initial vital signs. Explain reasons for variations and appropriate nursing interventions. Identify those situations in which the Pediatric House Officer/NICU must be involved immediately.

- Describe normal findings/appearance of the newborn at the initial screening assessment. Discuss variations from the normal and appropriate nursing interventions. Again, identify those situations in which the Pediatric House Officer/NICU must be involved immediately.

- Discuss newborn stabilization needs and nursing interventions in the immediate, postdelivery phase, related to warmth, maintenance of airway, safety, identification, eye/vitamin K prophylaxis, and attachment to parents.

- Discuss the appropriate procedure for suctioning with a bulb syringe, with a De Lee mucous trap and with wall suction—state the indications/contraindications for each method.

- Explain the proper procedure for identification of a newborn.

- Discuss the medication AquaMephyton (Vitamin K) given to the newborn for prevention of hemorrhagic disease of the newborn—include mechanism of action, route/site/timing of administration, normal dosage and side effects/contraindications.

- Discuss the medication Erythromycin Opthalmic Ointment given to the newborn for prevention of opthalmia neonatorum—include mechanism of action, method/timing of administration, normal dosage and side effects/contraindications. Relate the impact of this procedure on facilitating maternal-newborn attachment.

- Explain the proper procedure for obtaining and sending cord bloods/cord blood gas (arterial/venous) to the lab.

- List the indications and explain the appropriate procedure for obtaining a BG chemstrip on a newborn in the immediate, postdelivery period. State the normal range of results and appropriate interventions for abnormal results.

- List the signs of placental separation and discuss nursing interventions to assist with this process.

- Discuss the medications Pitocin and Methergine/Ergotrate combination given to the mother as oxytocics on delivery of placenta—include mechanism of action, route/site/timing of administration, normal dosage and side effects/contraindications.

- Discuss the procedure for examining the placenta, membranes and cord after delivery—describe the normal appearance of these structures, including the number of vessels normally found in the cord.

- Explain the proper procedure for disposal of the placenta.

- Discuss the procedure for assisting with perineal repair, including what suture materials are commonly used for repair.

- List the nursing priorities, in order of priority, during this stage.

- Discuss patient education related to this stage.

- Discuss nursing documentation required during this stage.

CONCEPT 6: FOURTH STAGE OF LABOR/RECOVERY

- Define the fourth stage of labor.

- List the key points involved in maternal assessment during this stage.

- State the policy for assessing and recording maternal vital signs and assessing maternal fundus, lochia, perineum, and bladder status during this stage.

- Distinguish normal from abnormal findings in maternal vital signs. Explain possible reasons for variations and appropriate nursing interventions.

- Describe normal tone/location of uterus, color/amount of lochia, appearance of perineum and location/status of bladder during this stage. Discuss alterations from the normal and appropriate nursing interventions.

- Discuss the proper technique for uterine massage—in particular, explain the rationale for providing uterine support during massage.

- Outline patient needs and nursing interventions related to diet/hydration, ambulation, elimination, hygiene, comfort, and attachment with newborn during this stage.

- Discuss initial behaviors which signal positive parent-newborn interaction and early nursing interventions which promote this process.

- List the nursing priorities, in order of priority, during this stage.

- Discuss patient education related to this stage.

- Discuss nursing documentation required during this stage.

*Admission procedures for the newborn should begin during this stage of recovery—please see Newborn Concept 1 for specifics on the admission process.

CONCEPT 7: COMPLICATIONS/SPECIAL SITUATIONS RELATED TO LABOR AND DELIVERY

- State the Birth Center policy for emergency transfer of a laboring patient to Labor and Delivery.

<u>Vaginal Birth after Cesarean (VBAC)</u>

- List contraindications and complications for VBAC.

- Discuss the criteria for trial of labor and nursing assessments necessary for VBAC patients on admission and during labor.

- Outline the protocol for management of VBAC patients, including required procedures and nursing interventions/documentation.

- Identify the s/s of uterine rupture and the appropriate nursing interventions and procedures to be followed.

- Discuss the important points related to patient education in this area.

<u>Premature Rupture of Membranes</u>

- Define PROM and the risk factors associated with PROM.

- Describe s/s of PROM and the nursing assessments necessary for PROM patients on admission and during labor.

- Outline the protocol for management of PROM, including required procedures and nursing interventions/documentation.
- Discuss the important points related to patient education in this area.

Mitral Valve Prolapse

- Define MVP and the risk factors associated with MVP.
- Describe s/s associated with MVP and the nursing assessments necessary for MVP patients on admission and during labor.
- Outline the protocol for management of MVP, including required procedures and nursing interventions/documentation.
- Discuss the important points related to patient education in this area.

Induction/Augmentation of Labor/Artificial Rupture of Membranes

- Define induction.
- Differentiate between medical and surgical induction and between induction and augmentation.
- State the Birth Center policy for management of patients requiring Pitocin induction or augmentation of labor.
- Explain the procedure for assisting with AROM induction.
- Discuss the nursing interventions required after AROM.
- Discuss the important points related to patient education in this area.

Meconium-Stained Amniotic Fluid

- Explain the possible reasons for fetal passage of meconium during labor.
- Discuss the various types/patterns of meconium passage (particulate vs non-particulate) and their significance to neonatal outcome.
- Discuss the protocol for management of meconium during labor, including required procedures and nursing interventions/documentation.
- Discuss the important points related to patient education in this area.

Prolapsed Cord

- Define prolapsed cord—discuss the causes/predisposing factors of a prolapsed cord and the nursing assessments necessary for identifying these risk factors.
- State the s/s of a prolapsed cord—relate the pathophysiology of prolapsed cord to fetal oxygenation.
- Discuss the protocol for management of prolapsed cord, including required procedures and nursing interventions/documentation.
- Discuss the important points related to patient education in this area.

APPENDIX S • INTRAPARTUM CARE

<u>Postpartum Hemorrhage</u>

- Define PPH and identify the causes/predisposing factors for PPH.

- Discuss the s/s of PPH and the nursing assessments necessary for identifying PPH.

- Review the protocol for management of PPH, including required procedures and nursing interventions.

- Discuss the medications Pitocin/Methergine/Ergotrate given to the mother for management of uterine atony following delivery—include mechanisms of action, routes/sites of administration, normal dosage, and side effects/contraindications.

- Discuss the important points related to patient education in this area.

<u>Neonatal Resuscitation</u>

* Please see Newborn Concept 6 for specifics on neonatal resuscitation immediately postdelivery and during the first few days of life.

CONCEPT 8: MEDICATIONS DURING LABOR AND DELIVERY

- State the five rights of medication administration.

- Discuss the nursing policy for administration/documentation of medications.

- Discuss the mechanism of action, route of administration, common dosage parameters and maternal/fetal side effects/contraindications of the following medications:

Amyl Nitrate	Bupivacaine
Ansef/Kefzol	Fentanyl
Gentamicin	Human Immune Globulin
Demerol	Methergine
Nubain	Narcan
Phenergan	Nembutol
Pitocin	Ampicillin
Ergotrate	Lidocaine
Terbutaline	Terbutaline

- Discuss patient education related to medications during labor and delivery.

- Discuss nursing documentation related to medications during labor and delivery.

University of Rochester - Strong Memorial Hospital
OB/GYN Nursing
Orientation/Crosstraining Program
LABOR AND DELIVERY SKILL COMPETENCY/LEARNING SUMMARY

Instructions: Completed by preceptor and learner with date and initials of preceptor in appropriate column. Returned to NM/NL when completed.

Learner: _____ Date: _____

	Reviewed Concept	Applies Concept to Practice	Observed/ Assisted Preceptor	Performs Satisfactorily
ADMISSION				
Admission Data Collection/Procedures				
Review of maternal record for care plan				
Maternal vital signs				
Fetal heart rate				
- fetascope				
- doptone				
- electronic fetal monitor/ external + internal				
Leopold's maneuvers				
- presentation				
- position				
- size				
Assessment/palpation of contractions				
- frequency				
- intensity				
- duration				
Assessment of membrane status				
- Nitrazine test				
Assessment of "show"				
Assessment of edema/reflexes				
Admission Hct				
Urine dipstick/SSA				
Admission vaginal exam				
- station				
- effacement/dilatation				
- presenting part				
Assistance with sterile speculum exam				
Initiation of IV access				
Patient/family orientation to BC				
Admission nursing documentation				
- nursing history				
- labor record				
- triplicates				

APPENDIX S • INTRAPARTUM CARE

	Reviewed Concept	Applies Concept to Practice	Observed/ Assisted Preceptor	Performs Satisfactorily
FIRST STAGE OF LABOR				
Latent Phase				
Assessment of latent phase				
- maternal vital signs				
- fetal heart rate				
- contraction pattern				
- rate of effacement/dilatation				
- rate of descent				
- behavior/sources of discomfort				
Nursing interventions				
- diet/hydration				
- activity				
- elimination				
- hygiene				
- comfort/support				
- family involvement				
Patient education				
Nursing documentation				
Assessment of true vs false labor				
Discharge instructions/Nursing documentation for undelivered patient				
Active/Transition Phase				
Assessment of active phase				
- maternal vital signs				
- fetal heart rate				
- electronic fetal monitor/ external + internal				
- in whirlpool				
- contraction pattern				
- rate of dilatation/descent				
- vaginal exam				
- Friedman graph				
- fluid/hydration status				
- behavior & sources of pain/discomfort				
Nursing interventions				
- (following) SROM				
- hydration				
- activity				
- elimination				
- comfort/support				
- whirlpool				
- psychoprophylaxis				

APPENDIX S • INTRAPARTUM CARE

	Reviewed Concept	Applies Concept to Practice	Observed/ Assisted Preceptor	Performs Satisfactorily
- family support/involvement				
Analgesia/anesthesia				
- IM/IV analgesics				
- epidural anesthesia				
Patient education				
Nursing documentation				
SECOND STAGE OF LABOR OF NEONATE				
Assessment of second stage				
- maternal vital signs				
- fetal heart rate				
- contraction pattern				
- rate of descent				
- behavior/sources of pain				
Nursing interventions				
- breathing/pushing techniques				
- suprapubic/fundal pressure				
- pain relief/support				
- maternal positioning				
- birthing bed				
- family support/involvement				
Preparation for/Assistance with delivery				
- routine set-up of equipment/ supplies/delivery cart				
- spontaneous delivery				
- forceps-assisted delivery				
- vacuum-assisted delivery				
Patient education				
Nursing documentation				
THIRD STAGE OF LABOR OF PLACENTA				
Post-delivery assessment of newborn				
- Apgar score				
- initial newborn vital signs				
- initial newborn screening assessment				
Nursing interventions for newborn stabilization				
- warmth/thermoregulation				
- drying/wrapping techniques				
- skin-to-skin contact				
- radiant warmer				
- maintenance of airway/ suctioning				

APPENDIX S • INTRAPARTUM CARE

	Reviewed Concept	Applies Concept to Practice	Observed/ Assisted Preceptor	Performs Satisfactorily
- bulb				
- De Lee				
- wall				
- identification				
- bands				
- footprint sheet				
- BG chemstrip				
- Vitamin K				
- Erythromycin Ointment				
- cord bloods/cord blood gas				
- parental/newborn bonding				
Maternal assessment				
- placental separation				
Maternal nursing interventions				
- fundal pressure				
- Pitocin				
- examination of placenta/membrane/cord				
- disposal of placenta				
Assistance with perineal repair				
Patient education				
Nursing documentation				
THIRD STAGE OF LABOR/ RECOVERY OF MOTHER				
Maternal assessment				
- maternal vital signs				
- fundus				
- fundal massage				
- lochia				
- perineum				
- fluid/hydration status				
- bladder/voiding status				
Maternal nursing interventions				
- diet/hydration				
- ambulation				
- elimination				
- hygiene				
- perineal cleansing				
- application of belt/pad				
- comfort/pain relief				
- perineal ice packs				
- maternal/newborn bonding				
- family support/involvement				
Patient education				

APPENDIX S • INTRAPARTUM CARE

	Reviewed Concept	Applies Concept to Practice	Observed/ Assisted Preceptor	Performs Satisfactorily
Nursing documentation				
SPECIAL SITUATIONS/COMPLICATIONS				
Emergency transfer to L&D				
Use of NICU hotline				
Vaginal Birth after Cesarean				
Assessment of VBAC patient				
Management/Nursing interventions				
Patient education				
Nursing documentation				
Premature Rupture of Membranes				
Assessment of patient with PROM				
Management/Nursing interventions				
Patient education				
Nursing documentation				
Mitral Valve Prolapse				
Assessment of patient with MVP				
Management/Nursing interventions				
- antibiotics				
Patient education				
Nursing documentation				
Induction/Augmentation of Labor/ Artificial Rupture of Membranes				
• Assessment of need for Pitocin induction/augmentation				
Management/Nursing interventions				
Patient education				
Nursing documentation				
• Assistance with AROM				
Nursing interventions following AROM				
Patient education				
Nursing documentation				
Meconium-Stained Amniotic Fluid				
Assessment of meconium in labor				
Management/Nursing interventions				
Patient education				
Nursing documentation				
Prolapsed Cord				
Assessment/identification of prolapsed cord				
Management/Nursing interventions				
Patient education				

APPENDIX S • INTRAPARTUM CARE

	Reviewed Concept	Applies Concept to Practice	Observed/ Assisted Preceptor	Performs Satisfactorily
Nursing documentation				
Postpartum Hemorrhage				
Assessment/identification of PPH				
Management/Nursing interventions				
- fundal massage				
- Pitocin				
- Methergine				
- Ergotrate				
Patient education				
Nursing documentation				
MEDICATIONS				
Administration responsibilities/five rights				
Patient education				
Nursing documentation				
Common Medications for Labor & Delivery				
Demerol				
Morphine				
Nubain				
Phenergan				
Pitocin				
Methergine				
Ergotrate				

PRECEPTORS

SIGNATURE	INITIALS	SIGNATURE	INITIALS

UNIVERSITY OF ROCHESTER - STRONG MEMORIAL HOSPITAL
OB/GYN NURSING
ORIENTATION/CROSSTRAINING PROGRAM

INTRAPARTUM POST TEST

Return completed tests to: _____ by this date: _____.

INTRAPARTUM CARE

Circle the one best answer.

1. What statement most accurately describes the four stages of normal labor?

    a. Regular uterine contractions, dilatation of the cervical os, birth of the infant and expulsion of the placenta.

    b. Progressive dilatation of the cervix with effacement, full dilatation with delivery of the infant, expulsion of the placenta and one hour adjustment for both mother and infant.

    c. Active phase, transition, delivery and recovery.

    d. Onset of regular contractions, transition, delivery and placental expulsion.

2. Labor consists of each of the four P's **except**:

    a. Presentation
    d. Powers

    b. Personality/Psyche
    e. Passenger

    c. Passage

3. Fetal presentation and position in relationship to the maternal pelvis are described as:

    a. Fetal lie
    d. Both a and b

    b. Attitude
    e. All of the above

    c. Internal rotation

APPENDIX S • INTRAPARTUM CARE

4. Identify the statements that accurately describe uterine activity during normal labor:

   a. Resting tone is assessed during the lowest pressure recorded between contractions.

   b. Intensity refers to the strength of contractions at the peak of uterine activity and occurs in the anterior surface of the uterus.

   c. Interval or frequency of contractions is determined by monitoring the beginning of one contraction to the end of the next contraction.

   d. Both a and b.

   e. All of the above.

5. Initial admission assessment of the laboring woman should include all of the following **except**:

   a. Immediate vaginal exam.

   b. Determination of the presence of bleeding.

   c. Description of the membranes as intact or ruptured.

   d. Vital signs and determination of the fetal heart rate.

6. A laboring woman is lying in the supine position. The **most** appropriate nursing action is to:

   a. Ask her to turn to one side.

   b. Elevate her feet and legs.

   c. Take her blood pressure.

   d. Determine if there is fetal tachycardia.

7. All of the following statements are true about failure to progress in labor (FTP), **except**:

   a. Leopold's maneuvers should be utilized to readjust fetal positioning.

   b. Primary management of FTP is prevention.

   c. Nursing interventions include providing adequate fluids/nutrition and facilitating position changes and ambulation.

   d. Friedman's curve should be reviewed to determine the progress and pattern of labor.

8. In obvious umbilical cord prolapse, where the cord is visible at the introitus, the nurse is expected to:

   a. Place the patient in Trendelenburg position and administer oxygen.

   b. Elevate the presenting part off the pelvis with a sterile gloved hand.

   c. Check the FHR, either by feeling pulsations in the cord or by continuous electronic fetal monitoring.

   d. Contact the physician and if the woman is in early labor, prepare for cesarean delivery.

   c. Both a and c.

   d. All of the above.

9. Identify the statement that accurately describes premature rupture of membranes (PROM):

   a. Prolonged PROM refers to any rupture of the membranes that occurs prior to term gestation.

   b. PROM is spontaneous rupture of the membranes prior to the onset of labor and is sometimes associated with intrauterine or cervical infections.

   c. Amniotic fluid obtained during speculum exam will appear in a typical ferning pattern under microscopic exam and will test as an acid with nitrazine paper in PROM.

   d. Both a and c.

   e. All of the above.

APPENDIX S • INTRAPARTUM CARE

10. Which one of the following findings suggest transition to the second stage of labor?

    a. Decreased urge to push.

    b. Decreased bloody show.

    c. FHR accelerations.

    d. Bulging of the perineum.

11. Which of the following signs indicates that delivery is imminent?

    a. The mother has the desire to defecate.

    b. An increase in frequency, duration and intensity of uterine contractions.

    c. The patient begins to bear down spontaneously with uterine contractions.

    d. Bulging of the perineum occurs.

    e. An increase in the amount of vaginal blood-stained mucous.

    f. a, c, d.

    g. All of the above.

12. Examples of nursing problems/diagnoses during the first and second stages of labor include:

    a. Fluid volume deficit related to nausea and vomiting and increased metabolic demands of labor.

    b. Potential injury and/or tissue trauma related to fetal descent or rapid delivery.

    c. Potential for postpartum hemorrhage due to hypotonic uterus and/or lacerations.

    d. Both a and b.

    e. All of the above.

Mark the following statements as true or false.

13. ___ The FHR must be assessed after every push and documented q 5 minutes in the labor record.

    ___ Mechanisms of delivery include delivery of the head, shoulders, body and extremities.

    ___ Engagement occurs when the largest diameter of the fetal head enters the plane of the inlet, generally at 0 station.

    ___ Floating, or ballottable means the presenting part is loosely fixed near the pelvic inlet at - 1 station.

    ___ Mechanisms of labor include: engagement, descent, flexion, internal rotation, extension, restitution, external rotation and expulsion.

Complete the following.

14. When doing Leopold's maneuvers on a labor patient, you feel a firm, rounded object in the uterine fundus; a smooth surface along the right side of the uterus (mother's right side); a surface that feels more nodular on the left side of the uterus; and a body part that is rounded and even more firm just above the symphysis. The fetal presentation is _____ and the fetal position is _____.

15. State the intrapartum routine for VS and assessments on the OB Service:

    a. on admission _____

    b. first stage/latent _____

    c. first stage/early active _____

    d. first stage/active _____

    e. second stage _____

APPENDIX S • INTRAPARTUM CARE

NAME:_____

UNIVERSITY OF ROCHESTER - STRONG MEMORIAL HOSPITAL
OB/GYN NURSING
ORIENTATION/CROSSTRAINING PROGRAM

INTRAPARTUM STUDY GUIDE

This study guide includes key points in intrapartum nursing and requires the learner to complete answers to various topics. Please complete and return to: _____ by this date: _____.

OBJECTIVES: After completing this guide, the learner will be able to:

1. Define the stages of labor.

2. Outline the four "P" components of labor.

3. Describe the mechanisms of labor.

4. Outline the nursing admission history and physical exam of the laboring woman.

5. Demonstrate Leopold's maneuvers.

6. Compare characteristics of true and false labor.

7. List three common nursing diagnoses for the woman in labor and two nursing interventions for each.

8. Describe two methods of assessing failure to progress.

9. Describe two symptoms of prolapsed cord and the primary nursing responsibility associated with this complication.

10. Describe diagnostic criteria for PROM and medical management.

11. Differentiate the critical elements of nursing documentation for the intrapartum patient.

12. State the routine for intrapartum vital signs and assessments on the OB Service.

*NOTE: **Fetal monitoring information is covered through the Fetal Monitoring Education Program for OB/GYN Nursing.**

RESOURCES: AWHONN Crosstraining Videotape on Intrapartum Assessment/Care
OB/GYN Nursing Intrapartum Learning Module
Obstetric Vital Signs/Assessment Guide (card)

*NOTE: Most of the information in this guide is taken from the video - other references are cited where appropriate.

APPENDIX S • INTRAPARTUM CARE

I. STAGES OF LABOR

    A. First Stage -> begins with onset of _____ uterine contractions, accompanied by _____ dilation of the cervical os, until _____ dilation of the cervix is achieved.

        1) The first stage is divided into 2 phases:

            a) _____ phase, characterized by progressive _____ with _____ change in dilation or descent
            b) _____ phase, characterized by more rapid _____ and _____ of the presenting part

        2) The end of the active phase is called _____, characterized by _____ intensity and duration of contractions and _____ intervals of contractions. During this time, the patient exhibits _____, _____, and _____.

        3) Duration of the first stage:

            a) in primips, is _____ hours
            b) in multips, is _____ hours.

    B. Second stage -> is the period from _____ dilation of the cervical os to _____.

        1) Duration of the second stage:

            a) in primips, is _____
            b) in multips, is _____.

    C. Third stage -> is the period between _____ and _____.

        1) In the majority of patients, the third stage lasts _____.

    D. Fourth stage -> begins with delivery of the _____ and lasts for _____ as the mother's body functions begin to stabilize. Dramatic and rapid _____ occurs as the _____ contracts to prevent rapid/excessive _____.

NOTES:

APPENDIX S • INTRAPARTUM CARE

II. P'S OF LABOR

1. _____
2. _____
3. _____
4. _____

A. Passage -> is the mother's bony _____.

1) The bony pelvis is divided into the _____ and _____ pelvis by the iliopectineal line.

   a) The false pelvis _____ the pregnant uterus.
   b) The _____ and _____ of the true pelvis determine its adequacy for delivery.
   c) The true pelvis is divided into the _____, _____, and _____.
   d) The route through the true pelvis is in the shape of _____ _____.

2) The diameters of the pelvis are important to determine adequacy for delivery. These are called _____.

Pelvic inlet:

   a) The transverse diameter of the pelvic inlet is approximately 13.5 cm side to side at the widest point of the iliopectineal line.
   b) The anterior-posterior diameter of the pelvic inlet measures approximately 11 cm, from the upper inner border of the symphysis pubis to the sacrum.

Midpelvis:

   a) The midpelvis is the area between the inlet and the outlet.
   b) The transverse diameter of the midpelvis is approximately 11 cm and measures the distance between the ischial spines.
   c) The anterior-posterior diameter of the midpelvis is approximately 13 cm and is measured from the 4th and 5th sacral vertebral junction to the lower border of the symphysis pubis.

Pelvic outlet:

a) The anterior-posterior diameter of the outlet is measured from the inferior margin of the symphysis pubis to the sacrococcygeal joint and measures approximately 11.5 cm.
b) The transverse diameter is the distance between the ischial tuberosities and measures approximately 11 cm.

3) The pelvic soft tissues also assist with delivery of the fetus and placenta.

a) The pelvic _____ is connective tissue which fills in the space between the pelvic organs and forms _____ which support the uterus.
b) The _____ muscles are the deep muscle group of the pelvis and form a muscular _____ that provides major strength to the pelvic floor.
c) The superficial perineal muscles act as sphincter around the _____ and _____.
d) The _____ lies between the vaginal opening and the anal canal providing a point of insertion for the deep and superficial muscles and assisting in childbirth.

B. Passenger(s) -> are the _____ and the _____.

1) Overlapping of bones of the fetal skull to diminish its size and allow passage of the fetal head through the pelvis during labor is called _____.

2) The membranous spaces between the bones of the fetal skull are called _____.

3) The intersections of these sutures are called _____.

4) Suture lines and bones of the fetal skull are used to determine _____ and are defined as:

a) _____ - brow area
b) _____ - area between anterior and posterior fontanelles
c) _____ - area behind posterior fontanel
d) _____ - chin area

5) The anterior fontanel is a large diamond-shaped area at the intersection of the _____ and _____ sutures.

APPENDIX S • INTRAPARTUM CARE

6) The _____ fontanel is triangular shaped and lies at the intersection of the _____ and _____ sutures.

7) The _____ suture unites the parietal bones and runs between the fontanelles.

8) The diameters of the fetal skull vary with flexion and range from _____ to _____.

There are several ways by which the relationship of the fetus to the pelvis is defined.

1) The _____ is the relationship of the long axis of the fetus to maternal anatomy.

   a) _____ lie occurs in the majority of cases and occurs when the long axis of the fetus is parallel to the maternal spine.
   b) Transverse lie occurs when the long axis of the fetus lies _____ _____ the maternal spine.

2) _____ is the relationship of fetal parts to one another.

   a) _____ - chin on chest, back curved, extremities folded over
   b) _____ - head bent backwards, chest and abdomen arched
   c) _____ - neither flexion nor extension, head straight
   d) _____ - moderate extension of the head

3) _____ is that part of the fetus entering the pelvis first.

   a) _____ - occurs in the majority of cases, usually term
   b) _____ - occurs in a small minority, usually premature
   c) _____ - very infrequent

4) _____ is the relationship of the presenting part to the pelvis. Fetal landmarks are used to describe fetal position in relation to the patient's right or left side and anterior, posterior or transverse of pelvis.

   a) _____ is the landmark for vertex presentation
   b) _____ is the landmark for face presentation
   c) _____ is the landmark for breech presentation
   d) _____ is the landmark for shoulder presentation

The mechanisms of labor are a set of passive adaptive movements by which the fetus is delivered.

1) _____ occurs when the widest diameter of the fetal head passes through the pelvic inlet.

   a) _____ is the relationship of the presenting part to an imaginary line drawn between the ischial spines = 0 station, with a range of -1 to -5 to +1 to +5

   b) engagement is complete when the fetal head is at _____ station

2) _____ is the downward passage of the presenting part.

   a) _____ -> presenting part is freely moveable above the pelvic inlet or above -3 station

   b) fixed -> presenting part has entered the pelvis but is not quite engaged (note: this term is not usually used on the OB Service)

3) Flexion allows the fetus to present the smallest diameter of fetal head to the pelvis.

4) Internal rotation brings the anterior-posterior diameter of the fetal head in line with the anterior-posterior diameter of the pelvis.

5) Extension allows the fetal head to move beneath the symphysis pubis. Delivery of the head occurs with full extension.

6) Restitution and external rotation occur after delivery of the head as the head rotates 45 degrees to straighten and then another 45 degrees to align with the anterior-posterior diameter of the pelvis.

7) Expulsion is the delivery of the rest of the body.

C. Powers

1) Involuntary powers are _____ whose intensity is greatest in _____ surface of the uterus.

   a) resting tone or _____ is the lowest pressure recorded between contractions

   b) uterine activity may be measured _____ by an IUPC or externally by a _____ or _____

   c) intensity of contractions is described as:

   i _____ - easily indented, like chin

   ii _____ - only indented with firm pressure at peak, like nose

   iii _____ - cannot be indented, like brow

APPENDIX S • INTRAPARTUM CARE

        d)   interval of contractions = _____ of one contraction to _____ of next

        e)   duration of contractions = beginning of _____ to _____

2)   Voluntary powers are muscles of _____, _____, and _____. Their activity enhances involuntary powers through breathing and relaxation exercises and by pushing the fetus out.

D.   Personality/Psyche -> woman's response to labor and her ability to cope. It is influenced by many things including (name 6):

    1) _____
    2) _____
    3) _____
    4) _____
    5) _____
    6) _____

NOTES:

III.   ADMISSION ASSESSMENT FOR LABOR

    A.   Admission history should include (name 11):

        1) _____
        2) _____
        3) _____
        4) _____
        5) _____
        6) _____
        7) _____
        8) _____
        9) _____
        10) _____
        11) _____

APPENDIX S • INTRAPARTUM CARE

B. True vs false labor - onset of labor generally occurs between _____ weeks before and _____ weeks after the EDC.

List the differences between true and false labor below:

	true labor	false labor
contractions		
show		
intensity of contractions		
duration of contractions		
effect of walking		
cervical changes		

C. Admission Physical Exam - should include the following steps:

1) check VS and assess general level of anxiety
2) inspect abdomen to evaluate _____ and _____
3) determine fetal position by using _____
   a) identify the fetal part that occupies the fundus
   b) locate the fetal back and small parts
   c) determine which fetal part is presenting to the pelvic inlet
   d) outline the fetal head to determine position
4) check the FHR
5) assess lower extremities for _____ and _____
   - evaluate the DTR for _____.
6) perform a vaginal exam if there is no PTL with PROM - evaluate _____, _____, _____, _____ and _____.

NOTES:

APPENDIX S • INTRAPARTUM CARE

List the routine for VS and assessments during labor (note: please refer to the Obstetric VS/Assessment Guide for this piece:

1) on admission _____
2) first stage/latent _____
3) first stage/early active _____
4) first stage/active _____
5) second stage _____

NOTES:

IV. **NURSING PROBLEMS/DIAGNOSES AND INTERVENTIONS**

    A. Potential for infection

       Interventions include:

       1) monitor maternal BP and pulse q _____ unless elevated
       2) monitor temp q _____ until ROM, then q _____
       3) monitor FHR for rising baseline
       4) assess the uterus for tenderness
       5) assess odor of amniotic fluid

    B. Potential for increased fetal stress r/t decreased uteroplacental perfusion

       Interventions include:

       1) assess fetal well being by monitoring the FHR
          a) by intermittent auscultation (note: per AWHONN recommendations - see attached sheet)
          b) by continuous electronic fetal monitoring - evaluate a FM strip q _____ during the first stage, then q _____ during transition and second stage

       2) treat fetal distress <u>immediately</u> by:
          a) changing maternal position, side to side
          b) starting oxygen at 10 L/min via tightly fitted face mask
          c) starting/increasing IV fluid administration
          d) discontinuing pitocin
          e) notifying physician

C. Potential for injury r/t tissue trauma d/t rapid fetal descent, premature pushing or rapid delivery

Interventions include:

1) assess labor progress and maternal response q _____
2) assist patient in voiding q _____
3) confirm complete _____ before the patient pushes
4) support and facilitate pushing efforts

D. Potential for PPH d/t hypotonic uterus or lacerations

Interventions (during the 4th stage) include:

1) check uterine tone and massage uterus q _____ for first hour post delivery - assess amount of free flow and/or clots expressed
2) monitor BP and pulse q _____ during recovery

E. Fluid volume deficit r/t nausea and vomiting and increased metabolic demands of labor

Interventions include:

1) maintain adequate _____ with oral or IV fluids
2) measure I&O q _____
3) check urine for _____ q _____

F. Anxiety/fear r/t birthing process

Interventions include:

1) ensure the patient understands the purpose of _____ _____
2) involve _____ in care as desired
3) keep the patient and significant other updated regarding _____ _____ and _____.

G. Pain and discomfort r/t labor

Interventions include:

1) support and encourage the patient in her choice and use of _____ _____

APPENDIX S • INTRAPARTUM CARE

2) assist with comfort measures, such as (name at least 4-5):
_____
_____
_____
_____

3) administer _____ as the patient desires and as the physician orders
4) facilitate regional _____
5) monitor the patient's _____ to pain control measures.

NOTES:

V. COMPLICATIONS

A. Failure to Progress (FTP) -> alteration in the normal pattern of labor - the progress of labor is usually plotted on a graph/labor curve (Friedman curve)

Lack of progress is reflected in:

1) alterations in the character of _____
2) effacement and _____
3) _____ and expulsion of the fetus.

Fetal descent occurs at the rate of:

1) _____ cm/hr in the nullipara
2) _____ cm/hr in the multipara

Cervical dilation occurs at the rate of:

1) _____ cm/hr in the nullipara
2) _____ cm/hr in the multipara

Intensity, duration and intervals of contractions progress in a coordinated manner.

APPENDIX S • INTRAPARTUM CARE

Types/causes of FTP

1) presenting part advances _____ cm/hr - most common type
2) dilation progresses _____ cm/hr - in secondary arrest, the cervix remains unchanged for _____ during the active phase of labor or after complete _____
3) prolonged latent phase d/t hypertonic or discoordinate _____ _____ - this occurs with a 20 hour or > phase in the nullipara and a 14 hour or > phase in the multipara - it responds to analgesia-induced rest with interruption of the _____ _____
4) CPD - occurs in 50%
5) excessive sedation
6) fetal malposition or _____
7) multiple gestation.

The primary management of FTP is _____.

Nursing interventions include:

1) adequate _____ and _____ to maintain energy, hydration and fluid & electrolyte balance
2) position changes and _____

Medical management includes:

1) determining the cause
2) r/o CPD, then....
3) AROM, if the membranes are intact and the presenting part is engaged
4) _____ to augment
5) assisted delivery with _____, _____, or _____.

B. Prolapsed Cord -> cord protrudes ahead of the presenting part - occurs in 1:400 deliveries.

Occult cord -> cord lies alongside the fetus - it may be palpable but not visible - the EFM pattern shows a characteristic pattern with occult cord.

Etiology -> ill-fitting present part - a long cord also adds to the risk.

Diagnosis -> the cord is felt or seen at the _____ or there is _____ unresponsive to maternal position changes, O2 or fluids.

APPENDIX S • INTRAPARTUM CARE

Interventions include:

1) place the patient in _____ or _____ position
2) perform a _____ to lift the presenting part off the cord manually
3) determine fetal status by feeling pulsations in the cord or by continuous electronic fetal monitoring
4) if the cord is located outside the vagina, keep it _____ and _____
5) administer O2
6) a C/S is done if the patient is in the first stage of labor or in the second stage if delivery is not imminent.

C. Premature Rupture of Membranes (PROM) -> spontaneous rupture of membranes (SROM) prior to the onset of labor - it may be a normal variant or d/t some pathology - it occurs in 10% of patients.

<u>Prolonged PROM</u> -> rupture of membranes greater than 24 hours

<u>Preterm PROM</u> -> rupture of membranes before term

Etiology -> unknown, although many cases are associated with intrauterine or cervical infection, especially preterm PROM - with term pregnancies, the risk for infection increases the longer the patient is not in labor; with preterm pregnancies, this relationship doesn't hold.

Diagnosis is made by:

1) examination of the fluid under a microscopic -> if membranes are ruptured, you will see a _____ pattern typical of amniotic fluid
2) nitrazine paper test -> if the paper turns from orange to bright blue on exposure to fluid, this is indicative of the alkaline pH of amniotic fluid.

Medical management is dictated by gestational age, chorioamnionitis, fetal distress and status of labor. It includes:

1) hospitalization for evaluation
2) if 36 weeks or > gestation, delivery is the goal, either spontaneous or induced

APPENDIX S • INTRAPARTUM CARE

3) if < 36 weeks gestation, PROM is managed expectantly -> the patient is monitored for signs of infection, such as (name 3-4):

_____
_____
_____
_____

COMPLETE AND ACCURATE DOCUMENTATION IS CRUCIAL TO ASSURE THAT APPROPRIATE AND TIMELY INTERVENTIONS HAVE BEEN INITIATED FOR THE LABORING WOMAN.

NOTES:

Recommended Procedure for FHR Auscultation

- Palpate the maternal abdomen to identify fetal presentation and position (Leopold's maneuvers).

- Place the bell of fetoscope or Doppler over the area of maximum intensity of fetal heart sounds (usually over the fetal back).

- Place a finger on mother's radial pulse to differentiate maternal from fetal heart rate.

- Palpate for uterine contractions during auscultation to clarify relationship between FHR and uterine contractions.

- Count FHR during a uterine contraction for 30 seconds thereafter to identify fetal response.

- Count FHR between uterine contractions for at least 30-60 seconds to identify average baseline rate.

- If distinct differences are noted between counts, recounts for longer periods are appropriate to clarify the presence and possible nature of FHR changes, for example abrupt or gradual.

- In clarifying accelerations, recounts for multiple brief periods of 5-10 seconds may be particularly helpful.

(NAACOG, 1990)

NEWBORN CONCEPTS

CONCEPT 1: ADMISSION OF THE NEWBORN

- Discuss normal newborn adaptation to extrauterine life—respiratory, cardiovascular, hepatic, gastrointestinal, renal, neurologic, endocrine/metabolic, immunologic, hematopoetic and behavioral. Explain what findings you will observe in the newborn as a result of these adaptations.

- State the procedure involved in the following:
  - BC transfer to NICU
  - NICU transfer to BC
  - BC transfer to NBN
  - NBN transfer to BC
  - L&D transfer to BC

Admission Data Collection

- Identify pertinent facts from the maternal prenatal record, nursing history and labor and delivery record, which must be considered in planning newborn care. Explain the significance of each to newborn outcomes.

Admission Assessment/Procedures

- List the key assessments/procedures involved in admission of the newborn.

*Please see Concept 2 for specifics on assessment procedures.

- List the indications and explain the appropriate procedure for obtaining a BG chemstrip during the admission period. State the normal range of results and appropriate interventions for abnormal results.

- State the criteria for evaluating a newborn's readiness for an admission bath. Describe the procedure for completing an admission bath and for rewarming the newborn after a bath.

- Discuss use of the radiant warmer during the admission process.

- Discuss the rationale and appropriate procedure for applying triple dye to the cord.

- State the Birth Center policy for initiating feeding, including criteria for evaluating a newborn's readiness to eat.

- Discuss those situations seen during the admission period, which necessitate notification of the Pediatric House Officer and/or transfer of the newborn to NBN or NICU.

- Discuss the procedure for identifying and obtaining pediatric coverage by SMH, by OOT attending, and by private attending.

- Discuss parental education related to admission of the newborn.

- Discuss nursing documentation related to admission of the newborn.

CONCEPT 2: NEWBORN ASSESSMENT (VITAL SIGNS/PHYSICAL ASSESSMENTS)

- State the Birth Center policy for assessing and recording newborn vital signs during the first 6 hours after birth and then routinely during the hospital stay.
- Identify those factors which must be included in the admission physical assessment examination of the newborn. Compare this with what must be included in a routine daily assessment of the newborn.

Vital Signs

- Discuss the appropriate procedure for obtaining a temperature (rectal and axillary), heart rate, respiratory rate and blood pressure on the newborn—state the method of choice for obtaining a temperature on newborns.
- State the normal parameters for newborn vital signs and contrast what is seen in the first few hours after birth with what is seen thereafter.
- Define and discuss the significance of tachypnea/TTN, tachycardia/bradycardia, hypothermia/hyperthermia.

Weight/Measurements

- Discuss the appropriate procedure for obtaining weight, length, and head/chest/abdomen circumferences in the newborn.
- State the normal parameters for newborn weight and measurements and discuss changes in readings normally seen in the early newborn period.
- Describe the appropriate method for converting grams and centimeters to pounds and inches. State when each system of measurement should be used.
- Define and discuss the significance of abnormal weight loss, rapidly increasing head/abdominal circumferences.

Skin

- List what factors must be included in nursing assessment of newborn skin.
- Discuss the appropriate technique for assessing newborn skin.
- Discuss the normal appearance of newborn skin, as well as common variations.
- Define and discuss the significance of vernix, lanugo, pallor/plethora, jaundice, acrocyanosis/circumoral cyanosis/cyanosis, telangiectasis, erythema neonatorum ("newborn rash"), Mongolian spots, vesicles/pustules/petichiae, ecchymoses, hemangiomas ("strawberry mark").

Head

- List what factors must be included in nursing assessment of newborn head.
- Discuss the proper technique for examining the newborn head.
- Discuss the normal appearance of the newborn head, as well as common variations.
- Define fontanel—describe the size, shape and location of anterior and posterior fontanelles.

- Define suture—identify the location of frontal, coronal, sagittal and lambdoidal sutures. Discuss overlapping vs widely spaced sutures.

- Define molding. Compare and contrast the cause, timing, characteristics and complications of caput succedaneum vs cephalhematoma.

- Define and discuss the significance of hydrocephaly/microcephaly/anencephaly.

Face

- List what factors must be included in nursing assessment of newborn face.

- Discuss the proper technique for assessing the newborn eyes, ears, nose, and mouth.

- Discuss the normal appearance of these structures, as well as common variations.

- Define and discuss the significance of short/tight frenulum (r/t "tongue-tied"), epicanthal folds, nasal flaring, subconjunctival hemorrhage, strabismus/nystagmus, preauricular tags, Epstein's pearls, thrush, red reflex, cleft lip/palate, choanal atresia.

- Discuss newborn capabilities related to sight, hearing, smell and taste.

Chest/Neck

- List what factors must be included in nursing assessment of newborn neck and chest.

- Explain the proper technique for assessing newborn neck and chest.

- Discuss the normal appearance of these structures, as well as common variations.

- Define and discuss the significance of "webbed neck," torticollis, opisthotonos, "witch's milk," supernumerary nipple, see-saw respirations/retractions/grunting, rales/rhonchi, barrel chest, funnel chest, fx clavicle, "heart murmur."

Abdomen

- List what factors must be included in nursing assessment of newborn abdomen. Discuss the proper technique for assessing newborn abdomen.

- Discuss the normal appearance of newborn abdomen, as well as common variations.

- Define and discuss the significance of linea nigra, Wharton's jelly, umbilical/diaphragmatic/inguinal hernia, omphalocele, gastroschisis, scaphoid abdomen.

Back/Buttocks

- List what factors must be included in nursing assessment of newborn back and buttocks.

- Discuss the proper technique for assessing newborn back and buttocks.

- Discuss the normal appearance of newborn back and buttocks, as well as common variations.

- Identify and discuss the significance of pilonidal dimple/sinus, imperforate anus, anal fissure, meningocele/meningomyelocele, spina bifida.

Extremities

- List what factors must be included in nursing assessment of newborn extremities. Discuss the proper technique for assessing newborn hips, legs/feet/toes, arms/hands/fingers.
- Describe the normal appearance of these structures, as well as common variations.
- Define and discuss the significance of hip click, polydactyly/syndactyly, Simian crease, clubfoot (talipes equinovarus or calcanus).

Genitalia

- List what factors must be included in nursing assessment of newborn genitalia and the proper technique involved.
- Describe the normal appearance of these structures, as well as common variations.
- Define and discuss the significance of hypospadias/epispadias, ambiguous genitalia, pseudomenstruation, phimosis, hydrocele, vaginal tag, imperforate anus.

Reflexes

- Discuss the following reflexes, including the method to elicit the reflex, a description of normal response, and normal duration of the reflex: Moro response, startle reflex, rooting reflex, sucking reflex, palmar grasp, plantar grasp, Babinski reflex.
- Differentiate between newborn jitters, seizures, and a vigorous startle reflex.

Behavior

- Discuss the predictable behavior patterns seen in newborns called periods of reactivity.
- List and define the sleep/awake states seen in newborns.

Gestational Age

- Discuss the use of the Ballard and Dubowitz exams as assessment tools for determining gestational age, per Birth Center policy. List the components of each exam and the appropriate techniques involved in performing the exams.
- Define AGA/SGA/LGA and premature/term/postmature gestation.
- Discuss the appropriate method for assigning these classifications based on use of the Lubchenco graph.
- Discuss parental education related to assessment of the newborn.
- Discuss nursing documentation related to assessment of the newborn.

APPENDIX T • NEWBORN CARE

CONCEPT 3: NEWBORN NUTRITION/HYDRATION/FEEDING

- State the daily caloric and fluid requirements for a newborn.
- Identify the best indicators of hydration in the newborn.
- Relate mother's hydration status to baby's hydration status in the breastfed newborn.
- Discuss the s/s of dehydration and appropriate nursing interventions.
- Explain the proper procedure for weighing diapers and doing a urine specific gravity with a spectrometer. Relate results of these procedures to assessment of fluid status in the newborn.
- State the minimal number of wet diapers/24hrs. which indicates adequate hydration.
- State the percent of body weight loss from birth weight normally seen in the first few days of life. State when the newborn can normally be expected to regain birth weight.
- Describe newborn s/s of hunger.
- Relate feeding pattern to the presence of mucous.
- Describe the difference between regurgitating, bubbling, and vomiting/projectile vomiting and discuss necessary nursing interventions.
- Review the advantages and disadvantages of breastfeeding and bottlefeeding. Discuss factors which may influence parents' choice of feeding method.

Breastfeeding

- Briefly review the anatomy of the breast and the neurohormonal physiology of milk production.
- Define colostrum and discuss the importance of colostrum.
- Explain the phenomenon of supply and demand.
- Define "on demand" feeding schedule, including the recommended frequency and duration of feedings over the first few days of life, and the recommendations for night feedings.
- Discuss breastfeeding techniques, including various holds that may be used.
- Discuss breastfeeding aides, especially nipple shells, nipple shields and hand/electric breast pumps. Explain indications and contraindications for their use.
- Explain the proper technique for breast massage and hand expression of milk. Discuss when hand expression vs use of breast pump is appropriate.
- Define the following types of breastfeeding babies:
  - barracudas
  - excited ineffectives
  - procrastinators
  - gourmets
  - resters.
- Define "newborn who refuses to nurse" and discuss nursing strategies for managing this situation.

- Discuss supplementation with breastfeeding, including indications/contraindications for its use.
- Identify situations when it may be necessary to store breast milk. Outline nursing interventions related to collecting, storing and reheating milk.

Bottlefeeding

- Identify different types/brands of formula and discuss the advantages and disadvantages of each.
- Discuss when soy formula is used and the rationale.
- Define "on demand" feeding schedule, including the recommended frequency and amount of feeding over the first few days of life and the recommendations for night feedings.
- Discuss the appropriate technique for bottlefeeding a newborn, including positions for burping.
- Discuss parental education related to newborn nutrition/hydration/feeding. Discuss nursing documentation related to newborn nutrition/hydration/feeding.

CONCEPT 4: NEWBORN ELIMINATION

- Describe the normal variations in newborn voiding patterns—state the timeframe for expecting a first void and nursing interventions if this does not occur.
- Describe uric acid crystals and discuss their significance.
- Describe the normal variations in newborn stooling patterns—define and differentiate among the following type of stools: meconium plug, meconium, transitional, mature, breast vs bottle, bili stools.
- Identify causes and s/s of "bellyache"/abdominal distention and discuss nursing interventions for its relief.
- Define newborn diarrhea, state possible causes, and discuss nursing interventions for its relief.
- List reasons for bloody stools and discuss appropriate nursing interventions.
- Discuss parental education related to newborn elimination.
- Discuss nursing documentation related to newborn elimination.

CONCEPT 5: NEWBORN HYGIENE/SAFETY/SECURITY

Bathing/Dressing

- Discuss the daily bathing needs of the newborn in the first few days of life—contrast this with the admission bath.
- Review the appropriate procedure for bathing an infant at home.
- Discuss the techniques for swaddling and diapering a newborn.

Cord

- Describe care of the cord during hospitalization and at home.
- List s/s of wet/infected cord and discuss appropriate nursing interventions.
- Review the appropriate technique for removing a cord clamp.

Genitalia

- Discuss hygiene for female genitalia and for circumcised/uncircumcised male genitalia.
- Review the procedure for performing a circumcision.
- Discuss nursing interventions related to preparing for and assisting with a circumcision, including those instances when Lidocaine is used as a local anesthetic.
- List the contraindications for circumcision.
- Describe the special procedures related to a ritual circumcision.
- Discuss complications of circumcisions and appropriate nursing interventions.
- Describe diaper rash, identify possible causes and discuss nursing interventions for its relief.

Safety/Security

- Discuss newborn safety and security during hospitalization, especially related to OB/GYN policies for rooming-in, use of the holding nursery, interactions with siblings/visitors/family, and identification/release of the newborn to appropriate individuals.
- Discuss parental education related to newborn hygiene/safety.
- Discuss nursing documentation related to newborn hygiene/safety.

CONCEPT 6: NEWBORN COMPLICATIONS/SPECIAL SITUATIONS

- Discuss use of the newborn emergency cart and equipment. **This must be reviewed and signed off on skills checklist.**

Neonatal Emergencies/Resuscitation

- Identify the s/s of distress seen in the neonate immediately post delivery, which signal a need for support/resuscitation, and the nursing assessments which help in identifying this need.
- List the procedures and nursing interventions which should occur initially before or while calling NICU. Discuss the rationale and any technique involved for each.
- Review the techniques for performing CPR on the newborn.
- State the appropriate procedure for utilizing the NICU hotline/communicating with NICU in emergent situations.
- List the medications/supplies/equipment which may be needed during neonatal resuscitation.

- Discuss the protocol for a neonatal resuscitation—include procedures utilized and the rationale and sequence of procedures, as well as nursing interventions/documentation and the role of the BC nursing staff vs NICU nursing staff.
- Discuss the medication Narcan given to the newborn as a narcotic antagonist following delivery—include mechanism of action, route/site of administration, normal dosage, and side effects/contraindications.
- Discuss important points related to parental support/education in this area.

Hypothermia/Hyperthermia

- Identify normal range of temperature for the newborn.
- Discuss the process of thermoregulation in the newborn.
- Identify the four major mechanisms of heat loss and the environmental factors which contribute to them.
- Define hypothermia vs hyperthermia.
- Discuss possible causes, s/s and newborn responses to hypothermia.
- Outline the protocol for management of hypothermia, including required procedures and nursing interventions/documentation. Discuss use of the Isolette and radiant warmer for the management of hypothermia.
- Discuss possible causes, s/s and newborn responses to hyperthermia. Outline the protocol for management of hyperthermia, including required procedures and nursing interventions/documentation.
- Discuss the important points related to parental education in this area.

Hypoglycemia

- Identify the normal serum glucose level for newborns.
- Define hypoglycemia.
- Discuss the maternal and neonatal risk factors for hypoglycemia—relate hypoglycemia to IDM, SGA/LGA and preterm/postmature newborns.
- Explain the relationship between hypothermia and hypoglycemia.
- List s/s of hypoglycemia.
- Outline the protocol for management of hypoglycemia, including required procedures and nursing interventions/documentation.
- Discuss the important points related to parental education in this area.

Polycythemia/Anemia

- State the normal range of Hct seen in the newborn:
- Define polycythemia and anemia.

APPENDIX T • NEWBORN CARE

- Discuss the maternal and neonatal risk factors for polycythemia and anemia.
- Discuss the s/s of anemia and polycythemia and potential complications associated with both conditions.
- State the OB/GYN policy for hematocrits in newborns, including protocol for management of low and high hematocrits, indications for draw and required nursing interventions/documentation.
- Discuss the important points related to parental education in this area.

Prematurity/Postmaturity

- Identify the normal gestational range.
- Define prematurity vs postmaturity and describe the characteristic appearance of both.
- Differentiate between prematurity, SGA and IUGR.
- Discuss the impact of prematurity on vital signs/temperature, blood glucose, and feeding behaviors.
- Outline the protocol for management of the premature infant, including required procedures and nursing interventions/documentation.
- Discuss the impact of postmaturity on vital signs/temperature, blood glucose, and feeding behaviors.
- Outline the protocol for management of the postmature infant, including required procedures and nursing interventions/documentation.
- Discuss the important points related to parental education in this area.

LGA/IDM/SGA/IUGR

- Define LGA and SGA, referring to use of the Lubchenco graph used to determine these classifications.
- Discuss the impact of an SGA and LGA classification on vital signs/temperature, blood glucose and feeding behaviors.
- Discuss the protocol for management of an SGA and LGA newborn, including required procedures and nursing interventions/documentation.
- Define IDM and differentiate this term from LGA. Discuss the protocol for management of an IDM, including required procedures and nursing interventions/documentation.
- Define IUGR and differentiate this term from SGA and prematurity. Discuss the protocol for management of the IUGR infant, including required procedures and nursing interventions/documentation.
- Discuss the important points related to parental education in this area.

Hyperbilirubinemia (Jaundice)

- Define jaundice.
- List the risk factors which may predispose a newborn to jaundice. Differentiate between physiologic jaundice, pathologic jaundice, and breastmilk/breastfeeding jaundice, in terms of etiology, onset, and anticipated course/bilirubin levels.

- Define kernicterus.
- Explain the physiology of bilirubin conjugation and how this process is altered in a newborn with jaundice.
- Describe the signs of jaundice in progressive order.
- Discuss the appropriate method of assessing jaundice in the newborn and differentiate methods of assessment for fair-skinned vs dark-skinned newborns. List important factors to be considered when assessing for jaundice.
- Define total, direct and indirect bilirubin and describe the relationship among these three lab values.
- Outline the protocol for management of neonatal jaundice, including required procedures and nursing interventions/documentation.
- Review the protocol for use of phototherapy in the treatment of hyperbilirubinemia, including required procedures, nursing interventions/documentation, mechanism of effect and potential complications.
- Discuss the important points related to parental education in this area and list the informational resources available to parents.

Sepsis

- Discuss neonatal immunological defenses.
- Define sepsis neonatorum.
- Discuss the etiology of neonatal sepsis, including prenatal, intrapartal and postnatal predisposing factors/causes.
- List the earliest clinical signs of neonatal sepsis, as well as symptoms seen later in the clinical course.
- Review the procedure for a septic work-up, including the lab/diagnostic tests involved, normal vs abnormal results of tests and the nursing role in assisting with this procedure.
- Outline the protocol for management of neonatal sepsis, including required procedures and nursing interventions/documentation.
- Discuss the procedure for instituting and maintaining isolation precautions on the Birth Center.
- Discuss the important points related to parental education in this area.

Maternal Substance Abuse

- Define maternal substance abuse.
- List pertinent facts found in the maternal prenatal and labor and delivery record which alert caregivers to the possible presence of maternal substance abuse.
- Discuss the signs of drug dependence and withdrawal in the newborn, using the W.I.T.H.D.R.A.W.A.L. acronym.
- Identify fetal/neonatal complications associated with maternal substance abuse.
- Outline the OB/GYN policy for management of an infant of a suspected substance abusive mother, including required procedures, e.g., chemical dependency screen, and nursing interventions/documentation.

APPENDIX T • NEWBORN CARE

- Discuss the important points related to parental education/communication/support in this area—identify resources available to parents.

CONCEPT 7: NEWBORN LAB/DIAGNOSTIC VALUES/TESTS

- Distinguish normal from abnormal findings in the following newborn lab tests: Hct, Hgb, RBCs, retic count, WBCs, platelet count, blood glucose, blood calcium, Rh/type/Coombs, TB/DB, U/A, blood/eye/cord cultures, gastric aspirate. Discuss possible reasons for variations and appropriate nursing interventions.

*Please see Newborn Concept 6 for specific situations.

- State the purpose and procedure/technique involved for the following:
  - drawing blood on newborns via a heelstick
  - assisting with a central blood draw
  - assisting with blood cultures
  - obtaining a gastric aspirate
  - assisting with X-rays (on and off unit)
  - obtaining a urine specimen via U-bag
  - obtaining cord/eye cultures
  - obtaining a BG chemstrip.

- List the routine lab and biochemical screening tests done on all newborns before discharge, including the rationale for testing, the procedure for requesting/obtaining a specimen, and nursing follow-up/documentation involved.

CONCEPT 8: NEWBORN MEDICATIONS/IMMUNIZATIONS

- State the five rights of medication administration for newborns.

- Outline the OB/GYN policy for administering medications to newborns.

- Discuss administration responsibilities in terms of calculating/verifying dosage for age and weight, dilution procedure, and choice of site, needle gauge and length.

<u>Medications</u>

- Discuss the mechanism of action, route, dosage parameters, and side effects/contraindications/drug and lab interactions for the following medications:

Vitamin K	Erythromycin Opthalmic Ointment	Narcan
Amikacin	Polysporin Ointment	
Ampicillin	Gentamicin	

APPENDIX T • NEWBORN CARE

<u>Immunizations</u>

- Discuss the indications, route, dosage parameters, and side effects/contraindications for the following immunizations:

  Hepatitis B Immune Globulin (HBIG)   Hepatitis B Vaccine (Heptavax-B)

- Discuss parental education related to newborn medications/vaccines.

- Discuss nursing documentation related to newborn medications/vaccines.

*Please see Postpartum Concept 11 for additional specifics on parental education regarding the newborn, which is required before discharge.

University of Rochester–Strong Memorial Hospital
OB/GYN Nursing
Orientation/Crosstraining Program
NEWBORN SKILL COMPETENCY/LEARNING SUMMARY

Instructions: Completed by preceptor and learner with date and initials of preceptor in appropriate column. Returned to NM/NL when completed.

Learner: _____ **Date:** _____

	Reviewed Concept	Applies Concept to Practice	Observed/ Assisted Preceptor	Performs Satisfactorily
ADMISSION/TRANSFER				
Admission Data C Collection/Procedures				
Review of maternal record for newborn care plan				
Admission vital signs				
Admission weight				
Admission measurements				
• length				
• head circumference				
• chest circumference				
Admission physical assessment exam				
Ballard exam for gestational age				
• premature				
• term				
• posanature				
Weight classification by Lubchenco graph				
• SGA				
• AGA				
• LGA				
BG chemstrip				
Admission bath/rewarming				
• radiant warmer				
• isolette				
Triple dye				
Initial feeding/assessment of readiness to eat				
• breastfeeding				
• bottlefeeding				
Pediatric coverage				
• NICU				
• SMH and OOT attending				
• Private attending				
Parental education				
Nursing documentation				

APPENDIX T • NEWBORN CARE

	Reviewed Concept	Applies Concept to Practice	Observed/ Assisted Preceptor	Performs Satisfactorily
Types of Admission/Transfers				
Routine BC/NBN admission				
NBN/BC transfer to NICU				
NICU transfer to BC/NBN				
BC transfer to NBN				
NBN transfer to BC				
L & D transfer to BC				
NEWBORN ASSESSMENT				
Vital Signs				
Admission vs routine				
Temperature				
- axillary				
Heart rate				
Respiratory rate				
Blood pressure				
- 4 limb with Dinamap				
Physical Assessment				
Daily weight/measurements				
Skin				
Head				
Face				
Chest/Neck				
Abdomen				
Back/Buttocks				
Extremities				
Genitalia				
Reflexes				
Behavior				
Notification of pediatrician for abnormalities				
ROUTINE NEWBORN CARE				
Nutrition/Hydration/Feeding				
Assessment of fluid/nutrition status				
- diaper weighing				
- urine specific gravity with spectrometer				
- daily weights				
- skin turgor/mucous membranes				
Assessment of readiness-to-eat				
- mucous/regurgitating/vomiting				
Nursing interventions				
- bottlefeeding techniques				
- positioning				
- positions for burping				
- breastfeeding techniques				
- positioning				
- "newborn who refuses to nurse"				
- flat/inverted nipples				

APPENDIX T • NEWBORN CARE

	Reviewed Concept	Applies Concept to Practice	Observed/ Assisted Preceptor	Performs Satisfactorily
- breast massage/hand expression				
- breastfeeding aides				
- nipple shells/shields				
- hand breast pump				
- electric breast pump				
- supplementation with breastfeeding				
- cup				
- syringe				
- breast milk collection/storage				
Demand feeding schedule				
Parental education				
- advantages/disadvantages of breast vs. bottlefeeding				
Nursing documentation				
Elimination				
Assessment of voiding/stooling patterns				
Nursing interventions				
- abdominal distention				
- "diarrhea"				
Parental education				
Nursing documentation				
Hygiene/Safety				
Assessment of hygiene/safety issues				
Nursing interventions				
- daily hygiene/bathing routine				
- female genitalia				
- male genitalia				
- circumcised/uncircumcised				
- erythema toxicum/"newborn rash"				
- diaper rash				
- cord care				
- removal of cord clamp				
- "wet" cord				
- swaddling/diapering				
Preparation for/Assistance with circumcision				
- routine				
- routine with Lidocaine				
- ritual				
Newborn Protection Practices				
Parental education				
Nursing documentation				
SPECIAL SITUATIONS/COMPLICATIONS				
Use of NICU hotline/emergency button				
Newborn emergency cart/equipment				
Newborn Resuscitation (NRP)				
Assessment of need for resuscitation				
Management/Nursing interventions				
- suctioning				
- bulb				
- wall				
- tactile stimulation				

	Reviewed Concept	Applies Concept to Practice	Observed/ Assisted Preceptor	Performs Satisfactorily
- administration of O_2				
- green line				
- ambu bag				
- Narcan				
- use of NICU hotline/emergency buttons				
- emergency cart				
Parental education				
Nursing documentation				
Hypothermia/Hyperthermia				
• Assessment/identification of hypothermia				
Management/Nursing interventions				
- use of isolette				
- use of radiant warmer				
- skin to skin				
Parental education				
Nursing documentation				
• Assessment/identification of hyperthermia				
Management/Nursing interventions				
Parental education				
Nursing documentation				
Hypoglycemia				
Assessment/identification of hypoglycemia				
Management/Nursing interventions				
Parental education				
Nursing documentation				
Polycythemia/Anemia				
• Assessment/identification of low Hct				
Management/Nursing interventions				
Parental education				
Nursing documentation				
• Assessment/identification of high Hct				
Management/Nursing interventions				
Parental education				
Nursing documentation				
Respiratory Distress				
Assessment/identification of respiratory distress				
TTN				
Management/Nursing interventions				
Parental education				
Nursing documentation				
Prematurity/Postmaturity				
• Identification/assessment of premature infant				
Management/Nursing intervention				
Parental education				
Nursing documentation				
• Identification/assessment of postmature infant				
Management/Nursing interventions				
Parental education				
Nursing documentation				

APPENDIX T • NEWBORN CARE

	Reviewed Concept	Applies Concept to Practice	Observed/ Assisted Preceptor	Performs Satisfactorily
LGA/IDM/SGA/IUGR				
• Identification/assessment of LGA infant				
Management/Nursing interventions				
Parental education				
Nursing documentation				
• Identification/assessment of IDM infant				
Management/Nursing interventions				
Parental education				
Nursing documentation				
• Identification/assessment of SGA infant				
Management/Nursing interventions				
Parental education				
Nursing documentation				
• Identification/assessment of IUGR infant				
Management/Nursing interventions				
Parental education				
Nursing documentation				
Hyperbilirubinemia				
Identification/assessment of neonatal jaundice				
Management/Nursing interventions				
- phototherapy treatment				
- bili lights				
- wallaby				
- bilimeter				
- frequent feedings				
Parental education				
Nursing documentation				
Sepsis				
Identification/assessment of neonatal sepsis				
- septic work-up				
Management/Nursing interventions				
- IM/IV antibiotics				
Parental education				
Nursing documentation				
Maternal Substance Abuse				
Identification/assessment of neonatal withdrawal				
- chemical dependency screen				
- abstinence scores				
- Paregoric				
Management/Nursing interventions				
Parental education				
Nursing documentation				
HIV				
Identification of HIV affected infant				
Management/Nursing Interventions				
HIV Protocol				
- AZT				
Parental education				
Nursing documentation				

APPENDIX T • NEWBORN CARE

	Reviewed Concept	Applies Concept to Practice	Observed/ Assisted Preceptor	Performs Satisfactorily
LAB/DIAGNOSTIC TESTS/VALUES				
Procedure/Technique				
Heelstick blood draw				
Assistance with/Performance of central blood draw				
Assistance with/Performance of blood cultures				
Assistance with X-rays				
Urine specimen via U/bag				
Eye culture				
Cord culture				
Routine Lab/Screening Tests				
Blood type/Rh/Coombs				
Retic count				
Hct				
WBC				
BG chemstrip				
STAT BG				
TB/DB				
Ca++				
NYS metabolic screen				
MEDICATIONS/IMMUNIZATIONS				
Administration responsibilities with newborns				
- calculating/verifying dosage for age/weight				
- dilution procedure				
- choice of site and needle length/gauge				
Parental education				
Nursing documentation				
Medications				
Narcan				
Vitamin K				
Erythromycin Opthalmic Ointment				
IM/IV antibiotics				
Polysporin Ointment				
Paregoric				
AZT				
Immununizations				
Assessment of need for ENGERIX/HBIG				
Administration of ENGERIX/HBIG				
Use of Vaccine History and Immunization Record				

PRECEPTORS

SIGNATURE	INITIALS	SIGNATURE	INITIALS

APPENDIX T • NEWBORN CARE

NAME:_____

UNIVERSITY OF ROCHESTER - STRONG MEMORIAL HOSPITAL
OB/GYN NURSING
ORIENTATION/CROSSTRAINING PROGRAM

NEWBORN STUDY GUIDE
PART I - NORMAL/ROUTINE NEWBORN

This study guide includes key points in newborn nursing and requires the learner to complete answers to various topics. Please complete and return to: _____ by this date: _____.

OBJECTIVES: After completing this guide, the learner will be able to:

1. Describe the process of extrauterine adaptation and its major assessment tool.

2. Describe the components of a newborn examination.

3. Perform a head-to-toe assessment of the newborn.

4. Differentiate normal and deviations from normal characteristics of newborns.

5. List acceptable parameters for neonatal vital signs.

6. State the routine for neonatal vital signs, feedings and assessments on the OB Service.

7. Identify minor indications of illness.

8. Differentiate the elements of nursing documentation for the newborn.

*NOTE: **Breastfeeding information is covered through the Breastfeeding Education Program for OB/GYN Nursing.**
Neonatal Resuscitation is covered through the AHA/AAP Neonatal Resuscitation Program.
Newborn Protection is covered through the Newborn Protection Practices Education Program for OB/GYN Nursing.

RESOURCES: AWHONN Crosstraining Videotape on Newborn Assessment/Care
OB/GYN Nursing Newborn Learning Module
Obstetric Vital Signs/Assessment Guide (card)
Obstetric Patient Teaching Reference Manual

*NOTE: **Most of the information in this guide is taken from the video - other references are cited where appropriate**

APPENDIX T • NEWBORN CARE

I. **THE NEWBORN PERIOD**

The term, _____, refers to an infant during the first 28 days of life, who is adapting to life outside the uterus.

II. **EXTRAUTERINE ADAPTATION**

Moving from uterine to extrauterine life is a major physiologic transition. Changes occur in the newborn's circulatory, respiratory and temperature regulation systems. These changes occur at the moment of birth and continue for hours to days.

The _____ evaluates the newborn's early adaptation to extrauterine life. Assessment is done at _____ min. and _____ min. of life. This assessment identifies newborns at risk for extrauterine adaptation and possible resuscitation.

Apgar Score

Sign	0	1	2
Heart rate	Absent	Slow, < 100	_____
Respiratory effort	Absent	_____	Good crying
Muscle tone	_____	Some flexion of extremities	Active motion
Reflex irritability	None	_____	Vigorous cry
Color	Pale blue	Body pink, blue extremities	_____

NOTES:

APPENDIX T • NEWBORN CARE

III. NEWBORN ASSESSMENT

    A. Newborn History - a newborn's medical history is an important part of the admission/transition assessment. It is found in the _____ record, which should be reviewed for the following information:

        1) _____
        2) _____
        3) _____
        4) _____
        5) _____
        6) _____
        7) _____
        8) _____
        9) _____
        10) prenatal testing results, including serology.

In beginning a newborn assessment, resist the urge to touch or disturb the baby; instead, step back and observe the newborn in a quiet, resting state.

The newborn should be undressed and under a _____ to avoid cold stress. The lighting should be adequate.

When handling a newborn, always use universal precautions until after the first bath.

The newborn assessment comprises a number of elements. The order they are carried out in is generally not important, except to complete observation and then auscultation, especially the cardiac and respiratory assessments, before doing any manipulation, such as palpation and percussion, since these movements will disturb the newborn and change results of assessment. It is important, however, to establish a clear routine, so that all elements of the assessment are completed and recorded.

Any of these factors can skew an assessment if they are not properly controlled.

    B. General Assessment

        <u>Newborn proportions</u>

        1) The head-to-body proportions of a newborn are _____; the head comprises 25% of body size and the trunk/extremities comprise 75%.

        2) The newborn's body midpoint is the _____.

APPENDIX T • NEWBORN CARE

3) _____ is assessed by looking for any body part out of place, out of shape, or at unsymmetrical distance or position to other parts.

Extremities are normally _____ in a full term newborn. If one or more extremities are extended, the newborn should be further examined for _____, _____, or _____.

The newborn should be observed for symmetrical movement of extremities and head. Asymmetry points to possible _____, _____, or _____.

4) The chest should be round and not caved in. Anterior-posterior and bilateral diameters of the chest should be the same.

5) The abdomen should be round but not too full or enlarged.

Cry

1) The full term newborn's cry is strong and lusty. An unusually high-pitched or shrill cry may indicate a _____ or _____.

Tremors

1) The newborn should be observed for tremors which are not uncommon in newborns but which should disappear when touching the baby. Continuous or pronounced tremors may indicate _____, _____, or _____.

Vital Signs

All four quadrants of the chest should be auscultated for cardiac and respiratory sounds.

1) Respiratory rate/effort

   a) Observe respiratory rate and character. Always count for a full minute, since the newborn's breathing is irregular. The normal respiratory rate is _____ breaths per minute.
   b) Examine the character of the chest movement. Any pulling between the ribs (intercostal) or a the base of the sternum (substernal) indicates _____.
   c) A newborn's breathing is usually shallow and abdominal.

d) Grunting is not uncommon; some is normal. If it is continuous, it may indicate that the newborn is _____ or _____, especially if accompanied by flaring nostrils or cyanosis.
e) Tachypnea is common in the newborn because lung capacity is limited by residual amniotic and other fluids. This fluid is absorbed in the first _____ hrs. of life.

2) Temperature

a) Take an _____ temperature, which should be between 36.5 and 37.5 C.

3) Heart rate/sounds

a) Auscultate heart sounds - listen for the classic 2 sound cardiac rhythm (lub dub) with no _____ or _____.
b) Murmurs are common during the first _____ when the heart is transitioning from fetal to neonatal circulation. If a murmur is present, it should be assessed by medical staff.
c) A muffled sound indicates _____ which can sometimes occur spontaneously in well babies.
d) Heart rate range in the normal newborn is _____ bpm while alert and quiet, slightly higher when crying and 70-100 bpm while asleep.

4) Blood pressure (not checked routinely for newborns on OB Service)

a) Check the blood pressure on upper and lower extremities with a Doppler cuff. Use the antecubital and popliteal spaces. Cuff size selection is essential for accuracy. Its width should be 1/2 the circumference of the extremity. BP is usually _____ in the lower extremity but a difference of more than 20 mm Hg indicates possible _____.
b) Systolic pressure at birth ranges _____ and diastolic pressure ranges _____. As the newborn transitions to extrauterine life, the systolic pressure increases slightly with the norm ranging _____.

Physical measurements

1) Length -> crown-to-sole with legs fully _____

2) Head circumference -> at its widest occiput-frontal circumference

APPENDIX T • NEWBORN CARE

3) Chest circumference -> at _____ line, usually 2 cm. < head circumference

4) Abdominal circumference -> at midline

5) Weight -> normal weight for a newborn is _____
(5 lb. 8 oz. - 8 lbs. 13 oz.)

NOTES:

C. Assessment of Skin

Assessment of the skin is normally performed as a part of the overall head-to-toe examination.

1) Note any unusual condition, such as _____, _____, and _____. Newborn skin should be warm - cold, clammy skin is a sign of _____ or _____ and should be treated immediately.

2) Check the skin for proper turgor by gently pinching the _____ to see how quickly it returns to smoothness. Loose skin indicates _____ which can be extremely serious, or indicates that the newborn is _____.

3) Skin thickness and opacity are indicators of _____. The more translucent the skin, the _____ the newborn's gestational age. If veins can be clearly seen over the body, the newborn is _____. A post term baby's skin is dry and _____ with _____ and _____.

4) Newborns often have a ruddy skin tone known as _____, caused by an overabundance of _____ in fetal blood because of lower O2 saturation in utero. Plethora disappears _____ _____. If this beefy red coloring persists, it may indicate _____ requiring further blood studies.

5) A downy-like hair that covers the developing fetus, called _____, has almost disappeared at term, so any significant covering of lanugo is another sign of _____.

APPENDIX T • NEWBORN CARE

6) The best way to assess a newborn's color is to examine the _____ _____. The newborn may exhibit transient or slight cyanosis as circulatory transition is taking place and the vasomotor system is unstable. It's important to distinguish between this type of cyanosis and _____ cyanosis caused by _____ or _____ insufficiency, which must be treated with O2.

7) A bluish discoloration of the hands and feet, known as _____, is common, especially if the newborn is chilled. To make sure this isn't a symptom of true cyanosis, rub the sole vigorously - if color returns, acrocyanosis is caused by transient vasomotor instability, often because the newborn is losing _____ -> take measures to warm the baby and stop heat loss.

8) Jaundice or _____ is common, often seen by _____ day of life. It is caused by the yellow pigment, _____, a product of _____ breakdown as the newborn's body clears excess _____. If the immature liver falls behind in clearing bilirubin from the blood, the resulting build-up may threaten the newborn's health. To check for jaundice, press on _____ to flush the capillaries -> jaundiced newborns will exhibit a _____ color. Jaundice is generally not a concern unless is appears in the first _____ or persists beyond _____. Jaundice should be followed by blood bilirubin levels -> very elevated levels may require intervention at any time.

9) A whitish, waxy-like coating, _____, is composed of skin cells and sebaceous secretions and forms a protective layer over the newborn's _____. If the vernix is stained green or brown, this indicates _____, which indicates possible fetal distress.

10) _____, a bluish discoloration on the hips or buttocks, is common in _____ newborns. It may take up to _____ to disappear completely.

11) Both mottling and Harlequin sign are signs of _____.

12) Petechiae are often found over the _____. General petechiae may be a sign of _____ and should be reported.

13) Nevi are common on _____, _____, _____, and _____. They are also

called _____ and may take _____ to disappear.

14) _____, a rash of white vesicles on a red macular base, clears up quickly without intervention.

15) Milia, small white papules caused by _____ on face or upper torso, clear quickly by themselves.

16) _____, caused by birth trauma or forceps clear in days.

17) Birthmarks are noted, including _____, _____, _____, and _____. Strawberry marks and _____ disappear during the first few years of life. _____ do not fade over time.

NOTES:

D. Assessment of Head

1) Examine the head for _____ and _____. The newborn skull is soft and pliable. It probably has been molded by the stresses of delivery but corrects itself.

2) Palpate the head to feel the sutures and fontanelles.

a) Suture lines are usually mobile, allowing bones of the skull to move, making room for the rapidly growing _____. The bones may be overriding at the suture line as a result of _____ - this is not abnormal but should be noted.

APPENDIX T • NEWBORN CARE

It is abnormal for spaces to be closed because it compromises brain growth and later neurological development.

    b) There are 2 fontanelles:

        i. anterior fontanel, which is _____ shaped and _____ cm at its widest point.
        ii. posterior fontanel, which is _____ cm in diameter

Both should be flat and not depressed, a sign of _____ _____ or full and tense, caused by _____ and _____.

    c) _____ is swelling of soft tissues of the skull that crosses suture lines - it's caused by _____ _____ during delivery.

    d) Cephalhematoma is a hematoma of the head due to the pressures of labor - it generally does not cross suture lines, but may increase the risk of _____ and calcium deposits over the bone.

NOTES:

E. Assessment of the Eyes

    1) Examine the eyes for symmetry.

    2) Epicanthic folds at the corner of the eyes are _____ in Asian newborns, but in non-Asian newborns their presence may indicate _____. They may also be caused by _____.

    3) Examine the corneas for _____, _____, and _____.

    4) Check the color of the sclera and conjunctiva. Sclera may have a slight _____ color but a pronounced _____ is abnormal. Yellow sclera indicate _____.

APPENDIX T • NEWBORN CARE

Conjunctiva should be _____ color. Subconjunctival hemorrhages are caused by the birth process and disappear in _____.

5) Check the eyes for movement and response to light. Newborns can focus on an object at _____ cms. distance and follow movement to _____. Neuromuscular control is immature, leading to random, uneven movement and some transient _____. Shining a light into the eyes should produce _____ and _____. The pupils should react symmetrically.

NOTES:

F. Assessment of Ears

1) Examine the size and shape of the ears. The top of the ears should be in line with the newborn's eyes - low-set ears indicate possible _____. The shape and stiffness of the ears also indicates _____ - in a term infant, the pinna is flexible but _____ and will spring back into shape when folded down.

2) Check the hearing, by clapping hands near the newborn's head - the normal response is _____ (note: newborns receive a routine hearing screening test before discharge on the OB Service).

NOTES:

G. Assessment of Nose

1) Newborns are obligatory _____ breathers.

APPENDIX T • NEWBORN CARE

2) Check that the nares are _____, that the _____ is present and that there are no _____ in the nasal passages.

3) The nose should be on the midline of the newborn's face. If the bridge is flattened, it may indicate _____, especially if other facial malformations are present.

NOTES:

H. Assessment of Mouth

1) The newborn's mouth should be on the midline of the face.

2) Check for an intact _____ by sweeping the mouth with a gloved finger.

3) Check for nerve symmetry and tone in the muscles around the mouth and in the movements of the _____.

4) Any excessively tight tissue under the tongue, known as _____ is usually outgrown.

5) Some newborns are born with _____ teeth which are extracted because they are a threat to development of normal teeth and a risk for aspiration.

6) The mucous membranes of the mouth should be _____ and _____.

7) Small white spots on mucosa of the mouth, called _____, are normal and will disappear in _____.

8) The salivary glands are immature, so there shouldn't be an excess of saliva - excessive salivation may indicate _____ and should be reported.

9) Excess mucous in the mouth and nares can interfere with breathing and should be suctioned with a bulb syringe. Position the newborn on

APPENDIX T • NEWBORN CARE

_____ and suction first _____, then the _____ and finally _____.

NOTES:

I. Assessment of Neck

1) Examine the neck for _____ and _____ _____.

2) There should be no webbing or excessive skin at the sides of the neck - this is a _____.

NOTES:

J. Assessment of Chest

1) The chest should be _____ and _____.

2) Amount of breast tissue and nipples indicate gestational age - in the term newborn, tissue is _____ under the skin with _____ _____ nipples. If nipples are spaced wider than _____ of chest circumference, this indicates a genetic abnormality.

3) Breasts may be engorged in both male and female newborns because of _____. This condition, called _____, fades quickly.

4) Palpate the clavicles for evidence of _____.

5) Observe for clavicular and intercostal _____ which indicate respiratory distress, especially if accompanied by _____ and _____.

460

NOTES:

K. Assessment of Abdomen

1) Assess the abdomen for bulges or distension, especially of the _____.

2) Check the umbilical cord for signs of _____ and _____. Note the number of vessels - there should be 2 _____ and 1 _____ (AVA).

3) Palpate for the liver edge, which should be 2 cm below the _____ _____.

4) The edge of the _____ may be palpated just below the left costal margin, but it is not as prominent.

5) The newborn's kidneys are difficult to palpate and if detectable, feel like _____ on either side of the spine, just above the _____.

6) Check for strong bilateral _____ pulses.

NOTES:

L. Assessment of the Genitalia

1) Check if the genitals are fully developed. Note _____, _____, _____ and _____ of various structures and any irritation.

2) With male newborns, check for patency of the meatus, with no additional openings on the dorsal or ventral surfaces. Testes may not be completely descended but should be palpable at _____.

APPENDIX T • NEWBORN CARE

3) Female newborns may present with _____ vaginal discharge called pseudo menses, which is due to withdrawal of maternal hormones.

4) It's no longer standard practice to test anal patency - instead, note the passage of meconium stool, which should occur in _____ hrs.

NOTES:

M. Assessment of Extremities

1) Examine the extremities for extra digits, called _____ or fused digits, called _____.

2) A single crease, called a Simian crease, across the palm, may indicate _____.

3) Assess ROM of arms - trauma to the brachial plexus may cause _____, called _____. The affected area is tightly abducted and internally rotated at the shoulder and does not show normal _____, _____, or _____.

4) Assess ROM of legs - assess for hip dysplasia, using the _____ _____. Flex the knees, then move legs up and out in a smooth, uninterrupted movement - any _____ indicates a congenital malformation. Examine the legs for symmetry, even at the _____.

NOTES:

APPENDIX T • NEWBORN CARE

N. Neurologic Assessment

1) The newborn passes through several stages of reactivity - for most, the first stage immediately postpartum is a period of _____, followed by a period of _____.

2) The _____ reflex is a defensive response to a startling change in the environment. To elicit, hold the newborn in a _____ position and allow the head and trunk to fall back slightly. The characteristic response is _____, then _____ of both arms with fingers spread. The arms then return to an _____ position and finally relax.

3) Rooting, sucking, swallowing and gag reflexes are essential for infant feeding. Rooting is elicited by touching the newborn's cheek - the newborn responds by turning to stimulus, opening the mouth and beginning to _____. Swallowing and gag reflexes can be observed during _____.

4) The _____ and _____ grasp reflexes are similar responses to stimuli of the hands and feet.

   a) touch the newborn's palm with the ulnar surface of fingertip -> the infant's fingers will curl into a grasp firm enough to lift from surface
   b) place pressure on underside of toes -> infant will curl toes toward stimulus - the opposing movment, called the _____ _____ can be elicited by stroking the sole of the foot upward -> the toes hyperextend and the great toe is dorsiflexed

5) The tonic neck or _____ reflex is present during the first few weeks of life. It is elicited by turning the head quickly to one side - the newborn responds by extending the arm on that side, while the other arm is flexed.

6) Placing and stepping reflexes - the newborn makes crawling movements when placed on the abdomen and stepping movments when held in a standing position.

NOTES:

APPENDIX T • NEWBORN CARE

O. Gestational Age Assessment

1) Gestational age is based on a sum of scores (0-4) on a variety of criteria that include both _____ and _____ characteristics. Two versions of this assessment tool are the original Dubowitz score and the newer Ballard score. Gestational age can also be determined by looking at various obstetrical parameters, such as the mother's last menstrual period.

2) Gestational age is described in 3 terms:

   a) preterm or premature - 37 or less weeks gestation
   b) term - 38 to 41 weeks gestation
   c) post term or postmature - 42 or greater weeks gestation

3) Once gestational age has been determined, the newborn's weight, length and occipital-frontal head circumference can be plotted on growth charts (note: on the OB Service, weight is the only item plotted routinely by nurses) to arrive at a classification.

4) The major groups of classification are:

   a) SGA - small for gestational age, or weight falling below the 10th percentile for gestational age
   b) AGA - appropriate weight for gestational age
   c) LGA - large for gestational age, or weight falling above the 90th percentile for gestational age

5) A newborn will then fall into one of 9 groups:

   a) preterm SGA, AGA or LGA
   b) term SGA, AGA or LGA
   c) post term SGA, AGA or LGA

6) Identifying which group a newborn falls into is importaat because each group has been shown to be linked with certain risk factors. Care and assessments can then be designed to address the risk factors for each newborn based on his/her classification.

NOTES:

APPENDIX T • NEWBORN CARE

List the routine for VS, feedings and assessments during the 6 hour admission period for newborns on the OB Service (note: please refer to the Obstetric VS/Assessment Guide for this piece):

___

List the ongoing routine for VS, feedings and assessments after the admission period for newborns on the OB Service (note: please refer to the Obstetric VS/Assessment Guide for this piece):

___

List the items that must be documented on the newborn caremap at least every 8 hours (note: please refer to the Obstetric VS/Assessment Guide for this piece):

___

NOTES:

APPENDIX T • NEWBORN CARE

NAME:_____

UNIVERSITY OF ROCHESTER–STRONG MEMORIAL HOSPITAL
OB/GYN NURSING
ORIENTATION/CROSSTRAINING PROGRAM

NEWBORN POST TEST—*PART I*

Return completed tests to: _____ **by this date:** _____.

NORMAL/ROUTINE NEWBORN CARE

Circle the one best answer.

1. Assessment of the newborn includes:

    a. Maternal history.

    b. Labor and delivery history.

    c. Psychosocial history and assessment of family.

    d. Physical examination of the newborn.

    e. All of the above.

2. When assessing respirations:

    a. Take temperature and pulse first.

    b. Count for a fall minute.

    c. Stimulate the newborn to elicit crying.

    d. Count for 15 seconds and multiply by 4.

3. Jaundice is usually not a concern if it:

    a. Appears within the first 24 hours of life.

    b. Develops after the first week of life.

    c. Occurs 72 hours after birth.

    d. Is present at birth.

4. Gestational assessment of the newborn:

    a. Is an unnecessary examination.

    b. Is detemined by newborn weight.

    c. Can be determined without a physical examination.

    d. Assists in identifying premature and postmature newborns, as well as LGA/AGA and SGA newborns.

5. Caput succedaneum is:
   a. Caused by a precipitous delivery.
   b. A normal swelling of the tissue that crosses suture lines.
   c. An abnormal swelling of the tissue that crosses suture lines.
   d. A collection of blood over the bony portion of the skull.

6. Erythema toxicum is:
   a. A rash with white vesicles on a red macular base.
   b. Caused by clogged sebaceous glands.
   c. A bluish discoloration on the hips or buttocks.
   d. A congenital infection.

7. All of the following statements about newborn blood pressure are accurate except:
   a. Diastolic blood pressure ranges between 40 and 60 mm of mercury
   b. A difference of more than 20 mm/mercury between upper and lower extremities indicates circulatory obstruction.
   c. Usually is greater in the lower extremities.
   d. Size of the blood pressure cuff is not essential.

8. What do the physical findings of an unequal Moro reflex, crepitus at the neck and delivery history suggest?
   a. Torticollis.
   b. Cystic hygroma.
   c. Fractured clavicle.
   d. Erb's palsy.

9. At 1 minutes of age, a newborn has spontaneous respirations, a heart rate of 120 bpm, some flexion, is crying with stimulation and is acrocyanotic. The Apgar score is:
   a. 6.
   b. 7.
   c. 8.
   d. 10.

Mark the following statements as true or false.

10. ___ Vitamin K should be given within 1 hour of delivery.

11. ___ Using the Ballard assessment tool, distinctive deep plantar indentations over the anterior two-thirds of the foot would be scored 2.

12. ___ Conjunctival hemorrhages will usually disappear in 7–10 days.

13. ___ The reflex that is elicited when a newborn loses head support is the tonic neck reflex.

14. ___ Erythromycin ointment is instilled in newborn eyes after delivery to prevent ophthalmia neonatorum.

Complete the following.

15. State the routine for newborn <u>VS. feedings and assessments</u> on the OB Service:

    a. during the admission/transition period (first 6 hours after birth)

    _____
    _____
    _____

    b. beyond the first 6 hours after birth

    _____
    _____
    _____

POSTPARTUM CONCEPTS

CONCEPT 1: ADMISSION/TRANSITION OF THE POSTPARTUM PATIENT

- List the patient criteria for admission/transfer of a postpartum patient to the Birth Center.
- State the procedure for L&D postpartum admission to the Birth Center.
- Discuss criteria for patient placement/bed utilization on the Birth Center.
- Define the postpartum period and list the three phases of this period.
- Discuss normal maternal adaptations to the postpartum period—cardiovascular, reproductive, endocrine, hematopoietic, urinary, gastrointestinal, neurologic, musculoskeletal, integumentary, emotional/behavioral. Discuss what findings you will observe during the postpartum period as a result of these adaptations.
- Discuss normal adaptations of the family following the birth of a newborn.

Admission/Transfer/Transition Data Collection

- State the important factors/their significance, found in the patient's prenatal record, nursing history, and labor and delivery record, which must be considered when planning postpartum care.

Admission/Transfer/Transition Assessment/Procedures

- List the key assessments/procedures involved in admission/transfer of a postpartum patient to the Birth Center.

*Please see Concept 2 for specifics on assessment procedures.

- Discuss what orientation/information is necessary to prepare the postpartum patient/family for admission/transfer to the Birth Center.
- Discuss nursing documentation related to admission/transfer of the postpartum patient.

CONCEPT 2: MATERNAL POSTPARTUM ASSESSMENT (VITAL SIGNS/ 8 POINT CHECKS)

- State the Birth Center policy for assessing and recording maternal vital signs and eight point checks during the first 24 hours following delivery and then routinely during the postpartum period.

Vital Signs

- State the normal parameters for maternal vital signs in the postpartum period.
- Discuss the significance of elevated temperature, decrease/increase in blood pressure, decrease/increase in pulse, and respiratory changes.
- List the eight factors included in a routine postpartum assessment.

APPENDIX U • POSTPARTUM CARE

Breasts/Nipples

- State what factors must be included in nursing assessment of breasts/nipples.
- Describe the proper technique for breast examination.
- Discuss the process of lactation and how it differs between a primiparous and multiparous patient and between a breastfeeding and bottlefeeding mother.

Fundus

- State what factors must be included in nursing assessment of the postpartum uterus.
- Describe the proper technique for assessing fundal height, including rationale for supporting the uterus above the symphysis during examination.
- Explain the proper technique for uterine massage.
- Discuss the process of involution and how it differs between primiparous and multiparous patients.
- Discuss the significance of a soft/boggy uterus or a uterus found above/to 1 side of the umbilicus after the first 1–2 hrs. post delivery.

Perineum

- State what factors must be included in nursing assessment of perineum/episiotomy.
- Describe the proper technique for examining the perineum postpartally.
- Describe the normal healing process and appearance of the perineum during the early postpartum period.
- Describe the following and state what complications can occur with each:
  - episiotomy (median and mediolateral)
  - extensions
  - lacerations (1st to 4th degree)
  - periuretheral laceration
  - sulcus tears
  - vaginal hematomas
  - hemorrhoids

Lochia

- State what factors must be considered in nursing assessment of lochia. List the components of lochia.
- Describe the different types of lochia and when each normally occurs in the postpartum period.
- Discuss the significance of persistently heavy lochia, passage of large clots, foul-smelling lochia.

Homan's Sign

- State what factors must be included in nursing assessment of the lower extremities of a postpartum patient.
- Describe the proper technique for assessing Homan's Sign.

APPENDIX U • POSTPARTUM CARE

- Explain the significance of a positive Homan's Sign.

Bladder Status

- State what factors should be included in nursing assessment of the bladder/voiding status of a postpartum patient.
- Describe the proper technique for palpation of the bladder.
- State policy for what constitutes an adequate void and how many voids are routinely measured postpartally.
- Explain the significance of frequent, small voidings, inability to void/distended bladder, hematuria, burning on urination.

Bowel Status

- Explain the rationale for assessing bowel sounds after a vaginal delivery.
- Describe the proper procedure for assessing bowel status postpartally.
- Discuss the significance of constipation or a distended abdomen in the absence of bowel sounds.

Emotional Status

- State what factors should be included in nursing assessment of the emotional status of a postpartum patient.
- Describe Rubin's taking-in, taking-hold, and letting-go phases of maternal behavior.
- Discuss patient education related to assessment of the postpartum patient.
- Discuss nursing documentation related to assessment of the postpartum patient.

CONCEPT 3: POSTPARTUM NUTRITION/HYDRATION

- Describe the changes in appetite normally seen in a postpartum patient.
- Discuss the nutritional and fluid needs of the postpartum patient.
- Discuss the unique fluid and nutritional needs of the breastfeeding mother.
- State the cause of increased perspiration in the early postpartum period.
- List the s/s of postpartum dehydration and discuss appropriate nursing interventions.
- Discuss patient education related to postpartum nutrition/hydration.
- Discuss nursing documentation related to postpartum nutrition/hydration.

CONCEPT 4: POSTPARTUM ELIMINATION

- Describe the normal patterns of elimination seen in the early postpartum period.
- Identify the primary causes for inability to void/urinary retention in the postpartum patient and discuss nursing interventions to assist with voiding.

- State the complications which can occur with a distended bladder.
- Review the procedure for postpartum catheterization and list indications for this procedure.
- State the reasons for postpartum constipation and discuss nursing interventions for its relief.
- Discuss patient education related to postpartum elimination.
- Discuss nursing documentation related to postpartum elimination.

CONCEPT 5: POSTPARTUM ACTIVITY/REST

- Discuss the benefits of early ambulation in the postpartum period.
- State the physiologic reason for assisting the patient with first ambulation after delivery.
- Discuss the need for rest/sleep in the postpartum period and nursing interventions to facilitate this.
- Discuss patient education related to postpartum activity/rest.
- Discuss nursing documentation related to postpartum activity/rest.

CONCEPT 6: POSTPARTUM HYGIENE/COMFORT

Breast Care—Engorgement/Sore Nipples

- Discuss routine care of breast and nipples in the postpartum patient.
- State the causes of breast engorgement and describe its s/s.
- Discuss nursing interventions for relief of breast engorgement in the breastfeeding and bottlefeeding mother.
- Define natural and chemical lactation suppression and the advantages/disadvantages of both methods.
- Discuss the causes of sore nipples in the breastfeeding mother and nursing interventions to promote comfort and healing.

*Additional information is found under Newborn Concept 3.

Uterine Cramping/Afterbirth Pains

- Explain the cause of afterbirth pains and why they are more common/severe in a multiparous patient.
- Identify appropriate nursing interventions for relief of afterbirth pains.
- Discuss the cause of uterine cramping in breastfeeding mothers.

Perineal Care—Episiotomy/Hemorrhoids

- State the proper procedure for perineal care.
- List at least eight perineal comfort measures and the rationale for their use.
- Discuss nursing interventions for the relief of hemorrhoids.
- Describe Kegel exercises and state when it is appropriate to initiate these exercises.

Headaches/Muscle and Joint Pains

- Discuss the causes for headaches after delivery and state nursing interventions for their relief.
- Discuss the causes for muscle and joint pains after delivery and state nursing interventions for their relief.
- Discuss patient education related to postpartum hygiene/comfort.
- Discuss nursing documentation related to postpartum hygiene/comfort.

CONCEPT 7: POSTPARTUM COMPLICATIONS/SPECIAL SITUATIONS

Maternal Emergencies/Resuscitation

- Discuss use of the adult emergency cart and equipment. **This must be reviewed and signed off on skills checklist and personal Education/Inservice Record.**

Uterine Atony/Subinvolution

- Describe the proper technique for uterine massage.
- Discuss the causes and s/s of uterine atony/subinvolution, including the nursing assessments necessary for identifying uterine atony/subinvolution.
- Outline the protocol for management of uterine atony/subinvolution, including required procedures and nursing interventions/documentation.
- Discuss important points related to patient education in this area.

Spinal Headache

- Discuss the cause and s/s of spinal headache—distinguish between spinal headaches and general types of headaches.
- Outline the protocol for management of spinal headache, including required procedures and nursing interventions/documentation.
- Discuss important points related to patient education in this area.

Puerperal Infection

- Describe the risk factors which predispose a patient to puerperal infection.
- Identify the most common types of postpartum infection.
- State the s/s for each type of infection.
- Outline the protocol for management of puerperal infections, including required procedures and nursing interventions/documentation.
- Discuss the proper procedure for a "fever work-up."
- Discuss the Birth Center policy for accommodating a patient with known or suspected infection.
- Discuss important points related to patient education in this area.

Thrombophlebitis

- Describe the risk factors which predispose a patient to thrombophlebitis.
- State the s/s of thrombophlebitis.
- Outline the protocol for management of thrombophlebitis, including required procedures and nursing interventions/documentation.
- Discuss important points related to patient education in this area.

Preeclampsia

- Distinguish between preeclampsia, eclampsia, and PIH.
- Discuss the significance of preeclampsia in the postpartum patient.
- Identify the classic s/s of preeclampsia.
- Outline the protocol for management of preeclampsia, including required procedures and nursing interventions/documentation.
- State the proper technique for doing a urine SSA and for assessing reflexes.
- Define "tox precautions" and discuss the rationale for their use.
- Discuss important points related to patient education in this area.

Postpartum Tubal Ligation

- Discuss the preoperative/postoperative routines and nursing interventions/documentation for a postpartum BTL.
- Discuss important points related to patient education in this area.

CONCEPT 8: BONDING/MATERNAL-INFANT-FAMILY INTERACTION

Bonding

- Describe the postpartum bonding process which occurs between mother and newborn.
- Discuss mother-newborn interactions which signal positive attachment.
- Discuss the importance of promoting bonding in the first few hours after birth and identify specific nursing interventions for facilitating this.
- Discuss mother-newborn interactions which signal poor adjustment.

Postpartum Blues

- Define "postpartum blues" and discuss the difference between postpartum blues and postpartum depression.
- Identify nursing interventions which will assist the patient in coping with "the blues."

Grieving

- Describe the grieving process which occurs when there is a "less than ideal" birthing experience, e.g., baby in NICU/with an anomaly/under bili lights, stillbirth, transfer to L&D.
- Identify nursing interventions which can reinforce the patient's coping mechanisms.

Rooming-In/Family Centered Care

- Discuss the concepts of "rooming-in" and "family-centered care."
- State the Birth Center policy for maintaining safety during mother-newborn interactions.
- State the Birth Center policy for night rooming-in guidelines.
- State the Birth Center policy for family visitation.
- Identify resources available for patient/family support and discuss the appropriate procedures for accessing them.
- Discuss patient education related to bonding/maternal-infant-family interaction.
- Discuss nursing documentation related to bonding/maternal-infant-family interaction.

CONCEPT 9: POSTPARTUM DIAGNOSTIC/LAB TESTS/VALUES

- Distinguish normal from abnormal findings in the following lab tests during the postpartum period: Hct, Hgb, WBCs, neutrophils, platelets, clotting factors, U/A, urine SSA. Explain the possible reasons for variations and appropriate nursing interventions.
- Relate activation of clotting factors after delivery to increased risk for thrombophlebitis in the postpartum patient.
- Discuss the effect of hemoconcentration caused by postdelivery diuresis on Hct values.
- List the routine postpartum lab tests, including the rationale for testing, the procedure for requesting/obtaining a specimen and nursing follow-up/documentation involved.

CONCEPT 10: POSTPARTUM MEDICATIONS/IMMUNIZATIONS

- State the five rights of medication administration.
- Discuss the nursing policy for administration of medications.

Medications

- Discuss the mechanism of action, route, common dosage and side effects/contraindications of the following medications:
    - Pitocin
    - Methergine
    - Ergotrate
    - Prostin
    - Deladumone
    - Halcion
    - Nembutol
    - Anusol HC
    - Dulcolax

Parlodel	Common Antibiotics
Motrin	Ampicillin
Tylenol	Ancef/Kefzol
Codeine	Vancocin
Percocet	Unasyn
Feosol	Gentamicin
Ammonia Inhalant	Cefotetan
Morphine	
Vistaril	
Demerol	

Immunizations (Rhogam/Rubella Vaccine)

- State the indications for administering Rhogam.

- Review the mechanism of action, route/site/timing of administration, common dosage, and side effects/contraindications for Rhogam.

- State the indications for administering rubella vaccine.

- Review the mechanism of action, route/site/timing of administration, common dosage, and side effects/contraindications for rubella vaccine.

- Discuss patient education related to postpartum medications/immunizations.

- Discuss nursing documentation related to postpartum medications/immunizations.

CONCEPT 11: POSTPARTUM PATIENT/FAMILY EDUCATION

- List and discuss the educational topics which must be reviewed with patient/family prior to discharge, referring to the OB Teaching Tool and Birth Center Patient Education Resource Manual. Include patient education related to pre/post-op care for BTL, postpartum danger signs, nutrition/exercise, physical/emotional changes in the postpartum period, sexuality/contraception, sibling preparation, breast/bottlefeeding, newborn bath/cord care, circumcision care, newborn temperature-taking, newborn protection practices, newborn metabolic screening/jaundice, and infant abilities.

- Identify educational resources available to the patient:
  - discuss the "Strong Beginnings" Program
  - state the time, location and topics of "Strong Beginnings" classes
  - discuss the role of the nurse educators
  - identify booklets which must be given to patients before discharge
  - state the times, channel and topics for CCTV educational offerings
  - identify additional videotapes available on the unit for patient education and the process for accessing them
  - discuss the role of the Lactation Coordinator
  - discuss the purpose and use of the Breastfeeding Support Line.

- Discuss teaching strategies/resources for patients with communication deficits, e.g., language barriers, speech/hearing impairments.

- Discuss nursing documentation related to postpartum patient/family education.

CONCEPT 12: DISCHARGE OF THE POSTPARTUM PATIENT/FAMILY

- Discuss the criteria and procedure for early discharge from the Birth Center.
- State the average LOS for patients on the Birth Center.
- Discuss the procedure for routine discharge of postpartum patients/families from the Birth Center.
- Identify forms which need to be signed before discharge and discuss nursing documentation related to discharge of postpartum patient/family.
- Discuss patient education/teaching which must be completed on the day of discharge.
- Discuss the appropriate procedure to initiate a WIC, CHN or IHAP referral.

University of Rochester–Strong Memorial Hospital
OB/GYN Nursing
Orientation/Crosstraining Program
POSTPARTUM SKILL COMPETENCY/LEARNING SUMMARY

Instructions: Completed by preceptor and learner with date and initials of preceptor in appropriate column. Returned to NM/NL when completed.

Learner: _____   **Date:** _____

	Reviewed Concept	Applies Concept to Practice	Observed/ Assisted Preceptor	Performs Satisfactorily
Admission/Transition				
Admission/Transition Data Collection/Procedures				
Review of maternal record for care plan				
Admission/transition vital signs				
Admission/transition eight point check				
Patient/Family orientation to BC				
Nursing documentation				
Types of Admission/Transition				
Routine BC postpartum transition				
L&D postpartum admission to BC				
MATERNAL POSTPARTUM ASSESSMENT				
Vital Signs				
Admission/transition vs routine				
Tempteature				
- Filiac electronic thermometer				
- Tympanic thermometer				
Pulse rate				
Respiratory rate				
Blood pressure				
Eight Point Check				
Breasts/nipples				
- breastfeeding				
- bottlefeeding				
Fundus				
- primipara				
- multipara				
Perineum				
- episiotomy				
- laceration				
- vaginal hematoma				
- hemorrhoids				
Lochia				
Homan's sign				
Bladder status				
Bowel status				
Emotional status				
Patient education				

APPENDIX U • POSTPARTUM CARE

	Reviewed Concept	Applies Concept to Practice	Observed/ Assisted Preceptor	Performs Satisfactorily
Nursing documentation				
Notification of obstetrician for problems				
ROUTINE POSTPARTUM CARE				
Nutrition/Hydration				
Assessment of fluid/nutrition status				
- routine postpartum/bottlefeeding mother				
- breastfeeding mother				
Nursing interventions				
- postpartum dehydration				
Patient education				
Nursing documentation				
Elimination				
Assessment of elimination patterns				
Nursing interventions				
- inability to void/urinary retention				
- postpartum catheterization				
- constipation				
Patient education				
Nursing documentation				
Activity/Rest				
Assessment of activity/fatigue level				
Nursing interventions				
- first ambulation after delivery				
- promotion of rest/privacy				
Patient education				
Nursing documentation				
Hygiene/Comfort				
Assessment of hygiene/comfort				
Breast Care—Engorgement/Sore Nipples				
Nursing interventions				
- routine breast/nipple care/hygiene				
- cleansing of breasts/nipple				
- air drying of nipples				
- positioning				
- comfort measures for engorgement				
- cold packs				
- moist heat				
- bra/breast binder				
- manual expression				
- lactation suppression				
- analgesics				
- comfort measures for sore nipples				
- expression/application of colostrum				
- dry heat				
- air drying				
Uterine Cramping/Afterbirth Pains				
Nursing interventions				
- analgesics				
- warm packs				

APPENDIX U • POSTPARTUM CARE

	Reviewed Concept	Applies Concept to Practice	Observed/ Assisted Preceptor	Performs Satisfactorily
Perineal Care—Episiotomy/Hemorrhoids				
Nursing interventions				
- routine perineal care/hygiene				
- handwashing				
- peri-bottle				
- changing peri-pads				
- comfort measures				
- cold packs				
- sitz bath/whirlpool				
- Dermaplast spray				
- witch hazel compresses				
- Nupercairal ointment				
- foam donut				
Headaches/Muscle and Joint Pains				
Nursing interventions				
- analgesics				
- whirlpool				
Patient education				
Nursing documentation				
BONDING/MATERNAL-INFANT-FAMILY INTERACTION				
Bonding				
Assessment of bonding				
Nursing interventions				
Patient education				
Nursing documentation				
Postpartum Blues				
Assessment of blues vs depression vs grieving				
Nursing interventions				
Patient education				
Nursing documentation				
Rooming-In/Family-Centered Care				
Assessment of family interaction				
Newborn Protection Practices				
Utilization of resources				
- Social worker				
- Chaplain				
- Community support groups				
POSTPARTUM COMPLICATIONS/ SPECIAL SITUATIONS				
Adult emergency cart/equipment				
Uterine Atony/Subinvolution				
Assessment of uterine atony/subinvolution				
- uterine massage				
- initiation of IV access				
- Pitocin/Methergine/Ergotrate				
- pad weights				
- orthostatic BPs				
- Prostaglandins				
Patient education				
Nursing documentation				

APPENDIX U • POSTPARTUM CARE

	Reviewed Concept	Applies Concept to Practice	Observed/ Assisted Preceptor	Performs Satisfactorily
Spinal Headache				
Assessment of spinal headache				
Management/Nursing interventions				
- positioning				
- IV hydration				
- analgesics				
- blood patch				
Patient education				
Nursing documentation				
Puerperal Infection				
Assessment of puerperal infection				
Management/Nursing interventions				
- septic work-up				
- antibiotics				
- isolation precautions				
Patient education				
Nursing documentation				
Thrombophlebitis				
Assessment of thrombophlebitis				
Management/Nursing interventions				
- TED stockings				
- warm packs				
Patient education				
Nursing documentation				
Preeclampsia				
Assessment of preeclainpsia				
- blood pressure				
- urine SSA				
- reflexes				
- edema				
Management/Nursing interventions				
- tox precautions				
- positioning				
Patient education				
Nursing documentation				
Postpartum BTL				
Preoperative routine/Nursing interventions				
Postoperative routine/Nursing interventions				
Patient education				
Nursing documentation				
POSTPARTUM LAB/DIAGNOSTIC TESTS/VALUES				
Procedures/Techniques				
Fingerstick blood draw				
Venipuncture blood draw				
Assistance with septic work-up				
- blood cultures				
- intrauterine/cervical cultures				
Urine C&S				
Routine Lab Tests				
Postpartum Hct/CBC				

APPENDIX U • POSTPARTUM CARE

	Reviewed Concept	Applies Concept to Practice	Observed/ Assisted Preceptor	Performs Satisfactorily
POSTPARTUM MEDICATIONS/ IMMUNIZATIONS				
Administration responsibilities/five rights				
Patient education				
Nursing documentation				
Medications				
Pitocin				
Methergine/Ergotrate				
Colace				
Tylenol				
Codeine				
Percocet				
Feosol				
Ammonia Inhalant				
Antibiotics				
Halcion				
Nembutol				
MO/MOM				
Motrin				
Immunizations				
• Assessment of need for Rhogam				
Administration of Rhogam				
• Assessment of need for Rubella vaccine				
Administration of Rubella vaccine				
PATIENT/FAMILY EDUCATION				
Assessment of educational needs				
Review of topics				
- pre/post op care for BTL				
- postpartum danger signs				
- nutrition/exercise				
- physical/emotional changes				
- sexuality/contraception				
- sibling preparation				
- breast/bottlefeeding				
- newborn bath/cord care				
- circumcision care				
- newborn temperature-taking				
- home safety/Newborn Protection Practiner				
- newborn metabolic screening/jaundice				
- infant abilities				
Utilization of resources				
- "Strong Beginnings" classes/educators				
- informational booklets				
- CCTV/videotapes				
- Lactation Consultant/Breastfeeding Support Line				
- Interpreter				
Nursing documentation/OB teaching tool				

APPENDIX U • POSTPARTUM CARE

	Reviewed Concept	Applies Concept to Practice	Observed/ Assisted Preceptor	Performs Satisfactorily
DISCHARGE OF POSTPARTUM PATIENT/FAMILY				
Discharge Procedures				
Discharge nursing documentation				
- discharge orders				
- completion of discharge forms				
Discharge teaching				
Referrals				
- WIC				
- CHN				
- IHAP				
Types of Discharge				
Routine BC discharge				
Early discharge from BC				

PRECEPTORS

SIGNATURE	INITIALS	SIGNATURE	INITIALS

NAME:_____

UNIVERSITY OF ROCHESTER - STRONG MEMORIAL HOSPITAL
OB/GYN NURSING
ORIENTATION/CROSSTRAINING PROGRAM

POSTPARTUM STUDY GUIDE

This study guide includes key points in postpartum nursing and requires the learner to complete answers to various topics. Please complete and return to: _____ by this date: _____.

OBJECTIVES: After completing this guide, the learner will be able to:

1. Describe changes in the reproductive system immediately after delivery.

2. Describe changes in the endocrine system and hormones following delivery.

3. Describe changes in the cardiovascular system and the effect on fluid volume and electrolyte balance.

4. Describe changes in the appearance of lochia during the postpartum period.

5. Define key aspects of psychological adaptation that occur in the mother during the postpartum period.

6. State eight components of the postpartum assessment.

7. List five nursing diagnoses and applicable interventions for the postpartum patient.

8. Differentiate the elements of nursing documentation for the postpartum patient.

9. State the routine for postpartum vital signs and assessments on the OB Service.

10. List patient education topics to be reviewed with the postpartum patient.

RESOURCES: AWHONN Crosstraining Videotape on Postpartum Assessment/Care
OB/GYN Nursing Postpartum Learning Module
Obstetric Vital Signs/Assessment Guide (card)
Obstetric Patient Teaching Reference Manual

*NOTE: Most of the information in this guide is taken from the video - other references are cited where appropriate.

APPENDIX U • POSTPARTUM CARE

I. THE POSTPARTUM PERIOD

The postpartum period, called the puerperium, is the first _____ weeks after delivery. It is a vulnerable time of recovery, stabilization and adjustment with several rapid changes occurring, especially in the first _____ days.

II. CHANGES DURING THE POSTPARTUM PERIOD

   A. Reproductive system changes

   Uterus

   1) The fundus is _____ between the umbilicus and symphysis pubis immediately after delivery.

   2) During the first two days post delivery, the uterus remains approximately the same size. After that the uterus involutes rapidly, descending to the true pelvis with involution completed by the _____ day after delivery. At this point the uterus can no longer be felt above the level of the _____.

   3) The uterus returns to its non-pregnant size in _____ weeks. The entire endometrial lining is restored by the end of the _____ week.

   4) Intense uterine contractions continue after delivery, usually in response to rapidly diminished uterine volume. In the first _____ hours post delivery, uterine activity greatly _____ and stabilizes. Contractions may become discoordinate unless coordination is re-established by endogenous or exogenous _____.

   5) Afterbirth pains are _____ in the primipara because the uterus tends to remain in tonic contractions unless there are _____ or _____. In multiparas, the uterus often contracts and relaxes at intervals causing a painful sensation. Afterpains become more mild within _____ hours.

   6) Uterine atony is the failure of the uterus to contract and results in _____ bleeding.

   7) Early breastfeeding facilitates _____ and controls blood loss.

8) The cervical opening contracts slowly. For the first few days, it readily admits 2 fingers. By the end of the first _____, it becomes so narrowed, there is difficulty admitting 1 finger.

9) There are 3 types of postpartum lochia:

	Type	Color	Length of Time Expected
a)	_____	_____	_____
b)	_____	_____	_____
c)	_____	_____	_____

Sloughing of the endometrium may persist for _____ weeks postpartum.

Persistent lochia rubra may be the result of _____.

Continued lochia serosa or alba may indicate _____, especially if fever, tenderness or pain are present.

Malodorous lochia usually indicates _____.

** **INFORMATION ON AFTERBIRTH PAINS AND LOCHIA IS DISCUSSED LATER IN THE AWHONN VIDEO.**

<u>Placenta</u>

1) Immediately after delivery, the placental site becomes partially _____ by vascular constriction. Upward growth of endometrial tissue prevents _____ at the placental site.

<u>Vagina</u>

1) The vagina gradually returns to its pre-pregnant state by _____ weeks after delivery. Vaginal rugae appear _____ weeks post delivery. Vaginal mucosa thickens with the return of _____ function.

2) The introitus is initially reddened with edema, especially in the area of _____ or _____, but returns to normal in _____ weeks.

3) The vagina never returns to its nulliparous condition.

APPENDIX U • POSTPARTUM CARE

NOTES:

B. Abdominal wall and skin changes

1) The first few days after delivery, the abdomen _____ and gives a pregnant appearance. The abdominal wall returns to normal within _____ weeks after delivery.

2) The skin returns to its normal elasticity, but some _____ persist.

3) Returning muscle tone depends on previous _____, _____, and _____.

4) _____ and _____ ligaments are much more _____ than prior to pregnancy and require considerable time to recover.

NOTES:

C. Bladder changes

1) There is both _____ and _____ of the bladder.

2) The bladder has increased _____ and relative insensitivity, which results in incomplete _____, residual _____, and increased risk of _____.

NOTES:

D. Endocrine system changes -> effect on breasts/breastfeeding

1) There is a rapid decrease in _____ after delivery which is responsible for the many physiological postpartum changes.

2) Concentrations of the following hormones, which are responsible for breast development during pregnancy, rapidly decrease after delivery:

   a) _____
   b) _____
   c) _____
   d) _____
   e) _____
   f) _____

Return to pre-pregnancy levels depends on whether the woman is breastfeeding or not.

3) The precursor of breast milk, _____, is secreted from the breasts during the first few days after delivery.

4) Then breasts become engorged - _____, _____, and _____. Engorgement is the result of temporary distension of _____ and _____ and not the result of accumulation of milk. It generally resolves in _____ hours.

5) Intensity and duration of lactation depends on the stimulus of breastfeeding. Breastfeeding stimulates release of the posterior pituitary hormone, _____, which causes contraction of the myoepithelial cells of the _____ and _____, resulting in expression of milk. This is called the _____ reflex.

6) Prolactin levels decrease to pre-pregnancy levels within _____ weeks in the absence of breastfeeding or with anti-lactogenic medications. In breastfeeding women, the level of prolactin depends on the number of times _____ occurs each day.

7) Estrogen levels fall to 10% of pre-pregnancy levels within _____ hours of delivery, reach its lowest point in the first seven days postpartum and return to normal with _____.

APPENDIX U • POSTPARTUM CARE

8) Progesterone cannot be detected in the blood after the first _____, but production of progesterone returns with _____.

9) FSH and LH also decrease and are low in all women for the first _____ days after delivery; _____ will probably not occur during this time. Breastfeeding is not a reliable method of _____.

NOTES:

E. Cardiovascular system changes

1) Rapid cardiovascular changes affect _____ and _____.

2) Blood loss results in an immediate but _____ decrease in blood volume, which returns to normal levels within _____ weeks post delivery.

3) Mechanisms which protect the woman against postpartum blood loss include:

a) _____ -> decreases vascular bed by 10-15%
b) _____ -> decreases stimulation for vasodilation
c) _____

4) The hematocrit rises during the _____ days postpartum, as a result of a _____ in plasma volume and a _____ in red cell mass. It returns to normal non-pregnant levels by _____ weeks postpartum.

5) WBC count can increase from the normal leukocytosis of pregnancy of _____ to values of _____ in the first 10-

APPENDIX U • POSTPARTUM CARE

12 days post delivery. Neutrophils are the most numerous WBCs seen, with an increase in immature cells commonly referred to as a _____ shift. This leukocytosis, together with a _____ ESR, may confuse a diagnosis of acute infection during the first 2 weeks postpartum.

6) Blood clotting factors are greatly activated, placing the woman at an increased risk for formation of _____.

7) Normal pregnancy is associated with an increase in extracellular H2O of _____ liters. Postpartum diuresis is a reversal of that process and occurs _____ hours post delivery.

8) There is a loss of about _____ lbs. as a result of evacuation of the uterus and an additional loss of about _____ lbs. in the postpartum period, mostly from _____.

9) An increase in serum _____ reflects the increased H2O water to sodium (Na) loss, as well as decreased progesterone levels.

10) Potassium (K) levels _____ as a result of cellular breakdown from tissue involution.

11) Cardiac output _____ during the early postpartum period. Within minutes after delivery, output declines _____ to pre-labor levels. Women with previous cardiac history are at increased risk and need to be carefully monitored during this time.

12) Temporary bradycardia, with pulse rates as low as 40-50, caused by _____ cardiac output and stroke volume, can occur. The pulse returns to normal levels within _____ months of delivery.

13) BP is altered slightly, if at all.

14) VS will stabilize, but any rise in temperature needs to be assessed for development of an _____ process.

NOTES:

APPENDIX U • POSTPARTUM CARE

F. Respiratory system changes

1) Respiratory function returns to normal within _____ weeks after delivery.

G. Gastrointestinal system changes

1) After recovery from anesthesia, analgesia and fatigue, the postpartum woman's _____ and _____ function return quickly.

NOTES:

** **INFORMATION ON AFTERBIRTH PAINS AND LOCHIA ARE FOUND IN SECTION A.**

H. Psychosocial adaptations

Parents undergo many psychosocial adaptations as they attempt to balance their needs with their newborn's needs.

1) Parental tasks include:

   a) _____
   b) _____
   c) _____

2) Reva Rubin's three phases of maternal adaptation include:

   a) _____
   b) _____
   c) _____

3) During the taking-in phase, the mother has a therapeutic need for _____ and _____. It is a period of dependency and passive behavior. The mother needs mothering and

she has a definite past orientation, focusing on L&D experiences. She is receptive to _____ during this time.

4) During the taking-hold phase, the mother becomes very independent, focuses on regaining control of her body and assumes the _____ role. It is a time for recovering energy and asserting independence. She has a present orientation, becoming the caregiver instead of care receiver. It is normal for her to experience _____ at this time, which gradually subside over time.

5) In the _____ phase, the mother releases her old role and establishes new maternal role patterns, incorporating necessary changes. She separates from her baby to exclude her baby from some parts of her life, re-establishing the couple relationship with her partner.

Paternal adaptation follows a similar pattern.

NOTES:

III. POSTPARTUM ASSESSMENT

Postpartum assessment is part of a continuum from labor and delivery experiences through recovery to the postpartum period.

A. Delivery history is an important part of the admission/transition assessment and includes:

1) _____
2) _____
3) _____
4) _____
5) _____

APPENDIX U • POSTPARTUM CARE

B. Initial post-delivery assessment includes:

   1) _____
   2) _____
   3) _____
   4) _____
   5) _____
   6) _____
   7) physical assessment, including VS, amount of lochia, presence of edema, fundal height and firmness, status of perineum, bladder distension

   List the routine for VS and assessments for a new delivery over the first 24 hours (note: please refer to the Obstetric VS/Assessment Guide for this piece):

   _____
   _____
   _____
   _____

C. Ongoing postpartum assessment (although the BUBBLE assessment is mentioned in the AWHONN video, an eight point check is done on the OB Service - please follow these guidelines for this assessment)

   1) List the 8 parts of the postpartum assessment:

      a) _____
      b) _____
      c) _____
      d) _____
      e) _____
      f) _____
      g) _____
      h) _____

   2) **Breasts** should be observed for _____, _____, and _____. They should be palpated for warmth, edema and blockages. Nipples should be inspected for _____, _____, and _____.

   3) The **uterus** is best evaluated with the patient in a _____ position and with an empty bladder. The nurse should support the lower uterine segment just above the _____

493

and palpate the uterine fundus for degree of _____.
Fundal descent is measured in relationship to the _____
in fingerbreadths or centimeters. Fundal assessment should be
performed q _____ hours during the first day postpartum. The
patient should be taught to _____ and
report any increase in vaginal bleeding.

4) In assessing **bladder** status, the _____ of the abdominal wall should be observed and palpated for distension above the _____. Frequent checks are important as distension can aggravate _____.

5) In assessing **bowel** status, the nurse should observe the contour of the abdominal wall, auscultate for _____, and ask the woman about her normal bowel habits.

6) Assessment of **lochia** includes noting _____, _____, presence of clots and foul odor. Any clots are examined for _____. Endometritis is a late complication of retained placental fragments or difficult birth.

7) Assessment of the **episiotomy/perineum** should occur with the woman in lateral Sims (sidelying) position (even if there is no episiotomy, the perineum should still be assessed). The perineum should be observed for _____, _____, bruising, discharge, approximation of skin and hemorrhoids. **Unusual** perineal discomfort may be a symptom of infection.

8) A **Homan's Sign** is elicited in order to assess for _____. With the patient supine, each leg calf is passively dorsiflexed. Calf pain with dorsiflexion is a positive Homan's Sign and a symptom of thrombophlebitis. Legs and feet should also be inspected for any areas of redness, pain or swelling.

9) **Emotional status** is also assessed (note: please refer to Section H for this piece).

APPENDIX U • POSTPARTUM CARE

List the routine for ongoing VS and assessments beyond the first 24 hours after delivery (note: please refer to the Obstetric VS/Assessments Guide for this piece):

_____
_____
_____
_____

NOTES:

IV. POSTPARTUM NURSING DIAGNOSES AND INTERVENTIONS

    A. Alteration in health maintenance related to the end of a normal pregnancy

        Interventions include:

        1) By performing the _____, the nurse plays an important role in detecting postpartum complications.

NOTES:

    B. Potential for postpartum hemorrhage

        1) Postpartum hemorrhage is the leading cause of maternal death in the U.S.

        2) Postpartum hemorrhage can result from:

            a) _____
            b) _____
            c) _____
            d) _____
            e) _____

APPENDIX U • POSTPARTUM CARE

3) Hemorrhage is a blood loss of more than _____ ml or _____ % or more of body weight.

Interventions include:

1) Monitor BP, uterine tone and _____.

2) Monitor color, odor and _____ of lochia on admission and throughout the postpartum hospital stay.

NOTES:

C. Alteration in patterns of urinary elimination related to labor and delivery

1) This may be the result of:

    a) _____
    b) _____
    c) _____

Interventions include:

1) Monitor _____ pattern.

2) Assess for bladder status at least q _____ hours.

3) Ambulate ASAP.

4) Ensure adequate _____.

5) _____ are common and specific antibiotic therapy after a urine C&S is the treatment of choice.

NOTES:

APPENDIX U • POSTPARTUM CARE

D. Pain

1) Postpartum pain can occur from:

a) _____
b) _____
c) _____
d) _____
e) _____

Interventions include:

1) Monitor the patient's verbal and _____ cues.

2) Provide the following comfort measures (note: heat lamp is not used on the Birth Center):
a) _____
b) _____
c) _____
d) _____
e) _____

3) Teach the patient good perineal care, including proper cleansing after _____ and aseptic placement of _____ and stress good _____.

NOTES:

E. Alteration in tissue perfusion to the breasts

Interventions include:

1) Provide breast care for the bottlefeeding mother:

a) instruct to wear a snug, supporting bra

b) apply ice packs to reduce _____ and _____
c) assess breasts for _____

2) Provide breast care for the breastfeeding mother:

   a) remove oozing _____ with warm H2O
   b) keep breasts dry and clean
   c) relieve engorgement with _____ and by expressing milk by _____ or _____
   d) increase let-down reflex by:
      i) assuming a comfortable, relaxed position
      ii) using _____ on breasts before nursing
      iii) positioning newborn to nipple in _____ position so all quadrants of the breast are emptied

NOTES:

F. Knowledge and skill deficits related to self and newborn care

   Interventions include:

   1) Assess the patient's current knowledge and _____.

   2) Assess the patient/family's support _____.

   3) Review the following topics as part of discharge teaching (note: please refer to the Obstetric Patient Teaching Reference Manual for this piece):

      a) _____
      b) _____
      c) _____
      d) _____
      e) _____
      f) _____
      g) _____
      h) _____
      i) _____
      j) _____

k) _____
l) _____
m) _____
n) _____

NOTES:

G. Alteration in family process and the potential for growth in family coping

1) This is related to:

a) addition of new family member
b) developing a sense of _____ in the family unit

Interventions include:

1) Assess parents' _____.

2) Foster necessary parenting skills and provide _____, as needed.

3) Facilitate early and frequent parent/infant _____.

NOTES:

IMPORTANT ASPECTS OF POSTPARTUM DOCUMENTATION INCLUDE A COMPLETE ADMISSION/TRANSITION ASSESSMENT, CONTINUING OBSERVATION AND INTERVENTION, AND EVIDENCE OF PATIENT/FAMILY TEACHING AND PARTICIPATION IN CARE.

UNIVERSITY OF ROCHESTER–STRONG MEMORIAL HOSPITAL OB/GYN NURSING ORIENTATION/CROSSTRAINING PROGRAM

NAME:_____

POSTPARTUM POST TEST

Return completed tests to: _____ **by this date:** _____.

POSTPARTUM CARE

Circle the one best answer.

1. The postpartum period is often described as:
   a. The puerperium.
   b. Abrupt changes that are most dramatic during the first 10 days following delivery.
   c. Six weeks immediately following delivery.
   d. Both a and c.
   e. All of the above.

2. The following statements accurately describe <u>normal</u> changes in the reproductive system during the postpartum period <u>except</u>:
   a. The uterus involutes to its prepregnant size within 10 days to two weeks following delivery.
   b. Failure of the uterus to adequately contract generally results in atony and excessive bleeding.
   c. Breast feeding facilitates contraction and control of blood loss because oxytocin is released by the posterior pituitary as a result of nipple stimulation.
   d. The introitus may remain somewhat reddened and edematous, especially in the area of the episiotomy or laceration repair, generally returning to normal within two weeks.

3. Delivery of the infant and placenta result in dramatic changes in the endocrine system. The following accurately describes these changes in the lactating woman:
   a. Circulating levels of estrogen and progesterone drop suddenly and prolactin levels rise rapidly.
   b. Infant breast sucking stimulates milk production because it stimulates the release of both prolactin and oxytocin from the pituitary.
   c. Oxytoxin released from the posterior pituitary affects the myoepithelial cells of the mammary glands and result in the let-down reflex.
   d. Both a and b.
   e. All of the above.

APPENDIX U • POSTPARTUM CARE

4. Normal changes in the cardiovascular system during the puerperium include:

    a. Activation of blood-clotting factors placing the patient at risk for formation of thromboemboli.

    b. Initial rise in hematocrit as a result of decreased plasma volume and hemoconcentration.

    c. Decrease in white blood cell production increasing the maternal risk for potential postpartum infections.

    d. Both a and b.

    e. All of the above.

5. Select the physiological change that does <u>not</u> provide the postpartum woman with protection from blood loss:

    a. Return of extravascular water to the circulatory system.

    b. Increase in cardiac output in order to compensate for rapid physiological changes precipitated by delivery of the infant and expulsion of the placenta.

    c. Removal of the stimulus for vasodilation as a result of a loss of placental endocrine function.

    d. Reduction of the relative size of the vascular bed due to elimination of the utero-placental circulation.

6. In assessing for postpartum complications following vaginal or cesarean delivery, nursing care would include:

    a. Assessing and documenting amount of decidua in the lochia.

    b. Observing color, odor and quantity of flow.

    c. Instructing the mother to contact her provider for any bleeding that continues beyond two to three weeks because this would be considered abnormal.

    d. Both b and c.

    e. All of the above.

7. Nursing care provided during the puerperium includes:

    a. Fostering frequent bonding opportunities and providing support and assistance during family-newborn attachment.

    b. Teaching infant care, breast care and perineal care while providing support as the mother takes on new roles and tasks.

    c. Encouraging adequate rest, proper nutrition and hydration and appropriate activity, such as early ambulation or leg exercises for the woman confined to bed.

    d. Both a and b.

    e. All of the above.

8. The three phases of maternal postpartum changed described by Rubin include:

   a. Openness, independence and adaptation.

   b. Taking in, letting go and adaptation.

   c. Taking in, taking hold and letting go.

   d. Taking in, letting go and acceptance.

9. Per SMH policy, ongoing postpartum assessment includes:

   a. Uterus, bladder, breasts, laceration and episiotomy.

   b. Baby, uterus, bladder, breasts, lactation and edema.

   c. Breasts, uterus, blood pressure, lochia and elimination.

   d. Breasts, uterus, episiotomy, lochia, voiding, bowel movements/bowel sounds, Homan's Sign, emotional status.

10. Nursing diagnoses and/or problems identified by the nurse from ongoing assessment during the puerperium might include:

    a. Knowledge and/or skill deficit related to care of the newborn.

    b. Potential for postpartum hemorrhage related to uterine atony, lacerations, retained placenta fragments, hemolytic disorders and/or overdistension of the bladder.

    c. Alteration in family process and potential for growth in family coping.

    d. Both a and b.

    e. All of the above.

11. On day 2 following an uncomplicated vaginal delivery, the nursing assessment indicated the following findings. Which finding is considered abnormal?

    a. Uterus firmly contracted at the level of the umbilicus and shifted to the right.

    b. Lochia rubra and a moderate flow without clots.

    c. Diaphoretic state.

    d. Breast discharge that is clear and yellowish.

Mark the following statements as true or false.

12. _____ If no episiotomy has been performed, it is not necessary to assess the perineum during the postpartum hospital stay.

13. _____ At 1 hour after a normal vaginal delivery, you would expect the uterus to be located at the level of the symphysis pubis.

14. _____ The normal progression of postpartum vaginal lochia is rubra, then alba, then serosa.

INDEX

Page Numbers followed by a "d" refer to displays.

A

Abdominal examination
   of newborn, 90, 433, 461
   postpartum, 87
Accountability
   for unlicensed assistive personnel, 108
Acuity levels
   and requirements for nursing care, 112-113
Admission assessment
   intrapartum, 228, 398
      checklist on, 406
      medical record audit on, 10
      professional organization guidelines on, 4d
   of newborn, 431, 443-444
   postpartum, 469, 478
   during pregnancy, 4d
   skills checklists on, 228, 277
Adolescents
   age-specific elements in care of, 199, 210-211, 220
Advanced practice nurses
   in orientation and cross-training program, 19
Age-specific care, 198-222
   by Health Care Associate, 370
American Academy of Pediatrics (AAP), 2d
   guidelines and standards of, 3
      examples of, 4d, 5d, 6d
      on home care, 84
      on nurse-to-patient staffing ratios, 113
American Association of Critical Care Nurses (AACN), 2d, 34
American College of Obstetricians and Gynecologists (ACOG), 2
   guidelines and standards of, 3
      examples of, 4d, 5d, 6d
      on home care, 84
      on nurse-to-patient staffing ratios, 113
      in orientation and cross-training program, 16
American Nurses' Association (ANA)
   on unlicensed assistive personnel, 106, 107, 108
      and delegation of tasks, 108, 109
American Society of Anesthesiologists (ASA), 2d
   guidelines and standards of care of, 3
American Society of Perianesthesia Nurses (ASPAN), 2d, 34
Amniotic fluid
   meconium-stained, 404, 410
Analgesia/anesthesia care
   continuing education on, 40
   medical record audit on, 10
   professional organization guidelines on, 5d
   skills checklists on, 277-281, 288-289
Anemia
   in newborn, 438-439, 446
Antepartum care
   competence validation on, 228-237
      core competencies in, 178
   consortium approach to education on, 63
   cultural sensitivity in, 184, 185, 187-188, 189, 191
   patient census reporting in, 114
   in rural hospitals, 34, 35
Apgar scores, 317
Assistive personnel, 106-134, 363-397
   core competencies of, 119, 122d-124d
   current trends in use of, 107
   delegation and supervision of, 106-115, 116-117
   orientation of registered nurses to, 118-119
   description and regulation of, 107-108
   in HealthEast program, 98
   job descriptions of, 111, 112d, 119, 120d-121d
   nurse to patient ratios in, 107, 112, 113, 114
   orientation and competence validation of, 116-134
   in Patient Care Associate Training course, 118, 125-134
   pre-employment skills assessment of, 117
   proactive strategies for perinatal nurses in, 113-114
   professional accountability in, 108
   review of available data on, 106-107
   in successful nursing care models, 110-112, 111d
Association of Operating Room Nurses (AORN), 2d, 34
Association of Women's Health, Obstetric, and Neonatal Nurses (AWHONN), 2
   guidelines and standards of, 2-3, 33
      examples of, 5d, 6d
      on home care, 84
      in orientation and cross-training program, 16
   resources available from
      for continuing education, 39, 40
      on core competencies, 35, 36
   on unlicensed assistive personnel, 106, 107, 108
      and delegation of tasks, 108, 109, 110
      and nurse-to-patient staffing ratios, 113
      and patient acuity, 112-113
      and professional accountability, 108
Audit of medical records, 3-11
   benefits of, 11
   sample of, 8d-9d

B

Bilirubin serum levels
   in newborn, 439-440, 447
Birth. *See* Intrapartum care
Blood sampling
   competence validation on, 396-397
   in home visitation program, 355
Bonding process
   mother-infant-family interactions in, 474, 480
Bottle feeding, 436, 444
Breastfeeding knowledge, 312-316, 435-436
   checklists on, 312, 444-445
   competence validation on, 299-301, 312-316, 444-445
   cultural issues in, 184-185, 186, 188, 190, 191-192
   in home care program, 85, 87
      of York Hospital, 347-349
   in Performance Based Development System
      unit-based assessment of, 58-59
   post-test on, 314-316
Brigham and Women's Hospital
   competence validation in
      on antepartum and intrapartum care, 233
      on critical illness in pregnancy, 238-246

C

Cardiovascular skills
   in critical care during pregnancy, 239-244
   in newborn care, 324-325
   in post-anesthesia care, 278-279
Care planning exercises
   in Performance Based Development System, 49, 50
Care standards
   of professional organizations, 2-11, 33-34
Catheterization
   intravenous
      skill validation tool on, 333
   umbilical artery
      skill validation tool on, 330
Census reporting, 114
Certified nurses' aide, 117
Cesarean section
   culturally sensitive care in, 184, 186, 188, 190, 191
   perioperative skills validation in, 229, 283-287
   vaginal birth after, 403, 410
Chest examination
   of newborn, 90, 433, 460
Chest tubes
   skill validation tool on, 335
Circumcision
   cultural issues in, 185, 187, 189, 190, 192
Clinical Nurse Specialist
   in HealthEast model, 99, 102
Collaboration
   in consortium approach to perinatal education, 62-65
Comfort measures
   nursing skills checklist on, 280
   postpartum, 472-473, 479-480
Communication skills
   of Health Care Associate, 364
Competence validation, 17-18, 28-29
   age-specific assessment in, 198-222
   on analgesia/anesthesia care, 277-281, 288-289
   on antepartum care, 228-237
      core competencies in, 178
   for assistive personnel, 119, 122d-124d
      Health Care Associates, 363-372
   on breastfeeding knowledge, 299-301, 312-316, 444-445
   core competencies checklist in, 40, 177-180
   on critical care during pregnancy, 238-246
   on fetal monitoring, 228-229, 264-270
   for Health Care Associates, 363-372
   in HealthEast model
      age-specific considerations in, 202-222
      checklists in, 100, 101d, 102
      on critical thinking skills, 226-227
      on newborn care, 318-340
   in home care program, 84-85
      checklists in, 84, 87-95, 342-355
      of York Hospital, 342-355
   on interpersonal skills, 223-224
   on intrapartum care, 228-237
      core competencies in, 178-179
   medical record audit in, 3-11
   in Performance Based Development System, 46-56
      development of, 49-51
      format of, 53-54
      implementation of, 51-53
      unit-based assessment in, 49-54
   on perioperative procedures, 271-289
   on postpartum care, 290-311
   in rural hospitals, 40
   in Strong Memorial Hospital, 17-18, 28-29
Computer assisted instructional programs, 39
   sources of, 181
Conferences
   in continuing education programs, 40
Consciousness
   nursing care altered level of, 245
Consortium approach to perinatal education, 62-82
   course agenda in, 63, 66
   criteria for membership in, 63, 64, 78-80
   facilitators in, 64-65, 81

503

Consortium approach to perinatal education, *(Continued)*
    financial considerations in, 64
    job descriptions in, 67-77
    major services in, 63-64, 67-77
    organizational structure of, 64
    program evaluation in, 64-65
Continuing education programs, 35, 39-40
    consortium approach to, 64
    in HealthEast model, 98
    on home care, 85
    March of Dimes Nursing Modules in, 39, 358-362
    in network hospitals, 43-61
    in rural hospitals, 35, 39-40
    outreach program in, 40, 43-61
Core competencies
    of assistive personnel, 119, 122d-124d
    checklists on, 40, 177-180
    in Postpartum Home Visitation program, 342-355
    in rural hospitals, 35-36
    periodic validation of, 40
    in York Hospital Postpartum Home Visitation program, 341-355
Cost considerations, 43-44
    in consortium approach to perinatal education, 64
    in unlicensed assistive personnel use, 106
Course agenda
    in advanced program, 15-16
    in basic program, 14-15
    in consortium approach, 63, 66
    in Patient Care Associate training, 118, 125-134
    in rural hospitals, 35-36, 39
Critical illness
    in pregnancy, 238-246
Critical thinking skills
    of assistive personnel, 110
    in HealthEast model, 99, 225-227
    in Performance Based Development System, 47-49, 48d
    unit-based assessment of, 50, 52d-53d, 57-59
    preceptor weekly evaluation of orientee on, 356
Cross-training and orientation programs, 12-32. *See also* Orientation and cross-training programs
Cultural sensitivity in caregiving, 184-197
Customer service
    interpersonal skills in, 223

D
Data gathering activities
    assistive personnel in, 109, 110
Delegation of tasks
    to assistive personnel, 108-114, 116-117
    job description on, 111, 112d
    orientation of registered nurses to, 118-119
    professional accountability in, 108
Depression
    postpartum, 309-311, 474-475, 480
Dilatation and uterine evacuation
    critical elements in, 271-272
Discharge procedures
    postpartum, 477, 483
Documentation. *See* Medical records
Drug therapy
    intrapartum, 405, 411
    in newborn care, 327, 441-442, 448
    postpartum, 475-476, 482
    skills checklist for Health Care Associate on, 371

E
Education and training
    of assistive personnel, 116-134
    consortium approach to, 62-82
    continuing education programs in. *See* Continuing education programs
    cost considerations in, 43-44
    differentiation of wants and needs in, 45-46
    in HealthEast model, 96-104
    orientation and cross-training programs in. *See* Orientation and cross-training programs
    outreach programs in, 40, 43-61. *See also* Outreach education programs
    on perioperative procedures, 271-289
    philosophy in, 13d
Electrocardiography skills, 240-241
    of Patient Care Associate, 129-130
Electrocautery
    competency test on, 274-276
Electronic fetal monitoring. *See* Fetal monitoring
Elimination patterns
    of newborn, 91, 436, 445
    postpartum, 88, 471-472, 479
Emergency management
    nursing skills checklist on, 281
Emotional status
    postpartum, 309-311, 471, 474-475, 480
Endometritis
    postpartum, 295
Endotracheal intubation
    skill validation tool on, 336
Extremity examination
    of newborn, 91, 434, 462
    postpartum, 88

F
Face
    of newborn, 433, 457-460
Facilitators
    in perinatal education consortium, 64-65, 81
Fallopian tube ligation
    postpartum, 474, 481
Family interactions
    in home care program, 83
    competence checklists on, 93-94, 352
    Patient Care Associate Training course on, 118
    postpartum, 474-475, 476-477, 480
Feeding. *See* Nutrition
Fetal monitoring
    assistive personnel in, 110
    competence checklists on, 228-229, 264-270
    medical record audit on, 3, 7, 8d, 10
    monthly home study program on, 39, 247-263
    patient census reporting in, 114
    in Performance Based Development System, 57-58
    professional organization guidelines on, 5d
    in rural hospitals
    continuing education on, 39
    orientation on, 36
Filipinos
    cultural sensitivity in caregiving to, 184-185
Fluids
    nursing skills checklist on, 279

G
Gastrointestinal skills
    in newborn care, 325-326, 331-332
    gastric lavage in, 332
    gastric tube insertion and gavage feeding in, 331
Gavage feeding
    skill validation tool on, 331
Genitalia
    of newborn
    circumcision of, 185, 187, 189, 190, 192
    examination of, 90-91, 434, 461-462
Geriatric care
    age-specific elements in, 201, 222
Gestational age, 434, 439, 464
Glucose serum levels
    in newborn, 438, 446

H
Haitians
    cultural sensitivity in caregiving to, 185-187
Head
    of newborn, 90, 432-433, 456-457
Headache
    spinal, 473, 481
Health Care Associates, 363-384
    job descriptions for, 373-384
    licensed, 371, 379-384
    skills checklists for, 363-372
Health Department regulations, 33
Health promotion activities
    in home care program, 83
    competence checklist on, 93-94
HealthEast Perinatal Services
    age-specific considerations in, 202-222
    competence validation in
    age-specific considerations in, 202-222
    checklists in, 100, 101d, 102
    on critical thinking skills, 226-227
    on newborn care, 318-340
    critical thinking skills in, 99, 225-227
    definitions of terms used in, 97, 97d
    orientation and education program in, 96-104
    benefits of, 98, 99d
    development of, 96-98, 102-103
    identification of need for, 96
    philosophy of, 99
    special care nursery skills in, 318-340
Hemorrhage
    postpartum, 405, 411
    competence validation on, 294-295
HIV infections
    newborn care in, 447
Home care program, 83-95
    competence based orientation in, 84-85
    expected outcomes in, 84, 84d
    skills checklist on, 84, 87-95
    definition of, 84
    philosophy in, 83, 83d
    of York Hospital, 341-355
Hospitals
    admission assessment in. *See* Admission assessment
    competence-based orientation and cross-training program in, 12-32
    in consortium approach to perinatal education, 62-82
    rural, 33-41. *See also* Rural hospitals
Hygiene measures
    in newborn care, 436-437, 445
    postpartum, 472-473, 479-480
Hyperbilirubinemia
    of newborn, 439-440, 447
    phototherapy in, 338, 440
Hypertension
    pregnancy-induced, 297-298
Hypoglycemia
    in newborn, 438, 446

I
Immunizations
    in newborn care, 442, 448
    in postpartum care, 476, 482
Induction of labor, 3, 404, 410

Infections
    in newborn, 440, 447
    postpartum, 473, 481
Intensive care
    neonatal, 317-340
Interpersonal skills, 223-224
    in HealthEast model, 99
    in home care program, 92-93, 353
    patient feedback on, 224
    in Performance Based Development System, 49
        unit-based assessment of, 50, 53d, 59
    preceptor weekly evaluation of orientee on, 356
Intrapartum care, 398-430
    admission assessment in, 228, 398
        checklist on, 406
        medical record audit on, 10
        professional organization guidelines on, 4d
    assistive personnel in
        job description on, 120d-121d
        Patient Care Associate Training course on, 118
    competence validation on, 228-237
        core competencies in, 178-179
    in complications and special situations, 403-405
        checklist on, 410-411
    concepts in, 398-405
    consortium approach to education on, 63, 66
    cultural sensitivity in, 184, 185-186, 188, 189-190, 191
    in HealthEast model, 100
    induction of labor in, 3, 404, 410
    medical record audit on, 3, 7, 8d-9d, 10-11
    medications in, 405, 411
    patient census reporting in, 114
    in Performance Based Development System, 59
    performance criteria in, 234-237
    post-test on, 412-416
    professional organization guidelines on, 4d-6d
    in rural hospitals, 35
        orientation on, 36
    skill competency/learning summary checklist on, 406-411
    stages of labor in, 399-403
        checklist on, 407-409
    standards in, 234-237
    in Strong Memorial Hospital, 406-430
    study guide on, 417-430
Intravenous start
    skill validation tool on, 333

J
Jaundice
    in newborn, 439-440, 447
        phototherapy in, 338, 440
Job descriptions
    on assistive personnel, 107-108, 119, 120d-121d
        appropriate tasks in, 108-110
    in consortium approach, 67-77
    on Health Care Associates, 373-384
Joint Commission on Accreditation of Healthcare Organizations (JCAHO), 2, 33-34, 41
    on competence model of assessment, 46
    on HealthEast program, 98
    March of Dimes Learning Modules integrated with standards of, 361-362
    on unlicensed assistive personnel, 109, 111, 112
Journals
    in continuing education programs, 40

L
Labor. *See* Intrapartum care
Laboratory tests
    in newborn care, 441, 448
    in postpartum care, 475, 481
LATCH scoring system, 313
Lavage
    gastric
        skill validation tool on, 331
Learners, 20
    competence validation of. *See* Competence validation
    evaluation of program and preceptor by, 18, 30-32
    in HealthEast model, 99-102
    learning needs of. *See* Learning needs
    orientation needs of, 17, 24-25
    weekly evaluation of, 17-18, 28-29, 356-357
Learning needs, 17-18, 28-29
    of assistive personnel, 122d-124d
    competence model of, 46
    differentiated from educational wants, 45-46
    in HealthEast model, 100
        competence checklists on, 100-102, 101d
        pre-employment inventory of, 99
    in outreach program, 45d, 45-46
    in Performance Based Development System, 46-56
        and recommended learning options, 54, 55d, 60-61
        unit-based assessment in, 49-54
    in rural hospitals, 40, 45, 45d
Learning process, 20-22, 21d
Learning summaries, 18
    on intrapartum care, 406-411
    on newborn care, 443-448
    on postpartum care, 478-483
Leopold's maneuvers
    competency checklists on, 228, 270

M
March of Dimes Nursing Modules
    in continuing education, 39, 358-362
    in orientation, 36
Maternal care
    crosstraining competencies in York Hospital program, 290-311
    by Health Care Associate, 367
    at home, 83-95
        in York Hospital program, 341-355
    intrapartum. *See* Intrapartum care
    medical record audit on, 7, 8d-9d, 10-11
    postpartum. *See* Postpartum care
    professional organization guidelines on, 5d-6d
Mechanical ventilation
    skill validation tool on, 339-340
Meconium-stained amniotic fluid, 404, 410
Medical records
    audits of, 3-11
        benefits of, 11
        sample of, 8d-9d
    skills checklists on, 230-231, 238, 281
        for Health Care Associate, 370
Medications. *See* Drug therapy
Mentoring period
    in home care program, 85
Metabolism screen
    skills checklist on, 393-395
Mexican Americans
    cultural sensitivity in caregiving to, 187-189
Mitral valve prolapse, 404, 410
Mother-baby model of care, 35
Multidisciplinary approach
    unlicensed assistive personnel in, 110-111

N
Nasopharyngeal suctioning
    skill validation tool on, 337
National Association of Neonatal Nurses (NANN), 2d, 34
National Certification Corporation (NCC)
    for the Obstetric, Gynecologic and Neonatal Nursing Specialities, 39
National Council of State Boards of Nursing (NCSB)
    on unlicensed assistive personnel, 108
Nebraska Methodist Hospital Perinatal Outreach Program, 44-61
Neonatal care. *See* Newborn care
Neonatal Resuscitation Program, 38
Nervous system skills
    in critical care during pregnancy, 245
    in newborn care, 322-323
    in post-anesthesia care, 279
Network hospitals
    perinatal outreach programs in, 43-61
Newborn care, 317-340, 431-468
    admission assessment in, 431, 443-444
    age-specific elements in, 198, 208-209, 215-216
    Apgar scores in, 317
    in complications and special situations, 437-441, 445-447
    concepts in, 431-442
    consortium approach to education on, 63, 66
    core competencies in, 180
    cultural sensitivity in, 185, 187, 189, 190, 192
    by Health Care Associate, 368-369
    in HealthEast model, 100, 318-340
        skills validation tools on, 318-340
    at home, 83-95
        competence checklist on, 90-92
        in York Hospital program, 341-355
    hygiene measures in, 436-437, 445
    medical record audit on, 9d
    medications and immunizations in, 441-442, 448
    metabolism screen in, 393-395
    nutrition in, 91-92, 435-436, 444-445
        bottle feeding in, 92, 436, 444
        breastfeeding in. *See* Breastfeeding
    Patient Care Associate Training course on, 118
    physical examination in, 432-434, 444
        in home care program, 90-91
        study guide on, 451-465
    post-tests on, 466-468
    professional organization guidelines on, 6d
    resuscitation measures in, 38, 405, 437-438, 445-446
    in rural hospitals, 35
        orientation on, 36, 38
    safety measures in, 437, 445
    skill competency/learning summary checklist on, 443-448
    in Strong Memorial Hospital, 443-468
    study guide on, 449-465
    temperature regulation in, 326, 438, 446
    vital signs in, 90, 432, 444, 452-453
    in York Hospital program, 302-308
Northwest Regional Perinatal Outreach Program at University of Washington, 62-82
Nurse managers, 19
    in Patient Care Associate training course, 132
Nutrition
    gavage feeding in, 331
    for newborn, 91-92, 435-436, 444-445
        bottle feeding in, 92, 436, 444
        breastfeeding in. *See* Breastfeeding
    postpartum, 88, 471, 479

Nutrition,
  (Continued)
    skills checklist for Health Care Associate
      on, 365

O

Operating room procedures, 271-289
  competence validation on, 271-289
  critical elements in, 271-272, 282
  orientation on, 38-39
Organizations, professional. *See* Professional
  organizations
Orientation and cross-training programs, 12-32
  advanced level, 14, 15-16, 16d, 19
  for assistive personnel, 116-134
    Patient Care Associate Training
      course in, 118, 125-134
    and registered nurses, 118-119
  basic level, 14-15, 15d
  consortium approach to, 62-82
  content of, 14-16
  core competencies in. *See* Core competencies
  definition of, 13
  future initiatives in, 22-23
  in HealthEast model, 96-104
  on home care, 84-85
    competence checklist on, 84, 87-95
  learners in, 20. *See also* Learners
  learning process in, 20-22, 21d
  learning summaries in, 18. *See also*
    Learning summaries
  Performance Based Development System
    in, 46-56
  on postpartum care, 290-311
  post-tests in, 18. *See also* Post-tests
  preceptors in, 19-20. *See also* Preceptors
  program evaluation in, 22. *See also* Program
    evaluation
  resources for. *See* Resources for orientation
    and training programs
  in rural hospitals, 35-39
    examples of, 37-39
  structure of, 14, 15d, 16d
  study guides in, 18. *See also* Study guides
  tasks in development of, 13-14, 14d
  team of personnel in, 19-20
  time required for, 20
    in Patient Care Associate Training
      course, 118, 125-131
    in rural hospitals, 37
  tools in, 16-19, 17d
  weekly schedule of, 17, 26-27
  in York Hospital, 290-311
Outreach education programs, 40, 43-61
  competence model of assessment in, 46
  conceptual framework in, 45, 45d
  consortium approach in, 62-82
  of Nebraska Methodist Hospital, 44-61
  Performance Based Development System
    in, 46-56
Oxygen therapy
  skill validation tool on, 334
Oxytocin administration, 3
  medical record audit on, 3, 8d, 10

P

Palos Community Hospital (Palos Heights,
  Illinois)
  competence checklists in
    on antepartum/intrapartum
      care, 228-232
    on perioperative procedures, 271-272
Patient acuity
  and requirements for nursing care, 112-113

Patient Care Associate
  clinical evaluation of performance, 391-392
  training course for, 118, 125-134
Patient care technician
  skills checklist on, 389-390
Patient feedback
  on childbirth experience, 224
Pediatric care
  age-specific elements in, 217-219
Performance Based Development System, 46-56
  critical thinking skills in, 47-49, 48d
    unit-based assessment of, 50, 52d-53d,
      57-59
  development of, 49-51, 51d
  dimensions of, 46-47, 47f
  format of, 53-54, 54d
  implementation of, 51-53
  interpersonal skills in, 49
    unit-based assessment of, 50, 53d, 59
  learning options in, 54, 55d, 60-61
  modifications of, 54-56
  outline of components in, 50, 52d-53d
  program evaluation in, 54
  sample report on, 53, 57-61
  technical skills in, 49, 50d
    unit-based assessment of, 50, 53d,
      59-60
  unit-based assessment in, 49-54
Performance evaluation, 17-18, 28-29. *See also*
  Competence validation
Perioperative procedures, 271-289
  competence validation on, 271-289
  critical elements in, 271-272, 282
  orientation on, 38-39
Phlebotomy skills
  of Patient Care Associate, 127-128
Phototherapy
  in newborn care, 338, 440
Physical examination
  of newborn, 432-434, 444
    in home care program, 90-91
    study guide on, 451-465
  postpartum, 469-471, 478
    in home care program, 87-88
Polycythemia
  in newborn, 438-439, 446
Postmaturity, 439, 446
Postpartum care, 290-311, 469-503
  admission assessment in, 469, 478
  in complications and special situations,
    473-474, 480-481
  concepts in, 469-477
  consortium approach to education on, 63, 66
  core competencies in, 179-180
    in York Hospital Postpartum Home
      Visitation program, 341-355
  crosstraining competencies in York Hospital
    program, 290-311
  cultural sensitivity in, 185, 186-187, 188-189,
    190, 192
  diagnostic and laboratory tests in, 475, 481
  elimination patterns in, 88, 471-472, 479
  emotional status in, 309-311, 471, 474-475,
    480
  family interactions in, 474-475, 476-477
  in HealthEast model, 100
  at home, 83-95
    competence checklists on, 84, 87-95,
      342-355
    in York Hospital program, 341-355
  hygiene and comfort measures in, 472-473,
    479-480
  medical record audit on, 9d, 10-11

medications and immunizations in, 475-476,
  482
nutrition in, 88, 471, 479
patient census reporting in, 114
physical examination in, 469-471, 478
  in home care program, 87-88
post-test on, 500-503
professional organization guidelines on, 6d
in rural hospitals, 35
  continuing education on, 39
skill competency/learning summary checklist on, 478-483
in Strong Memorial Hospital, 478-503
study guide on, 484-499
vital signs in, 87, 469, 478
Post-tests, 18
  on age-specific care, 209, 211, 213-214
  on breastfeeding knowledge, 314-316
  on intrapartum care, 412-416
  on newborn care, 466-468
  on postpartum care, 500-503
Preceptors, 19-20
  in assistive personnel orientation program, 118
  in HealthEast model, 98, 100, 102
  learner evaluation of, 18, 30-32
  in rural hospitals, 36-37
  weekly evaluation of orientee by, 356-357
Preeclampsia, 474, 481
Pregnancy
  admission assessment in, 4d
  antepartum care in. *See* Antepartum care
  critical illness in, 238-246
  cultural issues in, 184, 185, 187-188, 189, 191
  hypertension in, 297-298
  substance abuse in, 440-441, 447
Premature rupture of membranes, 403-404, 410
Prematurity, 439, 446
Problem-Solving Algorithm exercise, 49
Professional organizations
  guidelines and standards of, 2-11, 33-34
    on home care, 84
    summary of, 4d-6d
    on unlicensed assistive personnel,
      106, 116
Program evaluation, 22
  in consortium approach, 64-65
  by learner, 17-18, 30-32
  in Performance Based Development
    System, 54
  in rural hospitals, 41
Published guidelines and standards
  of professional organizations, 2-3, 4d-6d
Puerto Ricans
  cultural sensitivity in caregiving to, 189-190

R

Reflexes
  of newborn, 434, 463
Registered nurses, 1-104
  competence-based orientation and cross-
    training program for, 12-32
  HealthEast's model on orientation and
    education of, 96-104
  in home care of mothers and infants, 83-95
  in perinatal outreach programs of network
    hospitals, 43-61
  professional organization guidelines on, 2-11
  regional consortium approach to education
    and collaboration of, 62-82
  in rural hospitals, 33-41
  and unlicensed assistive personnel, 106-115
    current trends in, 107
    nurse to patient ratios in, 107, 112, 113

orientation of nurses to roles of, 118-119
professional accountability in, 108
Rehabilitation skills
of Patient Care Associate, 129-130
Resources for orientation and training programs, 14-16, 181-183
in continuing education programs, 39-40, 358-362
on core competencies, 35-36
on fetal monitoring, 247-263
March of Dimes Nursing Modules in, 358-362
in Performance Based Development System, 47-49, 55d, 60
in rural hospitals, 44
self-study modules in, 38, 39, 55d, 60
sources of, 182
videotapes in. *See* Videotapes
Respiratory skills
in critical care during pregnancy, 244-245
of Health Care Associate, 365
in newborn care, 323-324
checklist on, 446
chest tube in, 335
endotracheal tube in, 336
mechanical ventilation in, 339-340
oxygen headbox in, 334
of Patient Care Associate, 128-129
in post-anesthesia care, 277-278
Resuscitation
maternal postpartum, 473
of newborn, 38, 405, 437-438, 445-446
Rupture of membranes
artificial, 404, 410
premature, 403-404, 410
Rural hospitals, 33-41
challenges in, 34-35, 43-44
continuing education programs in, 35, 39-40
outreach program in, 40, 43-61
core competencies in, 35-36
periodic validation of, 40
orientation and cross-training programs in, 35-39
examples of, 37-39
outreach education programs in, 40, 43-61
Performance Based Development System in, 46-56
program evaluation in, 41
Rural Wisconsin Health Cooperative, 36
Russians
cultural sensitivity in caregiving to, 191-192

S

Safety knowledge
of Health Care Associate, 364-365
in newborn care, 437, 445
St. Elizabeth Health Center
skills checklists on Health Care Associates in, 363-384
St. Francis Hospital (Litchfield, Illinois)
continuing education programs in, 40
orientation programs in, 37-38
program evaluation in, 41
St. John's Hospital
competence-based orientation and education in, 96-104
HealthEast Perinatal Services in. *See* HealthEast Perinatal Services
St. John's Mercy Medical Center (Saint Louis, Missouri)
assistive personnel in
clinical evaluation of performance, 391-392

core competence assessment tool on, 122d-124d
job description on, 120d-121d
and Patient Care Associate training course, 125-134
feedback from patients in, 224
St. Joseph's Hospital (Breese, Illinois)
interpersonal skills validation in, 223
orientation programs in, 38-39
perioperative skills validation in, 283-289
program evaluation in, 41
Secretary of unit
skills checklist on, 385-386
Self-assessments
on mother/child care, 291-308
in home visitation program, 342-355
sources of modules for, 182
Self-study modules, 38, 39
in Performance Based Development system, 55d, 60
sources of, 182
Sepsis
in newborn, 440, 447
Sioux Valley Hospital (Sioux Falls, South Dakota)
LATCH scoring system in, 313
preceptor weekly evaluation of orientee in, 356-357
Skin
of newborn, 91, 326, 432, 454-456
Specimen collection
skills checklists on, 396-397
for Health Care Associate, 365
for home visitation program, 355
Staffing resources
and accuracy in patient census reporting, 114
and nurse-to-patient ratios, 107, 112, 113, 114
professional organization guidelines on, 116
in unlicensed assistive personnel, 116-134
Standards of care
of professional organizations, 2-11, 33-34
Strong Memorial Hospital (Rochester, New York)
competence-based orientation and cross-training program in, 24-32
on intrapartum care, 406-430
on newborn care, 443-468
philosophy of, 13d
on postpartum care, 478-503
Perifax program of, 39
Study guides, 18
on intrapartum care, 417-430
on newborn care, 449-465
on postpartum care, 484-499
Substance abuse
maternal, 440-441, 447
Suctioning
nasopharyngeal
skill validation tool on, 337
Supervision
of unlicensed assistive personnel, 108-114, 116-117
orientation of registered nurses to, 118-119
professional accountability in, 108
Support technician
skills checklist on, 387-388
Surgical procedures, 271-289
competence validation on, 271-289
critical elements in, 271-272, 282
orientation on, 38-39

T

Technical skills
in HealthEast model, 99

in Patient Care Associate Training course, 118
in Performance Based Development System, 49, 50d
unit-based assessment of, 50, 53d, 59-60
preceptor weekly evaluation of orientee on, 356
Temperature regulation
in newborn care, 326, 438, 446
in post-anesthesia care, 279
Thromboembolism
postpartum, 296-297
Thrombophlebitis
postpartum, 474, 481
competence validation on, 296-297
Top Priority game approach, 47
Tracheal intubation
skill validation tool on, 336
Tubes
chest, 335
endotracheal, 336
gastric, 331

U

Umbilical arterial catheterization
skill validation tool on, 330
Umbilical cord
prolapse of, 404, 410-411
Unit-based assessment
in Performance Based Development System, 49-54
sample report on, 53, 57-61
Unit coordinators
in orientation and cross-training program, 19
Unit secretary
skills checklist on, 385-386
Unlicensed assistive personnel, 106-134, 363-397.
See also Assistive personnel
Urinary tract skills
in newborn care, 326
in postpartum care, 296
Uterus
activity assessment
medical record audit on, 3, 7, 8d-9d, 10
professional organization guidelines on, 5d
atony/subinvolution of, 473, 480

V

Venipuncture
skills checklist on, 396-397
Ventilatory support
skill validation tool on, 339-340
Videotapes
on antepartum and intrapartum care, 231-232
in continuing education programs, 39-40
on newborn care, 321
in Performance Based Development System, 47, 54, 55d
simulation of clinical problems in, 47, 51, 57
sources of, 181-182
Vital signs
of newborn, 90, 432, 444, 452-453
postpartum, 87, 469, 478

W

Weight measurements
of newborn, 432, 439, 447
"What if" exercises, 48, 51

Y

York Hospital
mother-child care competencies in, 290-311
Postpartum Home Visitation program of, 341-355